Understanding mental retardation

D0094260

To Eunice Kennedy Shriver,
in recognition of her effective
work in improving the lives of our
nation's retarded citizens

Understanding
mental retardation

EDWARD ZIGLER *and* ROBERT M. HODAPP
Yale University

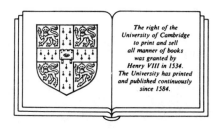

*The right of the
University of Cambridge
to print and sell
all manner of books
was granted by
Henry VIII in 1534.
The University has printed
and published continuously
since 1584.*

CAMBRIDGE UNIVERSITY PRESS

Cambridge
New York   Port Chester
Melbourne   Sydney

Published by the Press Syndicate of the University of Cambridge
The Pitt Building, Trumpington Street, Cambridge CB2 1RP
40 West 20th Street, New York, NY 10011, USA
10 Stamford Road, Oakleigh, Melbourne 3166, Australia

First published 1986
Reprinted 1988, 1991

Printed in the United States of America

Library of Congress Cataloging-in-Publication Data

Zigler, Edward, 1930–
Understanding mental retardation.
Bibliography: p.
Includes index.
1. Mental retardation.   I. Hodapp, Robert M.
II. Title.   [DNLM: 1. Mental Retardation.   WM 300 Z68u]
RC570.Z54   1986   616.85′88   85–31444

British Library Cataloguing in Publication Data

Understanding mental retardation.
1. Mental retardation
I. Zigler, Edward   II. Hodapp, Robert M.
616.85′88   RC570

ISBN 0-521-26809-5 hardback
ISBN 0-521-31878-5 paperback

Contents

v

Preface

Research on mental retardation can best be characterized as diverse but fragmented. Although workers have examined the functioning of retarded persons on many tasks and in many settings, it often seems that the various subdisciplines continue to be widely separated. Early intervention workers have little to say to those interested in the effects of institutionalization, who in turn care little about issues of definition, classification, or mainstreaming. In short, there remains a need for a unified treatment of the field of mental retardation.

The present volume is designed to provide at least a first attempt at such a treatment. By addressing several topics concerning mental retardation from the developmental perspective, we continually employ the theories of, and findings about, development in nonretarded children to inform work with retarded people. Through the application of such a broad-based approach, many disparate areas can be brought together within a single framework.

This book also serves the function of being both a summary of our own past work and a start on future ventures. For the past several decades, we of the Yale group have championed the developmental approach to mental retardation and extensively studied motivational and personality factors in the functioning of retarded individuals. This work has appeared in numerous articles and books, but has yet to be gathered together in one place, within one coherent format. One of our motivations in writing this book has therefore been to review, evaluate, and make accessible work that has appeared over the past 25 years. The book is not solely a review of past efforts, however. We feel that our extended discussions of the developmental approach toward retardation (Chapters 2 & 7), our ideas on the classification and prevalence of retardation (Chapters 4 & 5), and even some of our writings on miracle cures (Chapter 8), institutionalization (Chapter 10), and mainstreaming (Chapter 11), are original contributions. Many of these ideas will be further extended and studied in future years.

xi

Thus, this volume is on one hand a review of prior work, on the other an impetus to future efforts.

The organization of this book reflects the mixture of past and future orientations, as well as our desire to make work in the mental retardation field accessible to those only partially acquainted with the subject. The first part, consisting of two chapters ("What we do and do not know about mental retardation" and "The developmental perspective"), is introductory in both content and style. Although experienced workers may skip these pages, our efforts to present clearly the many controversies in mental retardation and the developmental approach toward these issues may be instructive. For students learning about mental retardation, such chapters should be indispensable. The second part explores the related issues of definition, classification, and prevalence. Although often discussed by professionals in mental retardation, these issues nevertheless remain unresolved. The third part involves our discussions of motivation and personality functioning in retarded persons. The fourth part is composed of three chapters, each of which examines a selected aspect of intervention with retarded individuals. The final part (before a short concluding chapter) deals with the issues of institutionalization and mainstreaming, and presents historical, philosophical, and research-based discussions of these two topics. The book thus examines a wide range of topics in the mental retardation field, all through the lens of the developmental perspective.

This book would not have been possible were it not for Grant HD 03008 from the National Institutes of Child Health and Human Development (NICHD), support from the John and Catherine MacArthur Foundation, and the hard work of many persons. Sally Styfco was responsible for editing drafts of most of the chapters, and W. M. Havighurst copyedited the manuscript; their meticulous work is much appreciated. David Evans spent countless hours tracking down, compiling, and revising references and in other ways assisting in the production of this manuscript. Nancy Hall and Christina Buchmann also helped in its preparation. Several other people have lent their advice, encouragement, and support throughout this endeavor; particular thanks go to David Caruso, Michael Faulkner, Marion Glick, Maren Jones, and Victoria Seitz. We would also like to extend our thanks to Susan Milmoe, David Longobardi, and Sophia Prybylski at Cambridge University Press; each has been thoroughly professional (yet at the same time friendly and supportive) in their treatment of this book and its authors.

Edward Zigler
Robert M. Hodapp

Part I

Introduction and background

1 What we do and do not understand about mental retardation

Compared to many of the physical sciences, the study of mental retardation is still in its infancy or early childhood. From the initial efforts of Seguin and Howe in the 19th century to the classic studies of Bayley, Spitz, and the Iowa group in the 20th, all of the advances in the mental retardation area have occurred in the past 150 years, and most within the last 50.

Thinking back to 1959 gives a sense of how recently the field has evolved. That was the year that Down syndrome ("mongolism" in those days) was found to be caused by an extra chromosome, thus leading to our present understanding of this familiar disorder. It was also the year when the American Association on Mental Deficiency (AAMD) published the first definition of mental retardation (Heber, 1959). Prior to this time workers had been guided by their own independent judgments; these judgments varied so much that mental retardation was not really a legitimate field or bonafide science. It seems only fitting that in reviewing the situation in this period, Masland, Sarason, and Gladwin (1958) should decry the lack of high-quality research in mental retardation.

Less than 20 years later, the situation had changed dramatically. In testimony before Congress, Zigler observed that "Current research in the mental retardation area is vibrant work of high quality, being carried out by methodologically sophisticated workers whose efforts are directed by a broad and rich array of theoretical formulations" (1977, p. 51). He further noted that "The general quality of America's major journal in reporting mental retardation research, the *American Journal of Mental Deficiency*, has improved so much over the past 20 years that it is hard to believe this is the same spotty journal that represented the field just two decades ago" (p. 51). These recent achievements have vastly improved our understanding of mental retardation, and additional knowledge accumulates at an astonishing rate.

Still, the extent of knowledge about mental retardation is and will remain limited until some basic issues are resolved. To begin at the most basic

3

level, how should we define mental retardation? Only when a consensus is reached can we more purposefully address the other big questions: How many retarded people are there? What causes mental retardation? How is it best treated? Can retardation be cured or prevented? Such issues have provoked passionate argument among professionals and laypeople alike. These rambling controversies are seen by some as a deterrent to further progress in the field. We choose to see them as catalysts to the maturation of a solid and seasoned discipline.

The purpose of this book is to examine critically the existing knowledge about mental retardation, to separate myth from fact, and to provide a unifying framework for understanding the phenomenon. In the process, we will expound ways of viewing retarded people that have helped us in our own thinking and research in the field. This is done not to impose our opinions but to encourage young workers to tackle difficult and crucial issues.

What we know about mental retardation

Subnormal intellectual functioning

The most salient characteristic of retarded people is that their intellectual level is lower than that of the average person in the society. Retarded persons are "slow" or "dull" in their abilities to learn and respond to the problems of everyday living. This is an obvious, commonsense observation, but a professional investigator must take a closer view and arrive at a more objective categorization.

What do we mean by "subnormal intellectual functioning"? Indeed, what is intelligence itself? Sternberg, Conway, Ketron, and Bernstein (1981) attempted to define intelligence from the perspective of the nonexpert, the person unacquainted with psychology. These investigators asked three groups of laypeople – college students in a library, commuters waiting for their trains, and shoppers at a supermarket – to list the behaviors they considered characteristic of "intelligence." Another group of nonexperts, as well as a group of professionals in the field, then rated these behaviors on the degree to which each reflects intelligence (e.g., on a scale of 1 to 9, to what degree is behavior X an "intelligent behavior"?).

Results showed that people unfamiliar with research on intelligence ranked highest those behaviors falling into three general categories: practical problem solving (e.g., reasons logically and well; identifies connections among ideas), verbal ability (speaks clearly and articulately; converses well), and social competence (accepts others for what they are; displays an interest in the world at large). The experts largely agreed with the nonexperts; they gave high ranks to verbal intelligence, problem-solving ability, and "practical intelligence" (e.g., sizes up situations well; determines how to achieve goals). Only this last factor, which was less social than the social competence category of the nonexperts, differed between the two groups. The point is that, while scholars have long argued about the definition of intelligence, most people have a fairly clear sense of the phenomenon.

A brief glance through several psychology texts provides a second source of information on the nature of intelligence. Kimble, Garmezy, and Zigler (1984) emphasize the function of intelligence as the "solving of real-life tasks." They note that "modern definitions of intelligence tend to emphasize cognition, the capacity to think, reason, remember and understand" (p. 227). In his textbook on mental retardation, MacMillan (1982) summarizes the attempts to define intelligence as having three general themes: "(1) the capacity to learn, (2) the totality of knowledge acquired, and (3) the adaptability of the individual, particularly to new situations" (p. 170). In the introductory chapter to Sternberg's *Handbook of Intelligence*, Sternberg and Salter (1982) define intelligence as "goal-directed adaptive behavior."

Combining the above elements, we are able to compose a general definition of intelligence: Intelligence consists of those mental operations, the accumulated knowledge, and the ability to learn that help one purposefully to solve real-life tasks. Intellectual functioning involves such cognitive processes as thinking, memory, and logical reasoning, and the knowledge of general information and vocabulary; many of these skills can be either linguistic or nonlinguistic in nature.

While this definition may seem general enough to satisfy everyone, it does step into some controversial ground. First, it omits physical, sensory, or personality attributes as features of intelligence, although some would argue that these traits influence cognition. Our definition also implies that intelligence consists of both general and specific mental abilities. Reasoning and the ability to learn are general features; they can be used to solve any number of problems faced by the individual. These types of processes enter into Spearman's g, or general intellectual factor. Accumulated knowledge and certain types of logical reasoning, on the other hand, are more specific in nature. These s factors involve specialized areas of knowledge and are contingent on a person's specific interests, environment, and experiences.

A debate has long raged over whether intelligence is a general ability underlying all mental functioning or a set of abilities that are independent of each other. The position that intelligence involves specific skills is based on the common observation that individuals have intellectual strengths and weaknesses. Someone may have superior mechanical aptitude but be illiterate, or be unable to balance a checkbook but able to do a *New York Times* crossword puzzle without an eraser. On a more scientific level, there have been some very complex and determined efforts to identify the specific skills that constitute intelligence. Guilford (1956) described no less than 120 distinct components of intellect and devised tests to measure most of them. More recently, Gardner (1983) proposed that there are separate "multiple intelligences" in the linguistic, musical, logico-mathematical, spatial, bodily-kinesthetic, and personal domains. Support for his theory comes from studies of persons who possess superior talent in one area while demonstrating little or no competence in other areas (the so-called idiot savant). The method used to isolate specific mental abilities is factor analysis, which indicates the degree of independence of the various traits. Arguments abound, however, over the appropriateness of different types of factor-analytic techniques, some of which may indicate a *g* factor while others, applied to the same data, do not.

The opposing view that intelligence is a single underlying entity also has supportive evidence. Jensen (1982), a strong proponent of *g*, writes that "Essentially the same g emerges from collections of tests which are superficially quite different. Unlike *all* other factors (i.e., factors found when intelligence tests are factor analyzed), g is not tied to any particular type of item content or acquired cognitive skill" (p. 133). Jensen also relies on evidence that people who score well on one type of mental ability test also generally score well on others, a fact that he calls "one of the most remarkable findings in all of psychology" (1981a, p. 52).

Since no resolution of this debate seems imminent at this time, our choice of definition reflects a middle-ground position: Intelligence consists of both general and specific abilities. The *g* and the various *s* factors combine to become the sum of "intelligence" for any particular individual. Our view of intelligence is similar to the "hierarchical models" of intelligence proposed by Vernon (1971), Snow (1978), and others. "In Vernon's view, for instance, intellectual abilities comprise a hierarchy, with a general factor (g) at the top; two major group factors, verbal-educational ability and spatial-mechanical ability at the second level; minor group factors at the third level; and specific factors at the bottom. Hierarchical models such as this one seem to account for much of the correlational data on the structure of intelligence" (Wagner & Sternberg, in press, p. 7). This mixture of general and specific abilities allows for strengths and weaknesses in an individual's intellectual functioning, while maintaining a basic intellectual "core" for each person.

Our view of intelligence also acknowledges the three general outlooks that currently pervade the intelligence field: the psychometric, the Piagetian, and the information-processing perspectives. Each of these emphasizes different aspects of the phenomenon. Psychometricians stress the differences among individuals on standardized measures of intellectual functioning, Piagetians concentrate on the development of cognitive operations, and psychologists working within the information processing perspective examine the microscopic processes that underlie the performance of any intelligent behavior (e.g., attention, encoding, memory). Thus, the first view is useful in defining mental retardation (because of its focus on individual differences), while the second teaches us about development, and the third about the mental processes by which individuals come to acquire knowledge. Thus these three seemingly divergent views complement each other by focusing on three different aspects of intelligence (Wagner & Sternberg, in press).

A second issue involves the specification of "subnormal" in the phrase "subnormal intellectual functioning." Obviously, such a determination must be arbitrary. There simply is no clear dividing line between normality and subnormality for almost any continuous human trait, and intelligence is no exception. For example, although different people will disagree about what constitutes a tall man (is it 6′, 6′2″ or 6′6″?), most would agree that tallness is a meaningful concept. There is likewise nothing in the nature of intelligence that clearly distinguishes those who have "normal" endowment from those who do not.

We will save the bulk of our remarks for the discussion of individual differences in a later chapter (Chapter 3). Suffice it to say here that subnormal intelligence is usually determined statistically, by means of standardized psychometric instruments. According to the current AAMD definition, a person's IQ score must be at least two standard deviations (*SDs*) below the mean of the population for that person to be considered retarded. In the 1960s the cutoff was one *SD*, indicating that even this statistical approach to definition is somewhat arbitrary.

It is also worth noting that intelligence tests themselves are not purely objective measures. Since there is no universal definition of intelligence, test constructors devise questions that tap processes represented in their own conception of intelligence. IQ tests were created to predict success in school (which they do quite well), but there is some doubt whether the abilities needed for academic achievement are the same as those needed for achievement in nonschool life. Other criticisms of intelligence tests are that they are too verbal in nature and that they are biased against minority and lower-class individuals, because they contain items "culture-bound" to middle-class, white American values. Responses to these criticisms have included attempts to develop restandardized, "culture-fair" and nonverbal tests. These efforts have to date met with only limited success. Thus, while standard intelligence tests are not perfect, they are the best we have at this time. Their use in the designation of mental retardation is justified by the view that diagnosis must be based on more objective measures of intellectual functioning than the subjective judgments of school administrators, physicians, or psychologists. Interested readers should consult Jensen (1980) and Vernon (1979) for reviews of this problem.

Some retardation involves known organicity, some does not

The typical image of a retarded person is that of a Down syndrome child with the striking features (pudgy face and limbs, protruding tongue) characteristic of the disorder. A casual observer might add that the child's speech might be slurred, that the child might have a pleasant personality, and that heart defects are possible. The presence of organic defects, and corresponding physical sequelae, are important to this general view.

This picture of retardation might be expanded by noting that organic insults are of three kinds: (1) those occurring prior to birth, either because of genetic anomalies or problems in utero (prenatal insults); (2) those occurring at or close to the time of birth (perinatal insults); and (3) those occurring at some time thereafter during the life span (postnatal insults). Examples of prenatal insults caused by genetic anomalies include Down syndrome, Fragile X syndrome, Tay-Sachs disease, and phenylketonuria; examples of insults that occur in utero are rubella syndrome and teratogenesis (e.g., thalidomide children). Perinatal causes include anoxia at birth and postnatal factors include head trauma and childhood encephalitis. Many of these organic insults (e.g., Down syndrome) seem to occur about equally across the socioeconomic spectrum (SES); others seem to affect certain ethnic, SES, or racial groups more than others (e.g., Tay-Sachs is peculiar to Ashkenazic Jews and retardation due to complications of prematurity occurs more often in children from low-SES mothers; see Cytryn & Lourie, 1975, for a description of the many etiologies of mental retardation).

Hidden from view, however, are all of those people who do not display any obvious organic etiologies but who are nevertheless retarded. This phenomenon has variously been called retardation due to sociocultural factors, familial retardation, retardation due to environmental deprivation, nonorganic retardation, and cultural-familial retardation. This group may comprise up to 70–75% of the total retarded population (see Chapter 4 for a fuller discussion of this issue). In general, IQ levels of this group tend to fall in the mild (IQ 55–70) and moderate (IQ 40–54) ranges of retardation.

As with many issues in mental retardation, a debate rages about the causes of retardation in these people. Have they been deprived in their early environments, are they offspring of parents with genes for lower intelligence, or do they in fact suffer from some as yet undiagnosed organic insult, an etiology that only future diagnostic procedures will discover? Or are several of the above factors working in concert to cause intellectual subnormality in this group? We simply do not know.

For now, let us say only that notwithstanding one's position on the cause of retardation in this group, all would agree that in some retarded people (probably less than half of all cases of retardation) a clear organic etiology can be specified. In other cases (probably over half of the total), no clear organic etiology is indicated.

Motivational and personality factors play an important role in life functioning of retarded people

We have all been impressed by the degree to which motivational and personality factors affect people we have known or read about. On one hand, there are persons who have driven themselves to career success. The example of Abraham Lincoln comes to mind, learning to read and write with little formal schooling, teaching himself the law, diligently studying famous authors to improve his own style of writing and speaking (Oates, 1977). The story of Lincoln is one of the Horatio Alger tales that have long been part of American folklore. On the other hand, we have all been equally impressed, or dismayed, by experiences with individuals who have not used their talents to the fullest. Countless men and women might have become great successes in any of a thousand careers, had they only tried. And yet, for some reason, they did not.

This is not to say that motivation conquers all. It is only one of a number of factors that help to determine success. Sociologists and historians have long argued about the degree to which success is due to the circumstances of one's birth and upbringing (e.g., social class, race) and the degree to which the individual's own initiative is involved. For example, few would argue that a black child born in dire economic circumstances will have a more difficult time succeeding than will a white child born of upper-class parents. The so-called privileges of birth – a stable and affluent home life, good schools, special tutoring, the best colleges – may be available to one child and not to the other. Similarly, one's historical epoch helps determine one's chances for career success. Becoming literate in the rural Midwest of the early 1800s (admittedly, not an easy task) gave young Lincoln a long head start on a legal and political career. It is not so clear that current social and economic conditions in most modern societies allow for such rises in social status.

Our point is simply that an individual's motivation and personality at least partially determine the degree of success attained. This point applies to retarded individuals as well. One retarded person with an IQ of 60 may differ greatly from another retarded person, also with a 60 IQ. The first may work, have a family, and live an independent life, whereas the other may be incapable of any of these achievements. It is unsettling to contemplate how often this simple fact is forgotten.

Similarly, those life experiences that affect normally intelligent people will also affect people who are retarded. Indeed, several negative life experiences that happen frequently to retarded persons may cause certain deficits that are falsely attributed to retardation itself. Consider the experience of failure, a common event for retarded persons (because of their lower levels of intellectual functioning). A fear of trying new tasks or a greater dependence on adults to solve problems may be more likely in retarded people not because of their lower intelligence, but because of repeated failures (Weisz, 1982). If put in situations that foster success, they may cease to show such behaviors altogether. One must also consider the effects of being institutionalized, of being labeled retarded, of being placed in a special class, and of being the lowest-functioning member of a mainstreamed class – all experiences common to retarded persons.

Most experts in the mental retardation (MR) field would agree to at least the three statements about mental retardation that are presented above. Mental retardation does involve subnormal intellectual functioning, some retardation involves known organicity and some does not, and motivational and personality factors play some role in the life functioning of retarded people. Beyond these facts, however, debate continues on a number of issues. We now turn to some of these areas of disagreement.

Issues in mental retardation about which experts disagree

The role of social adaptation in defining mental retardation

The current AAMD definition of mental retardation reads as follows:

Mental retardation refers to significantly subaverage intellectual functioning resulting in or associated with impairments in adaptive behavior and manifested during the developmental period. (Grossman, 1983, p. 11)

Three factors are involved in this definition: (1) subaverage intellectual functioning (i.e., IQ below 70); (2) impairments in adaptive behavior (as assessed by Vineland Scales or clinical judgments); and (3) impairments that are manifested during the developmental period (before 18 years of age). (For our present discussion, the third factor will be ignored, as it is in most discussions of the AAMD definition; see Grossman, 1983, p. 12.)

Disagreements arise when one considers the role of social adaptation in the definition of mental retardation. Social adaptation, as one outcome of the personality and motivational factors affecting each retarded and non-retarded person, is clearly important, but its role in defining who is and is not retarded is hotly debated.

On one side of this issue are those who argue that IQ tests discriminate against low-SES and minority groups. If one employs a definition based solely on the IQ criterion (IQ below 70) and administers IQ tests that are discriminatory, a greater proportion of minority children than nonminority children will be labeled retarded and placed in special-education classes. Indeed, the assignment of a disproportionate number of California black and Hispanic children to special-education classes led to the famous *Larry P.* decision (*Larry P.* v. *Riles*, 1974), forbidding California educators from using IQ tests in determining special-class placements (see MacMillan & Meyers, 1980, for a review of this issue).

On the other side of the debate are those (the authors among them) who claim that social adaptation should not be used to define mental retardation. We believe that social adaptation is not intrinsic to mental retardation (i.e., that the sole defining characteristic of mental retardation should be subnormal intellectual functioning) and that the social adaptation concept itself is not clearly defined or adequately measured. This does not imply that we are any less uneasy about the possible biases of intelligence tests, only that lower levels of intellectual functioning should be the sole criterion for defining retardation.

An important corollary to the two-factor definition of mental retardation, its effects on prevalence levels of retardation, also deserves mention. A two-factor definition in which both factors are weighted equally makes the prevalence levels of mental retardation dependent on the level of correlation between the two factors. However, Silverstein (1973, p. 380) notes that "correlations between various intelligence tests and the Vineland Social Maturity Scale (Doll, 1953), one measure of adaptive behavior, range from .00 to .90 for different samples (Leland, Shellhaas, Nihira & Foster, 1967)."

How many people are retarded, using the two-factor definition? Silver-

Table 1.1. *Prevalence rates using a two-SD cutoff in IQ and social adaptation, with varying degrees of correlation between the two factors*

Correlation	Number retarded in U.S.A. −2SD	Number retarded per 1,000 population −2SD
.00	104,000	.5
.20	274,000	1.4
.40	584,000	2.9
.60	1,100,000	5.5
.80	1,965,000	9.8
1.00	4,550,000	22.8

Source: Adapted from Silverstein (1973), p. 381, Tables 1 and 2.

stein (1973) concludes that, even using a definition that states that an individual must fall below two standard deviations from the mean on both social adaptation and IQ, the prevalence of mental retardation in the United States could range from as high as 4.5 million to as low as 104,000. Table 1.1 shows Silverstein's calculations of the prevalence of retardation, both nationally and per 1,000 population. The difficulties in having a prevalence figure that varies so widely demonstrate the problematic nature of the role of social adaptation in defining mental retardation.

The role of social systems in determining who is retarded

Throughout our discussion of mental retardation, we have assumed that retardation is an objective entity, that it exists independent of whether one examines it or of whether anyone is labeled retarded. Our view is based on the assumption that "intelligence" is a relatively stable underlying trait and that this trait is continuous. As a continuous human trait, there are people who are subnormal in their intellectual functioning, regardless of whether they are ever labeled retarded.

The concept of a trait, upon which our view of retardation is based, is found in many areas of psychology. Briefly, a trait is a relatively unchanging characteristic of an individual that is operative across a range of situations. For example, shyness might be thought of as a personality trait. The shy person of today does not get out of bed tomorrow and become the most outgoing person around. Similarly, one's level of intelligence is relatively stable from one situation to another. Thus there are individuals who are subnormal in their intellectual functioning, just as there are some who are supranormal. Trait theorists view mental retardation as an objective entity that exists whether or not it is formally identified or whether anyone is ever labeled retarded.

Other workers believe that intelligence is a situationally determined phenomenon dependent on the social systems in which people find themselves. A well-known proponent of this view, Jane Mercer, put it this way:

> Mental retardation is not a characteristic of the individual, nor a meaning inherent in [the retarded person's] behavior, but a socially determined status, which he may occupy in some social systems and not in others, depending on their norms. It follows that a person may be mentally retarded in one system and not mentally retarded in another. He may change his role by changing his social group. (1974, p. 31)

Therefore, "retardation exists . . . only to the extent that certain people persist in calling certain other people retarded" (Braginsky & Braginsky, 1971, p. 30). An example of such thinking is the notion of the "six-hour retarded child" (President's Committee on Mental Retardation, 1969), a child who is considered retarded in school, where demands on formal intellect are heaviest, but is perfectly capable outside the school doors. If it is true that one is "made retarded" by the demands of one's environment, then it follows that changing the environmental demands could produce less retardation. In fact, Mercer argues that since one's status as a mentally retarded person is tied to a specific role in a specific social system, "prevalence rates, in the traditional, epidemiologic sense, are meaningless" (1974, p. 30).

While the social systems perspective has made workers more aware of possible biases, it may ultimately not be helpful either to retarded persons or to the mental retardation field as a whole. Clearly, retarded persons often require help from society, and for this reason alone it is important to know just who is retarded and in need of help. Further, an exclusively social systems approach can hinder study of retarded people by denying the legitimacy of a whole class of scientific questions about mental retardation; even a problem as basic as the prevalence rate of retardation is "meaningless" according to proponents of this view. We will have more to say on this issue when we speak about the prevalence of mental retardation in Chapter 5.

How best to care for retarded people

Ideas about the best ways to care for retarded people have changed every few decades. At any one time, however, experts in mental retardation have been certain that the prevailing practice was the best, in fact the only, way

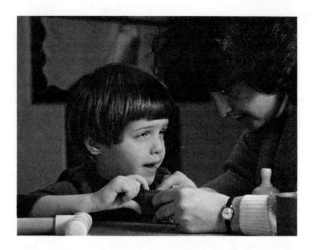

Photo 1. Tactile stimulation. (Photograph courtesy of Elwyn Institutes, Elwyn, Pennsylvania)

to treat retarded persons. Appeals have been made to the "humaneness" of the prevailing practice, to the practice's benefits to retarded persons, and to the good sense the practice makes to the society.

An example of a current fashion is the movement to mainstream retarded children. To mainstream handicapped children means to place them in regular school classes alongside nonhandicapped children. It is an effort to allow handicapped children to develop in as "normal" an environment as possible.

Although mainstreaming is considered by many to be the obvious best educational setting for retarded children, it is instructive to read samples from two major MR textbooks of the 1960s and 1970s on this issue. One can thereby judge the arguments previously advanced for special-class placements, the alternative educational option for most retarded children.

The consensus of special educators today definitely favors special class placement for the mildly retarded. This is true at least when sufficient facilities are available to make possible the homogeneous grouping of children by age and ability. (Robinson & Robinson, 1965, p. 436)

. . . the special class was thought to protect the EMR (educable mentally retarded) child from undue failure, peer rejection, and loss of self-esteem. Placing him in a class with a smaller enrollment supposedly afforded him more individualized instruction and a curriculum that would prepare him for the kinds of occupations he was likely to enter upon leaving school. While the advent of special classes probably brought a sense of relief among regular teachers, who were frustrated in trying to teach these children because they met with little success, special classes were created with the primary intent of helping the children. (MacMillan, 1977, p. 430)

A debate similar to the mainstreaming controversy has also occurred around deinstitutionalization, the practice of taking retarded persons out of large institutions and placing them into smaller community settings. Proponents of deinstitutionalization feel that the large institutions for the retarded are inhumane. They cite the abuses discovered at Willowbrook in New York and at other large institutions and conclude that no large institution can sensitively care for retarded persons. While not denying that certain institutions have provided (and some continue to provide) poor care for retarded residents, opponents of deinstitutionalization insist that large institutions may be necessary for some retarded individuals, and that blanket assertions about large institutions are unfair.

We will have much more to say about both the issues of mainstreaming (Chapter 11) and deinstitutionalization (Chapter 10) later in this book. For now, let us mention only that what seems humane today may not be considered so in future years. In addition, it is our contention that research, not slogans, should be employed to decide which are the best educational and living settings for retarded persons. For example, when considering the effects of institutions, one must examine such variables as institutional size, number of residents per living unit, cost per resident per day, percentage of employee turnover, professional staff per resident, and the number of volunteer-hours per resident (Zigler & Balla, 1977). Simple assertions that "large institutions are inhumane" are not enough. Care must first be taken to insure that a particular placement is indeed humane for a particular person, then an assessment of the effects of the placement on the individual's development must be performed. Only by this two-step process – first determining humaneness, then assessing effects on retarded individuals – is it possible to make enlightened and informed decisions as to the care and placement of retarded persons.

How best to intervene with retarded people

In the 1940s and '50s, experts believed that retarded persons suffer from an overly rigid cognitive system (Lewin, 1936; Kounin, 1948). Retarded persons were thought to be "stuck" in their ways; they supposedly lacked the flexibility to deal with new or unusual cognitive tasks. It followed from this belief that the best way to intervene with retarded persons was to give them monotonous, repetitive tasks. Numerous intervention programs consisted of training in stringing beads or counting and sorting materials again and again. Such boring tasks were thought to capitalize on the rigid programming inherent in the retarded person's brain.

Later critics derided such practices as not doing much to help the development of retarded persons, but the question of what does constitute the best method of intervention persists. The problem is a multifaceted one, involving at least the following issues: different views of how retarded people differ from nonretarded people; different views of human development; different estimations of what is and is not possible for an intervention to accomplish; and the entire issue of what constitutes an effective intervention (regardless of the specific program employed).

The first of these issues concerns the ways in which differences between retarded and normally developing individuals are conceptualized. We are referring here to the developmental–difference debate, which has been in the forefront of mental retardation research for the past 25 years. In short, the developmental position is that retarded persons, especially those who do not show evidence of organic involvement, are *delayed* in their development. They progress through the same stages of cognitive development as nonretarded individuals, but at a slower pace. The sequence of education for the two groups should be the same, but retarded children should be exposed to the same content areas at later chronological ages, and they should be allowed more time to learn specific skills.

In contrast, difference (or "defect") theorists contend that retardation is caused by one or a set of defects inherent in retarded people. Among the defects that have been postulated are rigidity and deficiencies in processes involving verbal mediation or attention. Whatever the specific problem, retarded people are viewed as basically different from nonretarded people. It follows from the difference position that the best type of intervention would be to improve behaviors closely associated with the defect.

A second issue concerns how one conceptualizes development itself. To developmental theorists such as Piaget, Werner, and Bruner, development involves a complicated interaction between an active organism progressing toward its mature state and an ever-changing environment. While any particular theorist may emphasize child or environment to a greater extent, the interaction between organism and environment is essential to all developmental theories.

An opposing view is that of behaviorist psychologists (e.g., Skinner), who tend to downplay the active nature of the organism and instead focus on the organism's reactions to environmental contingencies. According to these theorists, one's reinforcement history, or the sequence of positive and negative reinforcements since birth, determines present behavior. Taken to its extreme, behaviorist theories ignore the intrinsic nature of the organism and, some might say, the complicated nature of the environment itself. (See Overton & Reese, 1973, and Reese & Overton, 1970, for comparisons of developmental and behaviorist theories.)

Again, both viewpoints correspond to specific types of intervention program. Behaviorists have had their greatest impact on the *process* of intervention, especially with severely and profoundly retarded individuals. Through various reinforcement techniques they have succeeded in teaching adaptive behaviors such as toileting, feeding, and grooming to very low-functioning people.

Developmentalists have focused more on teaching behaviors in the areas of cognition, language, and social skills. The developmental perspective has helped provide the *sequence* of intervention in these domains, the order in which to teach skills to retarded children. However, the processes of teaching these behaviors (the so-called mechanisms of developmental change) have been less well-articulated. A blending of the developmental sequence and behavioral reinforcement processes may ultimately be the most advantageous method of intervention (see Chapter 7).

The third major question concerns the appropriate goals of an intervention program designed to help retarded people. From the very first remedial efforts, many interventionists hoped for nothing less than to make the retarded child normal. This lofty goals lives on, most notably in certain behavioral (e.g., Doman-Delacato) and medical (vitamin therapy) programs that we consider overpublicized and of dubious merit (see Chapter 9). Others argue that a more realistic goal of intervention should be to develop whatever skills the individual possesses to the highest level possible. Asking for "normality" only leads to frustrations for the retarded person, for his or her family, and for those trying to intervene.

If the goal of intervention is as nebulous as to help the retarded person to develop to the highest level possible, how can one distinguish a good from a bad program? How can one tell if a program is actually helping a retarded child to develop at all? This problem is compounded by the fact that mentally retarded children (and adults) often make only halting progress, and sometimes even regress. Indeed, the data on the stability of IQ scores for retarded children, especially those with the lowest IQs (Bayley, 1949; Lewis, 1976), indicate that quick progress of any type is difficult to achieve. Perhaps the most that can be expected is that the program increase the rate of development over that which the child previously demonstrated, not that the child progress as fast as a normally developing child. Several programs, most notably that of Hayden and Haring (1976), have aimed for this prudent criterion of success.

To further complicate the evaluation issue, certain important areas are often overlooked when searching for criteria of successful interventions (Zigler & Balla, 1982a). For one, better social adaptation for the retarded child – in school, at home, and with peers – may not affect the IQ but can make an important difference in the child's life. Parental adaptation to the retarded child is another neglected area, yet one where change certainly is possible and ultimately can lead to more optimal development in the child. For example, an intervention program might help the parents of a 2-year-old Down syndrome girl to accept the child's problem, to get over blaming themselves for her condition, and to communicate more productively with specialists working with her. Simple advances such as learning how to wean the girl from the bottle and onto solid foods would facilitate adaptation for both parents and child.

Finally, we note that the changing demographics of the retarded population have affected the range of necessary intervention programs. In particular, medical advances now allow most retarded persons to live longer (see Chapter 5), producing increasing numbers who need training in vocational and daily living skills. Such life-skills training poses new challenges to those working with and studying retarded people.

Summary

We have attempted to summarize, as fairly as possible, the state of the art in the mental retardation field. Of necessity, our list of facts and controversies touches only upon the major issues in mental retardation research, and ignores many lesser issues.

To reiterate, experts in mental retardation agree that retardation involves subnormal intellectual functioning, that some retarded persons show a clear organic cause for their retardation and others do not, and that motivational and personality factors play a role in the real-life functioning of retarded people. On the other hand, disagreements abound as to the appropriate role of social adaptation in defining mental retardation, the role of social systems in determining who is retarded, and how best to care for and intervene with retarded individuals. In our next chapter, we consider the developmental perspective, the basic framework that guides our thinking about mental retardation.

2 The developmental perspective

Defining the term *development* as it concerns human beings is not as straightforward as it may seem. On one hand, it is clear that the developing child is getting bigger, stronger, smarter, and increasingly like an adult. But it is not so clear just how far to extend the search for types of development. Are the many changes that occur in adulthood developmental in nature, or are they simply changes happening over time? Can changes in phenomena such as self-image or morality be looked at as development or simply as an individual's personal choice? And what causes all these changes? Are they a simple unfolding of some innate plan, or are changes determined by the environment? Such concerns have been grappled with in a fruitful approach to human growth called the developmental perspective. The general thrust of this approach was summarized by Zigler as follows:

The developmentally-oriented psychologist has always been struck by the phenomenon of growth and change and the orderliness, sequentiality, and apparent lawfulness of the transition taking place from the birth or conception of the organism to the attainment of maturity. The developmentalist's theoretical task has been one of constructing principles or constructs making such change comprehensible. Such principles clearly have little to do with time and much to do with those processes, involving the person and his environment, which give rise to changes in behavior. (1963a, p. 344)

As can be gleaned from this excerpt, the developmental perspective has its roots in the study of normal development. Through detailed investigation of the changes that occur in the "typical" individual, this approach has resulted in a solid body of knowledge and some sound theoretical formulations concerning the course of development. In this chapter we will first describe the developmental perspective, then show how the perspective can be applied to mental retardation and retarded people.

19

The nature of human development

Defining development

Let us begin by offering the following definition of development:

Development involves relatively predictable changes in internal mental structures (i.e., concepts) occurring over time, that lead the organism to its mature state; such change is partly due to the actions (mental and physical) of the organism itself, partly to the actions of a changing environment.

Notice that "change" is not synonymous with development. Indeed, many kinds of change are not developmental at all. Take the example of a child learning to push a bar after a light goes on in order to receive a candy reinforcement (or to push a button on a video game at the right time to score points). While the manner in which the child learns this response may be interesting to the psychologist (and may constitute a change in the child's behavior), this learning will not lead the child to maturity in any domain, the learned behavior may not be retained for long, and it does not involve a change in internal mental structures. Thus developmental psychology focuses on changes in the form or organization of responses over time and is not particularly concerned with the strength or accuracy of the response itself.

The need to specify a mature state is another important aspect of the definition of development. Piaget designates formal operational thought as the mature level of cognitive development, Werner and Kaplan (1963) specify the end point of the development of symbolization as "the contemplation of objects," and Freud envisions the genital stage as the highest level of psychosexual development. Each of these theorists provides a clear end point in the domain of interest. In short, developmental change is change directed toward a mature, adult form.

Having defined development in general terms, our task becomes one of characterizing developmental change. Here our discussion owes much to Heinz Werner (1948, 1957), probably the foremost among developmental theorists (for a retrospective review see White, 1984). According to Werner's "orthogenetic principle," development "proceeds from a state of relative globality and lack of differentiation to a state of increasing differentiation, articulation, and hierarchic integration" (1957, p. 126).

A few examples will serve to flesh out these rather esoteric terms. Consider the development of the human embryo, the original example of developmental change for most students of development. At conception, there is a single cell formed from two gametes. This cell then divides into two cells, the two cells themselves divide, and so on. This mass of cells is undifferentiated – no cell has a structure or function different from any other cell. Soon some cells will develop into the central nervous system, others into skin, still others into limbs and other parts of the body. Little by little, all cells assume specific structural characteristics as the embryo becomes increasingly differentiated. By the time of birth, the infant's complex systems are under the control of the brain. Not only do the specific parts exist independently and functionally, but each part is integrated into the whole. In this sense, "hierarchic integration at a higher level" has taken place.

The development of communication skills also illustrates the movement from a global and undifferentiated state to a differentiated and hierarchically organized state. At first, the infant's vocal and physical actions and the immediate contextual surroundings are completely bound together. Babies make their needs known by crying, but it is uncertain whether they know they are actually "communicating" or even if they understand more than that they are hungry, wet, etc. By about 8 or 10 months, however, there is a clear intention to communicate. An infant at this age might look to the mother while pointing to a desired object to get her to retrieve it. After the first year, words begin to emerge, often still accompanied by pointing or other gestures. This is the time when the child speaks in holophrases: One word or a word plus a gesture fills in for an entire sentence (e.g., "bottle!" stands for "I want my bottle!"). Finally, by around age 2, the child will put two or more words together in a sentence. Even with this ability, however, language is usually tied to the immediate context, or "the here and now" (R. Brown, 1973). Only gradually do children begin to speak about objects and events that they cannot see or that are in the past or future. The differentiation of communication from the context of action (e.g., crying or gesturing) and immediate environment now allows for symbolic communication through words that represent objects, events, and feelings. The movement of the child's communication from global and undifferentiated (action in context, not for the purpose of communication) to specific and hierarchically organized (words spoken within sentences for the purpose of communicating with others) is a good example of developmental change. Indeed, it is interesting to note that this application of the developmental perspective to language (from Werner & Kaplan, 1963) has been borne out by studies of infants in the first two years of life (e.g., Bates, Camaioni, & Volterra, 1975; Greenfield & Smith, 1976; Locke, 1979).

Notice from these examples that development to Werner is a positive process involving the emergence of ever greater adaptive abilities over time. Each successive stage is more effective, more useful in dealing with the world. For example, the child who can speak in sentences no longer requires that the adult follow his or her gaze or gesturing arm to infer the correct meaning. The child simply screams "Want juice!" and parents more than get the idea. Similarly, the child able to think in a formal operational manner can solve logical and hypothetical problems totally beyond the child in the earlier sensorimotor period. Such a positive progression is characteristic of Piagetian and Wernerian theories of development.

Piaget's cognitive-developmental theory

Although Werner played a major role in conceptualizing the general developmental perspective, the work of Jean Piaget has probably had a greater impact on the field of developmental psychology. From careful observations of his own and other children, Piaget delineated a specific series of stages in the development of cognitive functioning. Most importantly for the present discussion, Piaget's theories have been directly testable in ways not possible with Wernerian, Freudian, or other theories of development. Indeed, the testing, modification, and even the refutation of various parts of Piagetian theory have occupied a great many psychologists for the past three decades. While an extensive review of this literature obviously is beyond the scope of this book (see Brainerd, 1978), we will discuss a few selected aspects of Piaget's theory that are most relevant to the topic of mental retardation.

First, it is important to keep in mind that Piaget is primarily a cognitive developmentalist. While at various times he has addressed development in affective noncognitive domains (e.g., Piaget, 1981), his main contributions have been in detailing how children develop in the numerous areas of cognition. Even in his work on noncognitive phenomena, Piaget has emphasized their cognitive aspects, as in his study of children's developing understanding of rules as the basis of morality (Piaget, 1962). As might be expected, Piaget's theory has been criticized for underemphasizing the affective and motivational areas of children's functioning, such as their feelings, desires, and drives. Each of these factors can be very important in its own right, and each undoubtedly affects performance on tasks that seem purely cognitive. Later in this chapter we will attempt to expand cognitive-developmental theory to include motivation and other noncognitive phenomena.

Even with respect to cognition, Piaget's emphasis is almost exclusively on the processes, as opposed to the contents, of children's thought. In every instance, he examines children's responses to determine not what they think about (content), but rather the procedures involved in their thinking. It is therefore not unusual for Piaget to treat two widely divergent answers as stemming from a similar underlying mental process. For example, two boys may take opposite positions on a moral issue. One may justify his position by appealing to the authority of the police while the other appeals to the opposite authority of the gang leader. On the surface these answers suggest different types of social values, yet underlying this diversity may be a similarity of reasoning, a derivation of one's moral judgment from an external authority. It is this similarity of reasoning, the processes by which children arrive at their answers, that is of interest to Piaget.

A second issue concerns Piaget's interest in epistemology, or in how human beings come to acquire knowledge. Among Piaget's achievements is the categorization of the development of all of children's thinking processes into four identifiable stages (sensorimotor, preoperational, concrete, and formal operational). This strong point, however, is also a limitation in Piaget's theory. As Kessen noted, "Piaget has little interest in individual variation among children in the rate at which they achieve a stage . . . ; he is a student of the development of thinking more than he is a student of children" (1962, p. 77). This epistemological focus makes Piaget less interested in how children move from stage to stage, in the speed of cognitive development, in interventions aimed at increasing the speed of development, or in those extra-intellectual factors that affect performance on cognitive tasks, all areas of interest to those working with retarded children.

Finally, in recent years questions have arisen concerning the "cross-domain" nature of Piagetian cognitive stages. According to Piaget, each stage is a global characterization of the child's thinking; all areas of the child's cognitive functioning should indicate a certain level of reasoning. In addition, achievements in various domains should first occur at approximately the same time. Thus a child should display a particular substage in all cognitive domains simultaneously. However, this interrelationship of various cognitive subskills has not been borne out by research. Piagetian achievements that supposedly characterize a single underlying mental structure have often been found to develop at different times in individual children (Flavell, 1982). Such findings led Fischer to conclude that "unevenness is the rule in development" (1980, p. 510). Thus, while for any group of children various abilities may be acquired at a particular age, some children may be more advanced in one skill than in another, and for others the opposite will be true.

As a theorist interested in the cognitive growth of the prototypical child through a series of unified stages, Piaget has contributed greatly to our understanding of human development. But his focusing on the ideal child, his lack of attention to noncognitive phenomena, and the recently discovered difficulties with unified stages have caused many developmentalists to question parts of his formulation. Several psychologists (e.g., Fischer, 1980) have responded by proposing their own theories of cognitive development. Others (Flavell, 1982) have accepted some parts of the theory while rejecting others. Many have called for a broadening of cognitive-developmental theory, an issue to which we now turn.

Additions to cognitive-developmental theory

Piaget's cognitive-developmental theory can be expanded by attending to three sets of factors, environmental, motivational-affective, and endogenous. Each of these factors influences children in profound ways, and each helps to provide a more complete picture of the developing child.

In discussing the first of these factors, the effects of the environment on development, we first note that developmental theorists generally view developmental change as occurring through interactions between an active, "constructing" child and the environment. To Werner and Piaget, children are actively experimenting with their environments, forming new mental structures as they do so. In contrast, proponents of a mechanistic model (of which behaviorism is the main example) see all causes of change as external to the organism itself. The best example of such a behaviorist approach is Bijou and Baer's (1961; 1967) categorization of all of the child's behavior as consisting of either respondents (i.e., responses controlled by stimuli that precede them) or operants (responses controlled by stimuli that follow them). As summarized by Overton and Reese (1973), "In its ideal form the reactive organism model characterizes the organism as inherently at rest, and active only as a result of external forces" (p. 69).

These contrasting views of the source of change obviously affect how one envisions the role of the environment in promoting developmental change. While behaviorist theories have been criticized for overemphasizing environmental factors, developmentalists have been criticized for underemphasizing them. The issue of the environment is not altogether ignored in developmental theory, however. Werner (1948) refers to what he calls the *Umwelt*, the environment in the organism's terms. Thus, in viewing a room from the perspective of a dog, the areas of the strongest or most interesting smells might be considered most important. To an infant, the visual world is salient in the earliest months; after a year or so, the linguistic environment provided by others becomes increasingly important.

A compromise view of the role of environment in development appears in Sameroff's transactional model (1975). Troubled by the inability of tests of infant development to predict abilities at later ages, Sameroff came to the conclusion that both the child and the environment are developing – that each continually acts and reacts to interactions with the other. Examined in this way, there is no reason to expect early development to be predictive. A whole series of interactions from early infancy onward can deflect the child from his or her earlier course. To quote Sameroff,

> If developmental processes are to be understood it will not be through continuous assessment of the child alone, but through a continuous assessment of the transactions between the child and his environment to determine how these transactions facilitate or hinder adaptive integration as both the child and his surroundings change and evolve. (1975, p. 283)

This emphasis on a dynamic, developing environment is in harmony with the developmentalist's traditional view of an active and developing child.

We will return to this issue when dealing with intervention, but it is important to note here that Sameroff's model, and the idea of interaction in general (Bell, 1968), has spurred a large amount of work in developmental psychology in recent years. The areas of input language to children (e.g., Furrow, Nelson, & Benedict, 1979) and of mother–infant interaction (see Hodapp & Mueller, 1982) have especially flourished using this perspective. Indeed, by providing a more comprehensive view of the environment, the transactional model has opened up a whole new set of interesting problems to developmental research.

In discussing the environment, we must also be aware that it is not only changing as the child develops (the transactional perspective), but that it is also more extensive than is usually considered. For example, the average child develops within an environment that includes numerous adults (e.g., mother, father, neighbors, relatives), and other children (siblings, friends). In addition, children attend day-care centers, schools, and churches, and participate in clubs and sports. When discussing retarded children, several other environments must also be considered. Retarded children are often placed in special-education classes, mainstreamed classes, institutions, or sheltered workshops. The effects of each aspect of the total environment must enter into any discussion of children's development.

Surprisingly, most of the research on the so-called ecology of childhood has yet to be performed. Extensive research into the role of the father in the child's development, for example, only began in the 1970s (see Parke,

1979). Similarly, the effects of the birth of a baby on siblings and family functioning (Dunn & Kendrick, 1980) is a virtually unexplored area. Even the current focus on the family in child development (Bronfenbrenner, 1979) dates only from the late 1970s. Such ecological research is proliferating and promises new insights into development in the near future.

A second area, with a longer history of empirical interest, concerns the causes and effects of socioemotional factors. Such factors affect the child's performance on a variety of laboratory and everyday tasks in profound ways. For example, repeated experience with success or failure may influence how children feel about themselves (self-concept), whether they trust their own solutions to problems (inner-directedness) or instead feel dependent on adults for solutions (outer-directedness), and whether children feel highly motivated or wary about interacting with supportive adults (positive or negative reaction tendencies). These attitudes will color how, or even whether, children approach particular tasks in their environment.

Finally, there are several endogenous factors that influence development. A child's gender, race, and genetic inheritance are brought into whatever environment the child enters. Such biological givens may influence the child's rate of development, degree of social adaptation, and likelihood of being affected by any number of problems. For example, boys are somewhat more likely than girls to be retarded, as are lower-SES children and those whose parents have low IQs. Each of these groups also has a different experiential history, however, which brings us back to the notion that children and their environments influence one another.

The view that results from combining cognitive-developmental theory with environmental, motivational, and endogenous factors is that of a more complete, multidimensional child. This expanded version of the developmental perspective also provides for a more individualized person; the child's particular experiences, background, and personal characteristics are all considered.

This orientation is shown schematically in Figure 2.1. In contrast to the Piagetian cognitive-developmental view, a child responding to a question does not merely demonstrate a particular level of cognitive stages, but also shows idiosyncratic personal characteristics. For example, the retarded child accustomed to failure may not even attempt to solve a challenging problem (Harter & Zigler, 1974). The lower-class child, distrusting an unfamiliar tester, may produce monosyllabic answers well below his or her actual level of language (e.g., Labov, 1970). Both children end up performing far below their abilities. This distinction between a child's *competence* (what the child is capable of doing) and the child's *performance*

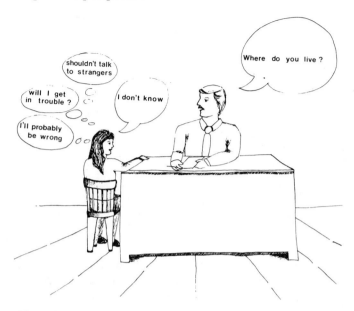

Figure 2.1. An example of the child's performance not reflecting the child's true competence. (Figure drawn by courtesy of Amy C. Cox)

(what the child actually does in a given situation) must be taken into consideration when one attempts to ascertain a child's level of functioning. Thus, in going beyond traditional developmental topics of cognitive and linguistic phenomena, serious attention must be paid to the many motivational, ecological, and endogenous factors that make up the whole child, a topic to which we return in Chapter 6.

The developmental perspective applied to retarded persons

The developmental perspective provides the researcher and practitioner with a broad conceptualization of children's growth. This approach has come to include all major influences on children, even in areas not normally associated with developmental (i.e., Wernerian or Piagetian) analyses. Obviously, the application of such a wide-ranging perspective to retarded individuals must itself be multifaceted, with different theorists, even those within the developmental camp, arguing among themselves about which aspects of the theory are appropriate to the study of retardation.

A preliminary question concerns whether all or part of the retarded population fits within the developmental framework. As we read in Chapter 1, some retarded individuals demonstrate clear organic etiologies while

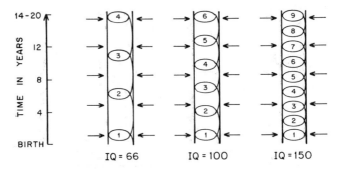

Figure 2.2. Developmental model of cognitive growth. The single vertical arrow represents the passage of time. The horizontal arrows represent environmental events impinging on the individual who is represented as a pair of vertical lines. The individual's cognitive development appears as an internal ascending spiral in which the numbered loops represent successive stages of cognitive growth.

others do not. We must briefly discuss some aspects of this issue before we can describe how the developmental perspective applies to the field of mental retardation.

Development in organic and familial retardation

Familial retarded persons, those who display no known organic etiology, are usually mildly or moderately retarded. Their IQs fall within the lower end of the Gaussian or bell-shaped distribution of intelligence. We view these individuals as normal in the sense that they possess the same basic cognitive equipment as those with IQs of 80, 100, or 120. Familial retarded persons differ only in their rates of development and, ultimately, in the highest mental levels attained. Thus the same principles of cognitive development that apply throughout the normal range of intelligence should also describe familial retarded persons.

This model is depicted in Figure 2.2, which shows the progression of developmental stages in familial retarded, average, and bright children. Children of higher intellect proceed at a faster pace and stop developing at a higher level, but the successive stages are identical. While we will present evidence for this developmental pattern in familial retarded children later, we should mention that this model has been supported for above-average children. That is, bright children have been found to perform at higher Piagetian stages than their average-IQ agemates in infancy (Gottfried & Brody, 1975) and for 5th and 7th graders (Keating, 1975).

The second type of retarded individual, the person who shows a clear organic etiology, is not so easily described in the same terms as his or her nonretarded peers. These people may not be a part of the normal (Gaussian) distribution of intelligence because their intellectual apparatus has in some way been damaged. Indeed, Zigler (1969) has called it "illogical" to extend developmental principles to individuals with organic defects, whatever their IQs may be: "If the etiology of the phenotypic intelligence (as measured by an IQ) of two groups differ, it is far from logical to assert that the course of development is the same, or that even similar contents in their behaviors are mediated by exactly the same cognitive process" (p. 533).

In contrast, other developmentally oriented workers are comfortable applying the developmental perspective to organically retarded people. Cicchetti and Pogge-Hesse (1982), for example, have attempted to apply developmental principles to children with Down syndrome and to children progressing through the early stages of cognitive development. These workers feels that all retarded children, regardless of the etiology of their retardation, do traverse similar stages of development and possess the same underlying structure to their intelligence as do nonretarded children (see Hodapp & Zigler, in press, for a discussion of the similar structure issue as it relates to organically retarded children). For the present, let us say only that the degree to which the developmental approach applies to organically retarded individuals is an open question. Our discussion below, then, concerns only familial retarded persons, although findings pertaining to those with organic etiology are noted when available.

General applications of the developmental perspective

In its most general form, the developmental view emphasizes the similarities between the functioning of nonretarded and retarded persons. Developmentalists conceptualize the cognitive growth of retarded children in three ways: (1) as progressing through the same cognitive stages that nonretarded children traverse (similar sequence hypothesis), (2) as having a similar structure of intelligence as nonretarded children at each level of development (similar structure hypothesis), and (3) as responding to environmental factors in the same ways in which all children respond. We now turn to each of these issues.

Similar sequence hypothesis. The similar sequence hypothesis predicts that retarded and nonretarded children traverse the same stages of cognitive development, differing only in the rate at which they progress and the ultimate ceiling they attain. In Piagetian terms, the sequence from sensorimotor to preoperational to concrete operational to formal operational thought is predicted to occur in retarded children, in exactly this order. A more rigorous test of the hypothesis occurs within each of the major stages. For example, based on Piaget's writings Uzgiris and Hunt (1975) identified a number of substages of sensorimotor development in six domains of infant intelligence. Similarly, universal sequences of development have been identified in numerous other areas examined by Piaget, and each of these sequences is open to test of the similar sequence hypothesis. (See Inhelder, 1968, and Woodward, 1979, for discussions of the application of Piagetian theory to retarded individuals.) Both Piaget (1956) and Kohlberg (1967) have argued that similarities in sequence should apply to all children, irrespective of cultural, intellectual, or neurological characteristics. Their arguments rest on their belief that such sequences are logically ordered, that the environment promotes development of such sequences, and that the human nervous system may be preprogrammed to develop according to these specific stages. Thus the similar sequence hypothesis should be applicable to both familial and organically retarded children. The bulk of the evidence to date confirms this. Summarizing 28 cross-sectional and three longitudinal studies of functioning in retarded children, Weisz and Zigler (1979) concluded that the great preponderance of the evidence indicates that the same stages of development appear in the same order in nonretarded and retarded persons, regardless of etiology.

Similar structure hypothesis. A second application of the developmental perspective involves the view that nonretarded and familial retarded persons have similar processes underlying their intellectual functioning. When the two groups are matched for general level of intellectual development (mental age, or MA), they should be similar with respect to the formal cognitive processes they employ in reasoning and problem solving. Defect theorists, on the other hand, hypothesize a different structure of intelligence in all retarded children. They argue that the defect that causes retardation should hinder functioning on tasks related to that defect. For example, if all mental retardation is caused by a defect in verbal mediation, then retarded children with a mental age of 6 years should show greater deficits on linguistic tasks than average 6-year-olds. This *MA-matched design* compares retarded and nonretarded children on a task thought to tap functioning in the area of hypothesized defect in the retarded group.

Although widely employed in mental retardation research, the MA-matched design has become controversial. Baumeister (1967) notes that "two people can have the same MA, but for entirely different reasons" (p. 874). He goes on to list other factors that might make differences between two MA-matched groups uninterpretable. These factors, including institutionalization, school experience, and SES, "deserve as much attention as MA" (p. 874). In short, Baumeister warns against a simpleminded matching strategy that does not account for other relevant factors affecting performance. He also advocates the study of retarded populations alone, without reference to normal individuals.

A second criticism of the MA-matched design is that it involves what statisticians call proving the null hypothesis. Statistically, it is easier to demonstrate that two groups differ than to show that they are the same. Indeed, there is a lively debate among statisticians over this issue: Some regard acceptance of the null hypothesis as inappropriate, whereas others argue that if the null hypothesis can be tested, it can also be accepted as valid (see Binder, 1963, and Grant, 1962, for discussions of this issue). "Given the preference of research journals for studies which report differences between groups, findings of 'no difference' between MA-matched retarded and nonretarded children may actually be underrepresented in the psychology literature. This may have been particularly true in the years prior to a clear articulation of the developmental position and its 'no difference' prediction (Zigler, 1967;1969), because the absence of a theoretical explanation for findings of no difference would, no doubt undermine the publishability of such findings" (Weisz, Yeates, & Zigler, 1982, p. 263). Thus, although tests of the similar structure hypothesis involve procedures thought unorthodox in some circles, they do have theoretical merit as one method of examining the structure of intelligence in familial retarded and nonretarded children.

Since organically retarded children show clear organic causes for their retardation, some argue that the similar structure hypothesis is relevant only for the familial retarded groups. Others (e.g., Cicchetti & Serafica, 1981) conceptualize development as "organized" across domains for nonretarded, familial retarded, and organically retarded children. For example, Woodward (1979) contends that the stage construct "may be useful in the case of those [retarded children] from whom only a small sample of behavior can be obtained" (p. 174), since if one knows that a child is capable of only a certain stage on one cognitive task, other tasks should show the child at an identical level. As noted above, however, the view that developments indicative of identical Piagetian mental structures develop simultaneously may not be correct, at least for development in nonretarded children.

Many studies have tested the similar structure hypothesis for both types of retarded children. These studies cover the entire spectrum of Piagetian tasks, including tests of conservation, role taking, sex identity, relative thinking, moral judgments, and color identity. In a review of 33 studies that matched nonretarded and familial retarded children on MA, 30 showed no differences between the groups, and only 3 showed the nonretarded group to be superior to the retarded sample. In general, then, there seems to be a similar structure of intelligence in familial retarded and in nonretarded children. In contrast, 22 of 71 studies showed differences favoring nonretarded children when etiology was uncontrolled (i.e., when the retarded group consisted of both familial and organically retarded children). Of the remaining 49 studies, 45 showed the two groups to be equivalent. Therefore, this summary of available studies does not provide support for the similar structure hypothesis as it concerns organically retarded children; instead, it may be that "organically impaired retarded persons are cognitively different from those not suffering from specific organic defects" (Weisz et al., 1982, p. 269).

A second method of testing the similar structure hypothesis, at least as it relates to familial retarded children, involves comparing them with nonretarded children on the profile of subtest scores on intelligence tests. The rationale is that, if a particular defect causes retardation in the familial group, then familial retarded children should perform lower on subtests tapping this particular ability, while tests of other abilities should remain relatively unaffected. For example, if a verbal mediation defect causes mental retardation, then verbal subtest scores of familial retarded children on an instrument like the WISC-R (Wechsler Intelligence Test for Children–Revised Version; Wechsler, 1974) should be lower than scores on performance subtests (which require less language). In one study of this issue, Groff and Linden (1982) examined subtests tapping three factors of the WISC-R, verbal comprehension, perceptual organization, and freedom from distractibility. They found that the profile of scores of older (aged 13–16) and younger (aged 8–11) familial retarded children was similar to that of nonretarded children aged from 8 to 11.

Profile analysis results offered no evidence of differences in the intellectual strengths and weaknesses of cultural-familial retarded and nonretarded groups of equivalent CA or MA. The findings are consistent with predictions from the developmental theory of retardation, which expects similar intellectual strengths and weaknesses for MA-matched cultural-familial retarded and nonretarded youth. (1982, p. 150)

Figure 2.3 shows the profiles on the three WISC-R factors for the three groups of children. (Similar results on the Stanford-Binet test were reported by Achenbach, 1970.)

A third method tests the similar structure hypothesis by experimentally manipulating the motivations that familial retarded and nonretarded chil-

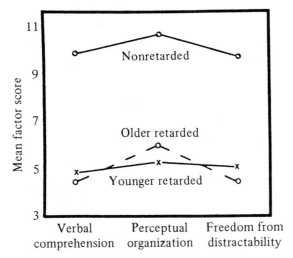

Figure 2.3. Profiles of WISC-R mean factor scores. Note how the two groups of familial retarded children show profiles similar to that of the nonretarded group.

dren have when attempting to solve cognitive tasks. For example, Zigler and deLabry (1962) gave familial retarded children concept-switching problems under two conditions. In the first condition, children were simply asked to sort cards (which could be sorted according to either form or color) for several trials. In the second condition, children were told that they would receive an attractive prize if they performed well. Zigler and deLabry found that retarded children less often switched their sorting principles (from color to form or vice versa) when no reinforcements were offered. When told that they could win a prize, however, the children switched sorting principles more frequently. This suggests that the so-called cognitive rigidity thought to be inherent in retarded children is the result of motivational factors, as the retarded children were capable of sorting flexibly when tangible rewards for good performance were offered.

In summary, studies using MA-matched designs, profiles of IQ subtests, and manipulation of motivations affecting performance on cognitive tasks, show that familial retarded children do seem to have an intelligence similar in structure to that of nonretarded children. But there does not seem to be a similar structure of intelligence in children who are organically retarded.

Similar responses to environmental factors. Developmental theorists emphasize the similarities between retarded and nonretarded people; they tend to believe both groups should react to environmental forces in like ways. But the environments of the two groups are usually not alike, as retarded persons tend to have peculiar experiential histories. They are more likely to attend special classes or special schools, to be the lower-functioning members of their peer group, and to experience failure in many situations. Considering just the latter case, a long history of failure may engender behavior patterns in retarded persons not commonly found in the nonretarded. Failure may teach one to act differently.

Studies of learned helplessness in retarded and nonretarded children provide one example of the power of experience in shaping behavior. Learned helplessness has three components: (1) the attribution of failure to factors over which one has no control (e.g., "I'm dumb" instead of "I could have succeeded if I had only tried harder"), (2) the lack of voluntarily initiated responses (e.g., not attempting to turn off a loud bell which has "accidentally" gone on while the experimenter is out of the room), and (3) the inability to persevere at a task at which one has failed. In one study of this phenomenon, Weisz (1978) examined the three components of learned helplessness in groups of retarded, average, and bright children matched on each of three MA levels (5, 7, and 9 years). Results showed that all groups demonstrated lesser amounts of "helpless" behavior with increasing MA. However, at the higher MA level, the retarded children were more helpless relative to the nonretarded group than they were at the lower MA levels. "This finding is in harmony with the view that retarded children learn helplessness over years of development, and, by extension, that successive failures and helplessness-inducing feedback play a causal role" (Weisz, 1978, p. 317).

Learned helplessness is but one of the behavioral effects that environmental forces can produce. Settings such as schools, families, and institutions can also affect behavior. Studies of such factors must include a simultaneous examination of changes based on increasing mental age and those due to the specific experiences that retarded children undergo. In addition, researchers must recognize not only that the effects of the environment are cumulative, but, as described above, that both the child and the environment are changing over time. See Chapters 6, 10, and 11 for further details of the effects of external experiences on the functioning of retarded persons.

The organic versus familial issue appears in the context of reactions to environment as well. In particular, the experiences faced by the two types of retarded person may differ radically, leading to different behavioral responses. For example, organically retarded children are found about equally in all socioeconomic levels, whereas familial retarded children come predominantly from lower-SES families. The experience of growing up as a retarded child in a middle-class family, with parents and siblings of normal intelligence, may differ greatly from the experience of a familial retarded child from a lower-SES family in which parents and siblings are themselves of low intelligence. Few studies have yet investigated the differential effects of such disparate environmental histories.

Practical contributions of the developmental perspective

The developmental perspective has allowed for a host of practical contributions to intervention and research with retarded persons. Armed with knowledge of normal development in the areas of cognition, language, and early social skills, workers have attempted to design interventions to foster similar development in familial and organically retarded children. For example, Carl Dunst (1980a) modified the Piagetian-based Ordinal Scales of Infant Development (Uzgiris & Hunt, 1975) so that they may be used to assess behavior in retarded and physically handicapped infants. In addition to providing a useful clinical instrument, the modified test, with its Piagetian scale of skills, serves as a basis for intervention. Teachers of retarded infants (or severely and profoundly retarded older children) can "teach to the test," secure in the knowledge that skills in object permanence, means–ends, causality, and imitation are necessary for later development (Bates et al., 1975; R. Brown, 1973; Curcio, 1978).

Other workers have focused on the naturalistic observations of development in various domains in order to see if retarded children do indeed progress along the "invariant stages of normal development." If it can be shown that retarded children develop along the normal sequence in a particular domain, all of the accumulated knowledge about normal development in that domain can be applied in an intervention program. One can then know whether or when to provide training in the sensorimotor domains of infancy, conservation training, language training, and even training in the stages of moral reasoning. Thus knowledge about normal development becomes the bedrock upon which to base intervention programs for retarded children. See Chapter 7 for a detailed description of behavioral interventions from a developmental perspective.

A second contribution of the developmental perspective as it relates to mental retardation is its emphasis on external forces. This focus now has a rich though recent history in the MR field. In response to early studies showing "defects" in retarded persons, Zigler decried the lack of attention paid to the atypical environments of such individuals (see Zigler, 1971; 1984 for reviews of these studies). Researchers acted as if a person's retardation overrides all other factors. Where and how a person lived were of little concern, only whether or not the person was retarded. For example, most studies compared home-reared nonretarded to institutionalized retarded children, then attributed differences between the two groups to the effects of retardation. Such designs obscured whether behavioral differences were due to something inherent in retardation, to motivational factors caused by different life experiences, or to some combination of these two forces.

Concerns such as these helped lead Zigler and his colleagues to explore the effects of institutionalization, failure, and social deprivation on the performance of retarded and nonretarded children. By now workers in mental retardation know a fair amount about such nonintellective factors. Indeed, this detailed account of the influence of external factors on the behaviors of retarded persons is considered "one of the richest legacies" of the developmental approach to mental retardation (Weisz, 1982).

A related issue involves research designs in studies of mental retardation. Before the developmental perspective was applied to retarded persons, work in the field was often of low quality (Zigler, 1977). Comparisons between retarded and nonretarded children of the same chronological age (CA-matched designs) were common, retarded groups were formed for study without consideration of etiology, and retarded children living in institutions were compared to nonretarded home-reared children. Currently, MA-matched designs are common, greater attention is paid to etiology, nonintellective determinants of performance are considered, and test scores are factor-analyzed to give more detailed comparisons of the structure of behavior in retarded versus nonretarded individuals. The application of many of these procedures to the retarded population is a direct outgrowth of developmental concerns.

Finally, we must mention the ways in which study of normal development informs work with retarded individuals, and vice versa. In general, "we can learn more about the normal functioning of an organism by studying its pathology and, likewise, more about its pathology by studying its normal condition" (Cicchetti, 1984, p. 1). Several benefits accrue from this cross-fertilization between developmental psychology and research in mental retardation.

First, research originally designed to answer developmental questions frequently provides knowledge about particular types of retardation. For example, consider Weisz et al.'s (1982) review of studies of the similar structure hypothesis discussed above. Analyses of the Piagetian task performance of any one etiological syndrome within the retarded group can tell us much about that particular condition. Even within a syndrome, subgroups can be discovered. Cicchetti and Sroufe (1976) found that Down syndrome infants progress through similar stages of cognitive development as do normal infants, but they also discovered that the most hypotonic of Down syndrome infants (i.e., those with the weakest muscle tones) were the lowest-functioning (a finding extended to early social and feeding behaviors by Cullen, Cronk, Pueschel, Schnell, & Reed, 1981). Similarly, Weisz and Zigler (1979) concluded that children who have severe electroencephalographic abnormalities (i.e., seizure disorders) may be the only organically retarded children who do not develop along the normal sequence of Piagetian stages. Each of these findings provides information as to the specific behavioral consequences (over and above retardation) of a particular syndrome. Information of this type is invaluable to anyone attempting to intervene with organically retarded children.

Second, atypical groups can help clarify the processes of normal development. For example, the entire issue of whether it is possible to have thought without language was answered in the affirmative through studies of deaf children. Indeed, Furth (1969) discovered numerous nonlinguistic children who nevertheless demonstrated cognitive abilities, up to and including concrete operational thought. Because retarded children progress through developmental stages at slower rates, the study of their behavior also allows for the examination of development in ways not possible with nonretarded children. For example, which sensorimotor developments are most important for the development of communicative skills, and which are least important? From studies of retarded (Kahn 1975; Mundy, Siebert, & Hogan, 1984), emotionally disturbed (Curcio, 1978), and language-delayed (Snyder, 1978) children, a clear picture emerges: Means–ends skills (use of an object or a person as a tool) and imitation skills are necessary, and object permanence and spatial skills unnecessary for further developments in this area. Research demonstrating which particular skills are necessary for the development of a later skill could not be performed using normal infants, in whom developments in related areas occur at roughly the same time.

Third, developmental psychology provides the current topics of interest for research in other areas. Historically, the field has undergone major shifts in orientation every decade or so. For example, the 1960s saw the Piagetian revolution, although the socialization model, studies of attachment, and linguistic studies based on Noam Chomsky's work were also prominent. The 1970s saw a greater emphasis on children's social-emotional development, the semantics and pragmatics of language, interaction between children and their parents, and the family focus. The 1980s have added life-span developmental psychology and expanded the emphases on several topics of the 1970s. While these examples do serve to illustrate the trendiness of developmental psychology, they also show how it provides the field with new sources of ideas and research problems.

Changes in the topics of interest in developmental psychology are also felt in the mental retardation field. For example, the 1960s focus on the development of grammar (reviewed by R. Brown, 1973) found expression in Lenneberg's (1967) attempts to demonstrate the innate unfolding of grammatical stages in retarded children. Later, when the hegemony of grammar was supplanted by semantics and pragmatics in developmental psycholinguistics, intervention programs for retarded children also began to emphasize these aspects of communication (e.g., MacDonald & Blott, 1974; McLean & Snyder-McLean, 1978). Similar extensions to research and intervention can be found in the current emphases in mental retardation research on mother-retarded child interaction (for a review of this research, see Marfo, 1984) and the role of the family in development (Blacher, 1984). Each is a topic of widespread interest in developmental psychology.

This is not to say that every fashionable idea in developmental psychology is automatically extended to work with retarded people, or that advances proceed only from developmental psychology to the mental retardation field. On several occasions current concerns in developmental psychology were foreshadowed by research in mental retardation. For example, work by Farber (1959) and Grossman (1972) on the families of retarded children predates work by Bronfenbrenner (1979) and Dunn and Kendrick (1980) on the families of nonretarded children. As the discipline with the smaller number of workers, however, the mental retardation field generally needs and benefits from the research and ideas of developmental psychology.

Summary

Development involves those changes in internal mental structures that lead the organism to its mature state. A general characterization of developmental change is provided by Werner (1957), who states that all development proceeds from a global and undifferentiated state to a state of differentiation, specification, and hierarchic integration. The role of the environment in promoting developmental change is controversial, with developmentalists viewing the child as the agent of change and behaviorists attributing all change to the environment. In Sameroff's transactional model, both the child and environment are seen as changing as a result of their ongoing interactions with one another. Our review of Piagetian cognitive-developmental theory emphasizes the need to study the motivational, ecological, and endogenous forces that affect children as they develop, in order to understand better the whole child.

Our application of the developmental perspective to retarded people emphasizes that retarded and nonretarded children go through a similar sequence of development, have a similar structure of intelligence, and react similarly to environmental forces. In tests of these hypotheses, the type of retardation must be considered, as familial retarded persons may differ from organically retarded persons in some or all of these areas.

The developmental perspective has contributed much to work and research involving mental retardation. First, developmental theories have provided meaningful ways to assess functioning and to intervene with retarded persons. Second, the perspective points to the need to examine external forces when attempting to understand the retarded person's behavior. Finally, the cross-fertilization between developmental psychology and the field of mental retardation informs work with retarded persons and provides knowledge about the processes of normal development.

Part II

Definition, classification, etiology, and prevalence

3 Definition and classification of mental retardation

Without a clear and universally accepted definition of mental retardation, efforts to understand its nature and to improve the lives of retarded people must be seriously compromised. Nowhere is the definitional void felt more seriously than in attempts to estimate the prevalence of mental retardation, whether throughout the United States or the world (see Chapter 5). Of course census data calculated for any condition will depend on how the condition is defined, the procedure for case identification, and the demographics of the geographic area under study. Studies done by different investigators in different places may vary on all these dimensions, making it difficult to interpret and generalize from research findings. If such figures were based on a common definition as well as on consistent reporting standards, there would be some reasonable basis for determining whether variations in social, political, medical, and educational practices have an appreciable impact on the prevalence of retardation in a society.

The lack of a soundly established definition also hinders classification *within* mental retardation, classification being the bedrock of any scientific field. Consider how even a simple, two-group categorization brings some order to the area of subnormal intellectual functioning. Individuals labeled mentally retarded might be assigned (with considerable agreement) to two distinct groups: those suffering known organic defects, and those with no evidence of organic pathology. This proposition leads immediately to insights concerning etiology, behavioral consequences, and prognosis for labeled individuals. Yet even this relatively straightforward typology is stifled by disagreement over who should be labeled mentally retarded, and even whether that label should be used at all. Theorists, researchers, clinicians, and educators are all caught in this definitional mire, which frustrates and complicates their efforts. Of course the real victims in all this

Portion's of this chapter appeared in the *American Journal of Mental Deficiency*. (1984, *39*, 215–230)

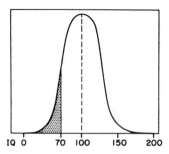

Figure 3.1. The normal or Gaussian distribution, as it is hypothesized to apply to the distribution of IQ scores.

are retarded persons, for whom society has good intentions thwarted by scientific indecision.

Elements of a basic classification system

The common approach to describing variations in human cognitive abilities relies on the normal or Gaussian curve to represent the distribution of intelligence (see Figure 3.1). Intelligence, as measured by intelligence tests, is viewed as having a distribution in which small segments of the population have either very low or very high IQs, with most of the population having intelligence levels falling around the mean score. Thus, intelligence is described as being distributed like other human characteristics such as height, strength of handgrip, and running speed. The pictorial distribution is thought to be little more than a representation of what is encountered in nature.

One thing *not* encountered in nature is the mean value of the distribution of 100. This particular value is nothing more than an outcome of test standardization practices and convention. Intelligence tests are constructed in such a way that the median score obtained in the standardization population is assigned the number 100. It is easy to forget that any number could have been assigned to the median test performance, and that many tests do not have a median (which in very large populations is the same as the mean) of 100. Scores on IQ tests having a mean of 100 can be converted to scores employing standard deviation (*SD*) units (i.e., how far in such units a person's score is from the mean). This alternative is mentioned here only to highlight the arbitrary nature of that powerful number, the IQ score.

Even more arbitrary is the line drawn in Figure 3.1 at IQ 70 to differentiate retarded from nonretarded people. The rationale for selecting this particular IQ cutoff is based on a statistical formula rather than on logic or sound classification procedures. For many years it has been customary to define mental retardation by IQ scores falling more than two *SDs* below the mean. Such a score depends on the psychometric characteristics of the IQ test employed. The most popular tests of intelligence are the Stanford-Binet and the Wechsler Intelligence Scales (WISC-R and WAIS). On each of these tests the *SDs* are approximately 15. Thus, the 70 IQ cutoff seen in Figure 3.1 reflects the widely accepted convention of applying the label "retarded" to those whose scores are more than two *SDs* below the mean.

But why two standard deviations? Why not one and a half, or three? The point must be made that computing an *SD* and employing the numerical result as the defining feature of mental retardation sheds no light on the phenomenon of intellectual subnormality. In fact, the practice of relying upon statistical criteria to define mental retardation has sometimes led to confusion rather than clarification. Consider what happened some years ago when our nation's leading professional and scientific organization in the field advanced the definition that all scores below one *SD* from the mean comprised the retarded range (Heber, 1961). Overnight, the prevalence of retardation jumped from approximately 3% to 16% of the population, increasing the ranks of retarded persons in our nation from approximately 6 to 32 million! The line was subsequently moved back to two *SDs* below the mean, where it remains today. This story suggests that where this arbitrary line is placed will change as a function of the time the decision is made and social propensities to offer more or less assistance. Regardless of how many times and to where the cutoff is moved, much knowledge about mental retardation will remain elusive.

A note on the goals of any classification system is in order at this point. While classification may have a number of purposes (Cromwell, Blashfield, & Strauss, 1975; Hobbs, 1975; Zigler & Phillips, 1961a), its primary goal is to enhance our understanding of the scientific area in which it is employed. Any useful and well-specified classification system has two major features. The first is the classificatory principle that provides the rules for placing an individual into one class rather than another. A good classificatory principle is one that allows for such placement with high agreement among different classifiers. The methodological issue here involves reliability: The better the principle, the higher the reliability of classification. The second important feature of a classification system concerns the number of meaningful correlates of class membership. That is, what do you know about an individual on the basis of the classification alone? The more you know (i.e., the more class correlates), the better the classification system. The methodological issue here concerns validity: The higher the number and statistical robustness of the class correlates, the greater the validity of the system.

A system could be established solely through the use of IQ as a classificatory principle. The principle would be based on scores obtained on well- standardized intelligence tests such as the Stanford-Binet or Wechsler. The reliability coefficient of such tests is so high (approximately .90) that the classification system would have considerable reliability. Individuals would be placed into categories on the basis of IQ, and then the task of mental retardation workers would be the systematic discovery of the behavioral correlates of each class. A very important collection of class correlates would consist of what individuals within each intelligence class can and cannot do. Such abilities and limitations would be age-related; for example, a child with an IQ of 45 may not be capable of a certain behavior at age 4 but would be able to perform the behavior at age 8.

The age aspect of this classificatory model is of crucial importance. The needs of planning for retarded persons give special value to class correlates that allow us to predict what behaviors a retarded individual will be capable of years after the classification has originally been made. Moving from contemporaneous to long-term prediction would be easier if one could assume that those in a particular IQ class at an early age will remain in the same class at a later age. This assumption touches upon one of the most problematic issues in the study of intelligence, namely the constancy of the IQ across the life cycle.

In the recent past it was fashionable to refer to the wandering IQ, viewing intelligence quotients as amenable to marked changes at different ages (Hunt, 1961). This notion of the plastic IQ represented a needed and perhaps healthy reaction to the fixed intelligence beliefs of the once-popular maturationists such as Arnold Gesell. As in the case of most conceptual reactions, however, this development probably went too far (see Chapter 4). The foolish heights to which the plastic view was carried can be seen in research reports that some minimal intervention early in life resulted in IQ increases in the range of 50–70 points (Hunt, 1971). Such interpretations blatantly ignored one of the soundest findings in the intelligence field: Developmental quotients (the IQ for infants) obtained in the first year of life are unrelated to intelligence quotients obtained a few years later (Bayley, 1955; Bayley & Schaefer, 1964; M. Lewis, 1976).

Discrepencies between infant and childhood test results are not surprising, given the absence of agreement on exactly what intelligence is (see Chapter 1). Thus, infant tests may not predict scores on later tests simply because the tests given at different ages gauge different collections of processes, with all collections labeled "intelligence." Making the constancy problem even more difficult is the accepted view that the growth of intelligence is essentially a developmental progression in which the processes and/or structures mediating intellectual behavior are always changing (Evans, 1973; Flavell, 1963).

The existence of such changes in IQ does not invalidate the system advanced in Figure 3.1. The IQ does appear to stabilize, and for large groups of children scores from about the age of 4 become relatively robust predictors of later IQs. After early childhood the IQ of any one child may change by as much as 20 points, but for most individuals the IQ remains relatively constant (Sontag, Baker, & Nelson, 1958; Vernon, 1979; Zigler, 1966). Furthermore, in the case of infants with severe physiological damage, one can say intelligence scores obtained in the first year of life do predict later intellectual behavior relatively well. When an infant obtains a very low developmental quotient such as 20, there is little doubt that throughout life he or she will evidence impoverished intellectual abilities. This is most evident in the extreme case of the anencephalic child whose developmental quotient may validly be ascribed as zero. Over the child's relatively short life span, intelligence will probably remain at this level.

A final caveat is in order before one accepts uncritically the notion that IQ scores do not wander far after the early years. Even if relative standing on intelligence tests is considered constant, this standing is defined in terms of changing criteria. That is, the individual must continue to meet the changing demands of the environment and the social expectancies of the culture in which he or she is a member. Thus, if an infant cannot crawl by 18 months of age, we label the child retarded. In an industrialized society a child who cannot talk by the age of 3 or manage to read by age 9 would also be considered retarded. The social component of our definition of intelligence immediately becomes apparent when we realize that in a society where no one reads, the failure to read by the age of 9 could not be used as an indicator of mental retardation. We thus see the arbitrariness of any classification system for intelligence that we might construct.

Relationships between IQ, CA, and MA

Another problem with the IQ-based system is that the emphasis on the classificatory principle of IQ gives the erroneous impression that the correlates of class membership are determined by the individual's IQ. In actuality, the IQ does not really determine anyone's abilities. The score is fundamentally a measure of the *rate* of intellectual development. The only

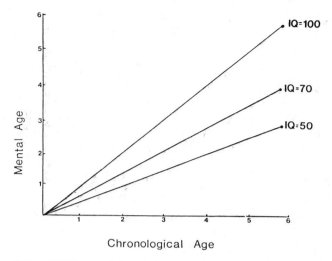

Figure 3.2. Slopes of changes in Mental Age over time at three IQ levels.

independent variables involved in assessing the child's relative intellectual standing are chronological age (CA) and mental age (MA). The MA is computed by awarding the child a certain number of months for the test items he or she is able to pass. Thus, the child's intellectual level is defined by the MA, the measure of what cognitive tasks the child is capable of doing. The CA informs us of how long it took the child to achieve this intellectual level. The IQ as a measure of rate of intellectual development can be seen clearly in Figure 3.2, which shows the relation between MA and CA for different IQ groups. The slopes of the three groups are markedly different, and a close examination should deter us from thinking that the low-IQ individual is invariably less capable than the higher-IQ individual. As can be seen in the figure, the 50-IQ child with a CA of 6 is at a higher intellectual level (as defined by MA) than a 100-IQ child with a CA of 2. However, the absolute difference in intellectual level between retarded and nonretarded children increases with age, because the abilities of those with lower IQs develop at a slower rate.

Confusing the issue further is the interrelation between the three measures (IQ, MA, and CA). A bit of simple arithmetic demonstrates that if CA is held constant, MA and IQ are correlated perfectly. Thus, in the classificatory model based on IQ, MA could be substituted for IQ as the classificatory principle so long as the MA classifications are limited to specific age groups. If validity is the primary goal of the system, then an argument could be made that both classification systems should be employed, one using MA and the other using IQ as the classificatory principle. MA is probably the best predictor we have of how well the child can do on the type of tasks found on IQ tests. However, like CA, MA is a constantly changing measure. Even severely impaired retarded children usually gain in their intellectual abilities. The IQ, which is relatively constant, therefore has a greater influence on how others perceive and interact with the child, although adults do modify their behavior in accordance with the child's level of ability (Brooks-Gunn & Lewis, 1984; Jones, 1980; Rondal, 1977). This interaction with adults, in turn, is another important determinant of the child's behavior. The low-IQ child whose social interactions have led him or her to feel inadequate will behave quite differently from a child at the same IQ level who has not developed such a negative self-image. There is thus a strong case for employing IQ as the classificatory principle, even if this gives the MA less status than we might like.

While IQ and MA have an extensive impact on behavior, the CA variable should not be overlooked. One interesting if iconoclastic formulation was advanced by Kohlberg (1969), who argued that certain behaviors partaking of cognitive development (e.g., role-taking ability) are influenced by the sheer number of exchanges that the individual has had with the environment. Since retarded children are older than nonretarded children of the same MA, they have had more of these exchanges. This would generate the prediction that in studies of retarded and nonretarded children matched on MA, the retarded group would perform more adequately. While an occasional finding supports this formulation (e.g., A. Brown, 1973), the bulk of the research in the field does not (Weisz et al., 1982; Weisz & Zigler, 1979).

Still, since CA is clearly a determinant of many physical behaviors, the issue remains as to which more psychological behaviors are influenced by CA and which are not. It is unlikely that CA would have much impact on the type of cognitive performance required on IQ tests or in studies that assess particular cognitive processes. Rather, CA probably does affect less cognitively demanding social behaviors and interests. Just as sex roles are learned in the socialization process, age roles are also inculcated. Through direct teaching, observation of others, and the omnipresent TV set, retarded people like everyone else learn that at certain ages one should engage in a repertoire of age-appropriate behavior. A 9-year-old boy should play baseball; a 16-year-old girl should wear makeup and have dates; a 25-year-old should be married. As long as the retarded person has the intellectual ability to perform the customary task, he or she is highly motivated to do so. This heightened motivation is understandable, since for many retarded persons behaving like others becomes evidence for their own normality and self-worth.

In addition to obvious age-role behavior (and consistent with the thinking of Kohlberg), there must be a wide variety of tasks whose performance is enhanced through sheer repetition or overlearning. We would of course be hesitant to tell a 7-year-old with an average IQ to catch a bus and go downtown. But such a task would be well within the ability of a 25-year-old retarded person with an MA of 7. In fact, the recent history of remediation efforts indicates that many retarded persons are more capable than commonly believed (Schroeder, Mulick, & Schroeder, 1979; Whitman & Scibak, 1979). Much of this capability may be due to CA, independent of MA and IQ effects. It is surprising that so little work has been done to determine which behaviors are particularly CA-sensitive. (See Podolsky, 1964, for an interesting effort in this direction.)

Nonintellectual determinants of behavior

The classification model based on IQ cannot account for the fact that two retarded individuals with exactly the same IQ may differ dramatically in everyday social competence. This oversight is not uncommon, as the importance of motivational factors in the adaptive ability of retarded people has long been underemphasized. To date many workers have focused exclusively on the intellectual inadequacy of retarded people, viewing all their behavior as a direct outgrowth of their lack of intelligence (although see Sternberg, 1981a; 1981b, for a consideration of both cognitive and personality factors in explanations of the behavior of retarded people). Within such a framework, the retarded child is treated as a cognitive being without emotions, desires, or a need for ego enhancement. The cognitive emphasis has been buttressed in recent years by the many advances in the field of cognitive psychology and the impact that this field has had on the study of mental retardation. This is despite a sizable and growing body of literature (see Chapter 6) that shows that because of atypical social histories, many retarded persons develop traits such as high needs for social reinforcement, strong social approach and avoidance tendencies, and permeating fear of failure. Such motivational factors have a pervasive influence on behavior and can attenuate performance much more than impoverished cognitive ability.

The tendency to focus on cognition may seem surprising in light of the official definition of mental retardation advanced by the American Association on Mental Deficiency (AAMD). The AAMD's diagnostic guidelines attempt to delineate differences in social competence that cannot be accounted for by differences in IQ level. As variations in adaptation even among individuals with the same IQ are likely to be shaped by differences in motivational structures, the AAMD (Grossman, 1977; 1983) adopted what is essentially a three-factor definition of mental retardation: (1) an IQ below 70; (2) a deficit in social competence, and (3) that these deficits arise in the developmental period (before the age of 18). Such a definition does acknowledge the significance of motivational factors in determining behavior. Yet by trying to avoid the IQ as the sole indicator of mental retardation, the AAMD definition appears to have created as many problems as it has solved. (These problems are discussed below.)

Classification by etiology

In a field where there is little clear agreement about anything, a bright spot is that workers generally recognize two basic types of mental retardation. The first involves organic damage, arising from inborn or prenatal phenomena such as Down syndrome, irradiation, and phenylketonuria, or postnatal events such as anoxia or lead poisoning that can harm the brain more or less seriously. These people are usually classified as suffering mental retardation due to organic causes. The second and larger group consists of retarded people who have no known organic defects; they are commonly referred to as *familial retarded*. While many other labels implying causation have been used (e.g., cultural-familial, sociocultural), we feel that the term *familial* is the only one that conveys an undisputed fact about this type of retardation – that it tends to run in immediate families. Familial retarded persons typically have IQs between 50 and 70 and at least one parent who is below average in intelligence. It is thought that the majority of retarded people are of the familial type, as we will discuss in Chapter 5.

Any agreement among workers ends when it comes to the cause of familial retardation. Briefly, some attribute familial retardation to genetic factors, others to environmental factors, and still others to some unspecified interaction between the two. A few even argue that all retardation is caused by organic damage (Knobloch & Pasamanick, 1961; Kugel, 1967; Richardson, 1981), but that the discovery of the exact problem causing familial retardation awaits advancements in diagnostic technology. For now, let us say only that each position is possible and that the many explanations advanced are the topic of Chapter 4.

There are also several influential workers (Bijou, 1966; Ellis, 1969; Ellis & Cavalier, 1982; Spitz, 1963) who continue to support the position that retarded people are best differentiated by differences in IQ alone. This view fits the system in which intelligence level is portrayed as the primary determinant of a retarded person's behavior. Thinkers of this persuasion maintain that differences in diagnoses or etiology have, at best, the status of a correlate of the classification principle. Of course it is true that organically retarded persons typically have lower IQ scores than those classified as familial. Yet this is certainly not always the case. Further, considerable research (Weisz et al., 1982; Zigler, 1969) has shown that there are important behavioral consequences of being retarded from organic causes rather than from nonorganic ones. Thus, given the importance of organicity as an independent determinant of behavior, we propose the classification system presented in Figure 3.3. This figure reflects the view that the etiology of mental retardation should be employed as a classificatory principle.

The importance of differentiating between the organically retarded and the familial retarded might become clearer in the context of the type of study that continues to advance our understanding of the nature of mental retardation. Assume a design in which groups of organic and familial retarded children, matched on IQ and CA, are selected at two IQ levels. If the task posed to them is a cognitive one, it would not be surprising to find that children of both diagnoses perform better at the higher than at the lower IQ level. However, at both IQ levels the performance of the familial groups may be superior to that of the organic groups. Such differences are actually found frequently when workers bother to separate their retarded samples by diagnostic status (see Weisz et al., 1982). While such findings pose their own problems of interpretation, these problems are compounded dramatically in the typical study in which the behavior of a heterogeneous retarded group is compared to that of a nonretarded sample. Studies like these shed little light on the nature of retarded functioning, since the organic and familial cases may differ in separate ways from those of normal intellect.

Another important difference in the classification systems based on IQ and on etiology should be noted. In the first system the basis for inclusion in each class is the same, namely IQ. In the second system inclusion in each of the three classes involves a different classificatory principle. For the organic group the principle is demonstrable biological etiology. This would involve subclasses based on different diagnoses (e.g., Down syndrome, anoxia). It would of course be preferable if membership in all classes was based on unequivocal knowledge about etiology. Yet etiology is often the last aspect discovered about a pathological phenomenon (Zigler & Phillips, 1961a), and classification simply cannot wait for such ul-

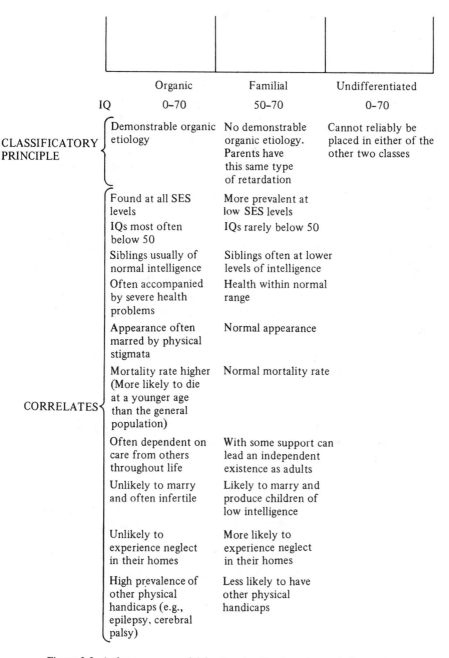

	Organic	Familial	Undifferentiated
IQ	0–70	50–70	0–70
CLASSIFICATORY PRINCIPLE	Demonstrable organic etiology	No demonstrable organic etiology. Parents have this same type of retardation	Cannot reliably be placed in either of the other two classes
CORRELATES	Found at all SES levels	More prevalent at low SES levels	
	IQs most often below 50	IQs rarely below 50	
	Siblings usually of normal intelligence	Siblings often at lower levels of intelligence	
	Often accompanied by severe health problems	Health within normal range	
	Appearance often marred by physical stigmata	Normal appearance	
	Mortality rate higher (More likely to die at a younger age than the general population)	Normal mortality rate	
	Often dependent on care from others throughout life	With some support can lead an independent existence as adults	
	Unlikely to marry and often infertile	Likely to marry and produce children of low intelligence	
	Unlikely to experience neglect in their homes	More likely to experience neglect in their homes	
	High prevalence of other physical handicaps (e.g., epilepsy, cerebral palsy)	Less likely to have other physical handicaps	

Figure 3.3. A three-group model for the classification of retarded persons.

timate discoveries. Indeed, the greatest single problem in the field of mental retardation concerns the etiology of the majority of the retarded population whom we have called familial. At this time the best we can hope for is a method of accurately classifying children whose retardation is not due to clear organic causes.

Our proposed system goes some way toward addressing this need. For example, take a child with an IQ of 60 who has parents of normal intelligence and no demonstrable organic defects. By using the correlates in Figure 3.3, it should be possible to construct an equation representing a probabilistic function of whether the child has either unknown organic impairment or has a low IQ due to polygenic factors (see Chapter 4). The more correlates the child has that are associated with the familial classification, the greater the likelihood that the child's intelligence is polygenically determined. Thus, a child with no physical stigmata and no health problems born to lower-SES parents of low intelligence is much more likely to have retardation due to polygenic factors than due to an organic defect. If the child has siblings in the IQ range 50–90, the classification is further validated. However, even with the application of all current knowledge concerning familial and organic retardation, we will still probably always need an undifferentiated category in our system of classification. Yet research directed at expanding our knowledge of class correlates should eventually allow more informed diagnosis.

The issue of labeling

The two-group approach to classifying mentally retarded people is neither new nor radical. In fact, such a dichotomy has been employed either implicitly or explicitly for several decades. This can be seen in the various terms that have been used to differentiate among retarded persons. Several of these labels are presented in Table 3.1, but this listing is by no means inclusive. Over the years the nomenclature has grown so large and confusing that the field has become a veritable Tower of Babel.

What possible use could there be for so many terms that describe the same phenomena? For one, the large number of labels reflects the little appreciated fact that mental retardation is not a phenomenon studied by a single discipline. Rather, it is a multidisciplinary field and legitimately falls within the interests of genetics, psychiatry, neurology, endocrinology, pediatrics, psychology, education, sociology, and anthropology. Of course each of these disciplines brings its own language to the study of mental retardation. Geneticists are comfortable speaking about a *polygenic curve*. Neurologists know exactly what they mean by the term *neurologically*

Table 3.1. *Former and current terms to describe retarded persons*

Organic	Familial
Organically involved	Cultural-familial retarded due to psychosocial disadvantage
Organismically impaired	Nonorganically involved
	Lower portion of the polygenic curve of intelligence
Moderate, severe, and profound	Mild
Exogenous	Endogenous
	Garden-variety
	Feebleminded
Imbecile, idiot	Moron
Trainable and subtrainable	Educable

Source: From Zigler, Balla, and Hodapp (1984), with permission.

involved. Given the professional demands made on them, educators are attracted to the *trainable–educable* distinction. And only within the field of psychology does the term *garden-variety retardation* have any particular meaning. These disciplinary semantics can easily confuse anyone who is forced to make translations between the different terms employed by the different professionals. The significance of this is that mental retardation workers have an inordinate difficulty in communicating with laypersons and decision makers who are responsible for committing resources to the cause of retarded people.

Labeling by ability

While a few of the labels shown in Table 3.1 are now historical oddities, the fuzzy and inexact nomenclature continues to be a major problem. The difficulties with many of our common terms are self-evident. Some are lacking in rigorous definition and are therefore confusing. For instance, where exactly does *training* end and *education* begin? In everyday usage both terms are roughly synonymous with *teaching*, so the distinction between trainable and educable groups is hidden. Of course IQs are markedly lower in the trainable than in the educable group. But if this is the only point we are trying to make, we would be well advised to forgo such unclear terms and simply employ the IQ-oriented classification system presented in Figure 3.1.

Actually, workers are trying to convey with the trainable–educable distinction something more than mere differences in IQ or intervention methods. The distinction has to do with the behavioral potential of the retarded groups and exactly what can be taught at a given potential. Those considered trainable are taught relatively low-level skills (e.g., personal hygiene and other self-help skills) and simple intellectual tasks (e.g., learning to direct one's attention). Educable individuals are taught more intellectually demanding tasks such as reading and simple mathematics – tasks that approach what is taught to slow-learning children whose IQs are not in the retarded range. The trainable–educable distinction causes problems because it can lead to a confusion between the classificatory principle employed to distinguish between individuals and the correlates of the classes thus established.

The correlates of a sound classification system should not only involve what can be accomplished by individuals at given IQ levels. Correlates should help to answer interesting and important questions such as "What can an individual in this category learn when exposed to other teaching methods?" A double assessment of what retarded individuals at different IQ and CA levels are capable of with and without educational programs would have a forceful impact on social policy. First, such catalogs of possible achievements could spur a healthy change of public attitude, inasmuch as recent intervention efforts have had rather amazing outcomes, demonstrating that retarded persons have much more potential than previously thought (Schroeder et al., 1979; Whitman & Scibak, 1979). The juxtaposition of lists of behavioral capabilities with and without intervention would also make clear just how much can be accomplished if the United States commits itself to available programs. American society continues to be reluctant to devote resources to human services. Such reluctance is more likely to be overcome if workers can present a clear case for the value of interventions rather than a continuing plea for more funds because it is the decent thing to do.

The retardation stigma

Much thinking concerning retarded persons has been unrealistically pessimistic. The stereotype of the retarded individual is of someone at a very low level of functioning who is capable of performing only the simplest tasks. Laypeople are surprised to learn that at least half of those classified as retarded (IQs below 70) are capable of marrying, being employed, and blending into society. This surprise is at least partially caused by the mistaken notion that many everyday activities require a high degree of intelligence. Some 30 years ago a survey by Whitney (1956) revealed that around one half of common occupations could probably be performed by people in the IQ range 60–80. As our society has become more mechanized and service-oriented, this proportion has undoubtedly increased. Indeed, success at many occupations is determined less by intellectual ability than by such personal characteristics as reliability, perseverance, and appropriate sociability.

Another reason why many underassess the competence of retarded persons has to do with certain peculiarities in intelligence testing. It sounds ominous to describe a 35-year-old whose IQ is 70 as having the mental capacity of a 12-year-old. The description becomes much less dramatic when we realize that in the scoring of IQ tests, the 35-year-old of normal intellect (IQ = 100) is assigned the mental capacity of a 16- to 18-year-old. This practice is based on the widespread assumption that most intellectual abilities level off at about 18 to 20 for individuals of all IQs.

Just as the label *mentally retarded* can lead to undue pessimism, so too can it not be taken seriously enough. Some theorists in the field (Baer, Peterson, & Sherman, 1967; Baer & Sherman, 1964; Bijou, 1966) have inherited from Skinner a distrust of genetic and other nonexperiential determinants of behavior. These workers seem to argue that most people have few limitations and can be raised in intellectual level if subjected to appropriate behavior-shaping procedures. They assert that our failure to make retarded people intellectually normal is likely to be due to the fact that we have not yet discovered the right behavioral technology. While not held in as extreme a form, this view appears to have permeated the normalization movement throughout the world. We will have more to say about it when we discuss the issues of institutionalization (Chapter 10) and mainstreaming (Chapter 11).

Labeling the unknown

In addition to the confusion precipitated by the labels in Table 3.1, some of these terms make assumptions and predetermine issues that are themselves difficult and cannot be resolved by a simple naming process. One is reminded of Maslow's (1948) warning that when people have a name for a phenomenon they feel they understand it and no longer give it the study it deserves. Consider the nosological category, "mental retardation due to psychosocial disadvantage." This term emanates from a simplistic environmental approach to intelligence and makes it sound as if the perpetual nature–nurture debate had been decided in favor of nurture for this group of retarded persons. In fact, although certain rare and extremely poor environments can produce low intelligence, there is no convincing evidence that less drastic differences in environment (such as those between working- and middle-class families) can impose great differences in ability (Vernon, 1979).

The fact remains that familial retardation (IQs 50–70) is much more likely to affect people of lower SES than those in the middle or upper classes. We are a long way from knowing whether this higher prevalence of mental retardation is due to the impoverished environment or to poorer genetic potential for individuals in the lower-SES population. Adoption studies (studies of children born to lower-SES parents but adopted into higher-SES families) suggest that both genetic and environmental factors are at work (Scarr & Weinberg, 1979; Vernon, 1979). The danger in associating SES and IQ is that it easily leads to the incorrect generalization that most people of low socioeconomic status are of low intelligence. The truth is that the vast majority of children born into a low SES level are not intellectually retarded, even to a mild degree.

Not only lower-SES people, but a variety of cultural groups are demeaned if we insist on viewing variations in intelligence as the product of variations in upbringing environments. This insult is exacerbated when the term *cultural-familial* retardation is used in preference to the single *familial* designation. True, the schools have applied the label *retarded* to differential percentages of children from different ethnic groups (see Berk, Bridges, & Shih, 1981; Heller, Holtzman, & Messick, 1982; Mercer, 1973a, 1973b). At least three explanations of this phenomenon can be advanced. One is that different groups produce children with different intellectual capacities, so that in fact more minority-group children are retarded. The second interpretation is that standard IQ tests are not valid measures of the actual intelligence of minority-group children, since these tests are biased in favor of the values and practices of the majority culture (Mercer, 1973a, 1973b). This likelihood may have influenced the AAMD to expand its definition of mental retardation to require a low IQ *plus* social inadequacy in everyday activities. A third interpretation is that there is a greater propensity to apply the label retarded to minority- than to majority-group children, even though there may be no difference in their intelligence levels. While Mercer's position is that too many minority children are labeled retarded, this last explanation suggests that too few majority-culture children are so labeled.

It is our position that, whatever mental retardation is, it is best conceptualized as a stable characteristic of the person who is retarded rather than a creation of social agents who apply descriptive terms to children. Theorists of labeling argue that retarded behavior is prompted by the act of assigning the label to a child. If intellectual subnormality is so suggestible, then the problem of mental retardation could be diminished by withholding use of the label. Since this would not bring much help to retarded persons, we would be better off making the inclusion rules of the classification very demanding. The field did something on this order by shifting the definition from one to two standard deviations below the population mean. Yet as we have seen, such maneuvers do not influence at all the real occurrence of mental retardation *if the condition is conceptualized in terms of actual cognitive functioning*. Such a conceptualization renders extraneous such phenomena as everyday social competence and the age at which the intellectual shortcomings are first detected. What become central to and definitive of mental retardation are the quality and nature of cognitive functioning and a pattern of cognitive abilities that necessitates the use of descriptive terminology.

The prevalence of mild mental retardation in the United States and Sweden

The implications and consequences of how mental retardation is defined are vividly seen in an actual cross-cultural comparison. Scientists at the Kennedy Foundation were struck by the very low prevalence of mild mental retardation in Sweden reported by Grunewald (1979). U.S. estimates were seven to fifteen times greater than the rates reported for Sweden. The estimates of prevalence rates for severe mental retardation (IQ below 50) in the two countries were comparable.

The Kennedy workers advanced a number of hypotheses to explain this national difference (Kennedy Foundation, 1981). Their most intriguing suggestion was that the many social programs mounted in Sweden have resulted in the prevention or amelioration of a large number of cases that in a different society would have been placed in the mildly retarded category. The nomenclature currently prevailing in the field lends plausibility to this hypothesis. If mild mental retardation is due in part to"psychosocial disadvantage," then its prevalence should be lessened in any society that has successful programs to do away with conditions that contribute to such disadvantage. Being a social welfare state, Sweden is certainly a likely candidate for such a society. Evaluation of the Swedish prevalence rates is facilitated by the fact that in Sweden the government keeps a registry of all individuals officially designated as retarded. A person can be placed in this registry at any time between birth (in the case of severe retardation) and the end of the school year. Placement in the registry excuses males from required military service. Benefits also accrue to registered individuals in the form of a variety of programs directed toward aiding their adaptation to society.

The Swedish prevalence rates and the Kennedy Foundation's analysis were brought to the attention of the U.S. President's Commission on Mental Retardation. The decision was made to send a small scientific contingent to Sweden to scrutinize further the Swedish statistics.[1] The American workers, headed by Dr. Robert Cooke, entertained both obvious and hypothetical possibilities. One was that the Gruenwald data were artifactual, a misleading result of the Swedish use of out-of-date standardized IQ tests. If similarly old tests had been given to U.S. children, the mean would have been well above 100 with a commensurate reduction in the number of individuals in the 50–70 IQ range (Gallagher, 1985). Another possibility was that the gene pool for intelligence in the Swedish population contains more high-IQ genes, but there is no convincing evidence on this point.

The Swedish scientists were themselves divided in their interpretations of the Gruenwald data. One viewpoint was that the entire intelligence distribution in Sweden had in fact been moved upward, resulting in a genuine reduction in the incidence of mild mental retardation. Another position was that the prevalence rate for mild retardation in Sweden is the same as that in all industrialized nations, including the United States, but in Sweden many more individuals with IQs between 50 and 70 are never designated as mentally retarded. Others pointed out that the many health screenings beginning in infancy made it unlikely that so large a group of mildly retarded persons would remain undetected.

An examination of the ethos within which Sweden deals with retarded persons does lend credibility to the underdetection hypothesis. While the Swedish method of handling severely retarded cases is very much like that in the United States, the two nations diverge markedly in their approach to less dramatic intellectual variations. American practices do appear much more likely to result in the formal identification of mild retardation. For example, the United States has many psychologists who do a great deal of testing both in and out of schools. Sweden has very few psychologists and as a society has become disenchanted with tests of all sorts, including IQ tests. In the United States, labels are employed routinely, whereas distinctions between individuals appear to be made only grudgingly in Sweden. In the field of mental retardation, Sweden is much more committed to principles of normalization than is the United States. There it is taken for

---

[1] This group consisted of Robert Cooke, James Gallagher, Denise Horton, Nancy Robinson, Miron Straf, and Edward Zigler.

granted that all but severely retarded persons can successfully adapt to school as children and to the society as adults, provided that they receive support through an array of social services (see Kennedy Foundation, 1981; Gallagher, 1985). Thus, if a child does not do well in school, blame is more likely placed on the inadequacy of school services than on the child's intellectual shortcomings. Application of the retardation label to a child is perceived as some sort of failure of both the school and the society. The entire nation consequently has a viewpoint toward mental retardation that may lead to the underidentification of large numbers of mildly retarded people.

Some empirical evidence that the Swedish prevalence of mild mental retardation is underestimated comes from a study by Granat and Granat (1973). In Sweden, 19-year-old males are tested during their mandatory induction into the armed forces. Those who are included in the Swedish registry as either severely or mildly retarded (approximately .71% of the 19-year-old male population) are excused from the induction tests and from military service. Those who are tested have therefore never been labeled retarded. Nevertheless, Granat and Granat reported that about 1.5% of Swedish males scored below 70 on the IQ test. Combining this figure with that of the registered retarded men, the overall prevalence of Swedish males who have IQs below 70 is 2.21%. This rate is similar to that found elsewhere.

In a follow-up study, Granat and Granat (1978) investigated the adjustment of young men who scored below 84 on the induction IQ test, including some who scored below 70. Of the total sample, 50% were found to be well adjusted and 50% were poorly adjusted. Interestingly, a sizable group of those whose poor adjustment showed up in the workplace had also had problems in school. This study suggests some of the dangers of not identifying below-average individuals while they are in their school years, as assistance would have been available to them much sooner.

It is of interest that a nation as committed to normalization as Sweden does not admit retarded persons into the armed forces, despite evidence that many mildly retarded individuals make a perfectly adequate adjustment to military life (Weaver, 1966). As in Granat and Granat's follow-up, the adjustment of retarded soldiers appears to have more to do with personal characteristics than with their IQ scores. This notion can be carried too far, however. Influenced by the popular study by Baller, Charles, and Miller (1967), a view has developed that the postschool adult status of mildly retarded persons is not particularly bleak (Willerman, 1979). A common assertion is that half of mildly retarded persons merge completely

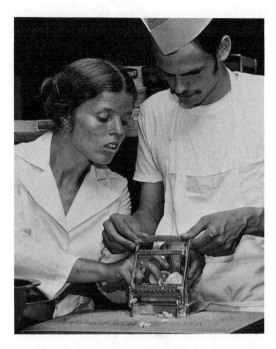

Photo 2. Dietary training. (Photograph courtesy of Elwyn Institutes, Elwyn, Pennsylvania)

into society in their postschool years. This belief has some basis in fact, in that the reported prevalence of mental retardation is much greater for those of school age (Gruenberg, 1964; Zigler, 1966a). Yet the Granat and Granat (1978) follow-up should lead us to be less sanguine about the adult adjustment of mildly retarded persons. Although it is reassuring that 50% of their below-average sample were well adjusted, it is disturbing to discover that even in a social welfare state like Sweden the other half were having adjustment problems. It would not be surprising that in a less supportive society such as the United States, an even greater percentage of low-IQ people would be having difficulty in social adaptation.

The heart of the matter remains: Is it better to label an individual with an IQ between 50 and 70 mentally retarded, or should the label be avoided if at all possible? The nature of the labeling debate in the United States (Hobbs, 1975; Mercer, 1973a, 1973b) has commonly emphasized the downside risks of labeling. There should be little disagreement that if nothing of value befalls the labeled person, then the label should never be employed. What is underemphasized is that the label may result in advantageous consequences such as helpful interventions and social services. The potential liabilities of labeling must be weighed against potential assets.

When a Swedish person is labeled mentally retarded and placed in the national registry, he or she is eligible to receive special vocational training that should eventually make it possible to obtain employment. What about mildly retarded children who are never labeled and who are promoted from grade to grade in the schools? Besides the adjustment problems suggested by Granat and Granat (1973), one Swedish educator pointed out that many of these individuals find themselves unemployable upon graduating from school – the same situation experienced by U.S. students who have received "social promotions." However, in Sweden these individuals can request the status *mentally retarded* in order to qualify for special vocational education. No such recourse exists in the United States. We must strongly suggest that this current tendency not to employ the mental retardation label, evident in both the United States and Sweden, is harmful.

Resolving the definitional problem

Definitions cannot be right or wrong, or true or false, but only useful or not useful. A useful definition of mental retardation would aid in the construction of a classification system that has two major goals: (1) to benefit those classified by being helpful to their clinicians and service providers, and (2) to bring much-needed order to the knowledge in the field, while directing workers to important issues in need of further study. A worthy definition should be as parsimonious as possible and should be based on the bedrock essence of the phenomenon being defined. As we have suggested, the essence of mental retardation is a cognitive system in which many of the cognitive processes are less efficient than those found in the average person in the society. Starting with this premise, the construction of a definition requires only a set of agreed-upon operations to determine how poor the formal intellectual processes of an individual must be in order for the individual to be classified retarded.

There are currently two major approaches to the assessment of intelligence: (1) the psychometric approach, which relies on the use of standardized intelligence tests, and (2) the cognitive-developmental approach, based on measures of the nature of cognitive processes that are associated with such theorists as Piaget, Vygotsky, and Bruner (Cronbach & Snow, 1977; Sternberg, 1981a). (A third approach, information processing, has not generated as much work in testing per se.) Both approaches attempt to assess the same phenomena, namely the formal cognitive structure and its information-processing characteristics. Thus it is not surprising that scores on the two types of assessment are highly correlated (Kaufman & Kaufman, 1972; Zigler & Trickett, 1978). There has been some rapprochement between these two schools of thought. In particular, Laurendeau and Pinard (1962), Tuddenham (1971), and Uzgiris and Hunt (1975) have attempted to apply traditional psychometric procedures to the scaling of cognitive processes emphasized by cognitive-developmentalists. Refinement of this promising method of intellectual measurement is many years away, but the need for the definition and classification of mental retardation is pressing. Currently we have no alternative but to utilize scores obtained on standard measures such as the Binet and Wechsler in the operational definition of mental retardation.

This reliance on IQ-test performance runs headlong into the current ethos of American psychology, where it has become fashionable to bemoan the inadequacies of IQ scores (e.g., McClelland, 1973; Mercer, 1973a, 1973b). The truth is that in the history of psychology the IQ is probably the most theoretically and practically important measure yet devised. More than 75 years of sound work and study have gone into its development. The result is that the IQ score has more correlates than any other known measure (Kohlberg & Zigler, 1967) and has predictive power across a wide array of situations (Mischel, 1968). Thus, while the IQ score is hardly a perfect measure of intelligence (nothing could be, since there is no agreement on what intelligence is), it is not at all that inadequate either.

Given the nature of IQ tests, a definition of mental retardation based solely on IQ scores would not be problem-free.[2] In view of the possibility of error in measurement, an individual should certainly be tested at least twice before the label *retarded* is applied. The additional tests might include a cognitive-developmental measure, a different IQ test, or a specific area assessment. So confirmed, the IQ score would become the basis for classification and would free us from the dangers of false positives and false negatives. That is, obtained IQ scores would stand as factual indicators, since there would be no criterion for mental retardation other than the IQ score itself.

The only remaining issue is where on the IQ score continuum should we draw the line to separate mentally retarded from nonretarded persons. Here we must keep firmly in mind that such a selection process is completely

[2] A definition based solely on IQ scores would classify as retarded many individuals who suffer primarily from a disorder other than mental retardation, e.g., autistic children, the senile aged, and decompensated schizophrenics. The nomenclature for such cases might highlight the primary disorder (e.g., schizophrenia) with the added notation of whether the condition exists along with mental retardation. Such dual diagnoses are fairly common in the characterization of a variety of disorders.

arbitrary. Given current conventions and the history of the field, it would appear best to adopt a cutoff point of two standard deviations and define as retarded all individuals who score below 70 on the Binet or Wechsler. Most professionals are by now comfortable or at least familiar with this cutoff; if it became a standard they would be assured of communicating about the same phenomenon. A lower cutoff would deny services to mildly retarded persons, who have proved quite responsive to available programs. A higher dividing line, when adopted in the 1960s, did not work because it made the retarded population too heterogeneous, with needs in some cases indistinguishable from standard educational practices. Thus the two-*SD* cutoff, though totally arbitrary, does appear to have some practical benefits.

Social adaptation abandoned as a defining characteristic of mental retardation

The exclusive reliance on IQ scores to define mental retardation is in opposition to the definition of the AAMD and to the views of certain prominent workers in the field (e.g., Leland, 1969). The AAMD definition requires that regardless of IQ, no individual can be labeled retarded unless he or she displays a deficit in adaptive behavior. In the everyday practice of those working with retarded people, however, exclusive reliance on IQ scores to define mental retardation is routine. Smith and Polloway (1979) found that most researchers use IQ as the sole criterion for defining and classifying their retarded samples, a practice that the editor of *AJMD* accepts "with some regret" (Robinson, 1980, p. 107). Physicians and psychologists also primarily employ the IQ when making diagnoses of retardation, a practice that continues despite criticism (e.g., Adams, 1973).

Why do professionals generally avoid social adaptation indicators in defining mental retardation? Perhaps because social adaptation is itself undefined and simply too vague to have any utility in a classification system (Zigler, 1966a; Zigler & Trickett, 1978). For example, a child with an IQ of 65 who fails in school might be considered maladapted and labeled retarded. Yet with some added services, perhaps as minimal as an understanding teacher, the child might succeed in school and no longer meet the definition of retardation. The child's cognitive processes would not have changed. All that would have changed is the response of others in his or her social environment. A similar situation can be drawn in the case of low-IQ adults assessed against a definition of social adaptation that is as straightforward as whether or not one is employed. The 65-IQ man who holds a job is not retarded. Yet if he is laid off, on the day his employment terminates he becomes retarded.

Obviously social adaptation is a variable trait and it leads to a classification system that allows individuals to flit from category to category. For the adaptation concept to have any definitional value, one would have to catalog and analyze every social situation that could be encountered. This impossible task has been finessed by the construction of social adaptation scales, but they do not begin to be comprehensive enough. And while the definition of intelligence may remain elusive, workers are light years away from agreeing on the ultimate defining feature of social adaptation. Suggestions range from the commonplace, such as school and job success or whether a person gets and stays married, to one analysis in which social sensitivity and facility with social niceties are deemed the crux of social competence (Greenspan, 1979). Since the concept of social adaptation is so far from basic definition, measures to assess it necessarily lack validity. Such a vague foundation for such an important classification system is inadequate and unacceptable.

Dropping social adaptation from the definition of mental retardation does not imply that the concept is unimportant. On the contrary, the discovery of the relation between IQ level and performance in many situations is a crucial branch of investigation. What is being proposed here is that information on adaptation be included in the correlates of class membership rather than in the defining features of class inclusion.

It should be noted that there may be little relation between IQ and many measures of everyday social competence. For example, consider the common notion of the genius as a highly intelligent but maladapted person. More typical are the children of normal intellect who are considered underachievers in school (a label that means only that their school performance is not commensurate with their measured abilities). There are simply too many nonintellective determinants of social competence to expect the IQ to be a particularly robust predictor of everyday behavior. This should not dissuade us from appreciating the value of social adaptation. Making the IQ central to the definition of mental retardation is predicated only on our view that the behavioral sciences currently have no better measure to assess intellectual functioning.

Conclusion

The proposals offered in this chapter revolve around two conclusions. The first is that the essence of mental retardation involves inefficient cognitive functioning; hence, mental retardation should be defined solely by subaverage performance on measures of intellectual abilities. Second, we believe that classification of individuals defined as retarded cannot adequately describe the heterogeneity within the retarded population unless etiology is given clear recognition. Differences in various subject characteristics (e.g., SES, motivational and personality traits) between the two diagnostic groups, possibly extending to a difference in the structure of intelligence, lead us to champion etiology as a classificatory principle.

The proposed definitional system is simple and workable, but it is by no means the final word. We must vigilantly continue to ask whether it is better to label individuals with IQs between 50 and 70 mentally retarded or if the label should be avoided if at all possible. If our society does not provide needed services, children within this IQ range may be better off being called slow learners, which describes their school behavior adequately. The problem is that although the label *slow learner* is probably less stigmatizing than the label *retarded*, it is not a label that conveys much of the need for special care or added help. We should not be so worried about stigmatizing as to lose sight of the general needs of retarded people. Some years ago there was a movement to substitute the term *exceptional* for the term *retarded*. Workers soon learned that Americans who were quite willing to pay for services for *retarded* children were not prone to spend money for children labeled *exceptional*. We thus see vividly that our classification systems and nomenclature have a forceful impact on the daily lives of individuals of low intelligence.

4   Familial retardation and the nature–nurture controversy

Having considered the basic problems of definition and classification of mental retardation, we now turn our attention to a further examination of familial retardation. Our analysis of this subject will, we hope, also shed light on the entire nature–nurture issue and suggest some new directions for mental retardation research.

As we have seen, from the beginning of this century mental retardation has typically been separated into two diagnostic categories: retardation with a known organic etiology, and cases of unknown or uncertain etiology. In the first type, a specific organic cause is present. In the second type, no organic determinants can be identified. Since retarded individuals of the second type are typically offspring of low-IQ parents and often are raised in poor environments, both genetic and environmental agents are implicated. Such labels as *sociocultural*, *familial*, *sensorily deprived*, and others sampled in Chapter 3 indicate the disagreement among workers about the cause of this type of retardation. Yet this group is thought to comprise the majority of the retarded population (see Chapter 5). Because of the large percentage of individuals involved, the etiology of the nonorganic group has been viewed as the single greatest mystery in the field of mental retardation (Zigler, 1967).

Despite the tremendous insufficiency of present knowledge, most workers have apparently been able to form a lucid picture of familial retardation. The following description by a major worker in the field conveys the typical point of view:

I shall be talking about those retardates in whom currently available biomedical technology cannot demonstrate significant physical or laboratory pathology; in whom no specific, single somatic etiologic agent can be made significantly accountable for the condition; in whom the diagnosis often disappears at young adult age; who are normal in physical appearance; whose morbidity and mortality rates do not differ greatly from those of the average population; in whom the retardation is usually mild, with the difference between average parental IQ and that of the index case often rather small; who generally come from socially, economically, and educationally underprivileged strata of our society. (Tarjan, 1970, pp. 745–746)

In diagnosis, as well, there is a fairly common framework used to identify familial retarded individuals: A medical examination reveals no physiological manifestations, and retardation of this same type exists in one or both parents. Level of intellectual functioning also enters into the diagnosis. Organically retarded individuals most commonly place at the lower end of the IQ distribution (IQs below 50), while familial persons are invariably mildly retarded (IQs 50–70). Thus, a mildly retarded child with no known organic pathology and a poor environmental background is likely to be diagnosed as familial retarded.

A major problem with our current classification methods now becomes apparent. As we will discuss shortly, the polygenic model is today accepted by many experts to explain variations in quantitative human traits such as intelligence. This model generates the prediction that parents of average and even superior intellect may produce children with IQs in the 50–70 range. Within the current classification system, however, there is no specific category for this type of mental retardation, i.e., mild retardation in children with no known organic pathology who are the progeny of nonretarded parents.[1] A basic question is whether such children actually exist and in what numbers.

This inquiry is unanswerable given our present classification structure. Indeed, how would a diagnostician classify a child with an IQ of 60 whose parents are of middle socioeconomic status and have average IQs? Given the current system, there would be no alternative but to place the child in the undifferentiated category (i.e., retardation due to unknown causes). While the exigencies of classification will always require the use of an undifferentiated class, the field should strive to make the number of individuals assigned to this group as small as possible. The existence of a sizable "unknown" category in a classification system represents a confession of conceptual inadequacy.

The purpose of this chapter is to propose a classification system that can account for virtually all retarded people. We will examine how the polygenic model of intellectual inheritance can help in conceptualizing and identifying individuals who display mental retardation without known organic causation. We will analyze the development of a strong environmental bias in the field, which has created an aversion to this model. This bias has not only resulted in a misconceptualization of a large class of retarded people, but also makes it likely that there is a large group in our society with IQs below 70 that is never labeled retarded. Our basic position is that mental retardation can be understood only by truly appreciating both genetic and environmental factors, a perspective that all espouse but few practice.

---

[1] We note, however, that the current Manual on Classification does include a little-used category (Other) for this type of retardation (see Grossman, 1983, p. 150).

The polygenic model

The theory of polygenic inheritance asserts that many human traits that are continuously distributed (e.g., intelligence or height) are determined by a number of genes that work independently and additively to produce the trait whenever normal environmental conditions prevail. In discussing this theory, a distinction must be made between the genotype (the genes inherited from parents) and the phenotype (the expression of the genotype, which is determined both by the genes and by the environment that the organism encounters). Polygenic models address the likelihood of particular gene combinations being inherited, not with how the environment impacts this genetic potential.

Probably the best-known example of the polygenic inheritance of intelligence is the Gottesman model. Gottesman (1963) postulated a five-gene explanation to account for IQ scores within the normal distribution of intelligence. He considered this normal range to be from IQ 50 to IQ 150. Each child receives five genes for intelligence. Since each gene consists of two alleles (one contributed by each parent), there are ten alleles that determine IQ. Every " + ," or good allele, boosts the child's IQ by 10 points above the baseline of 50. Table 4.1 shows the probabilities of parents with particular IQs producing children at each IQ level. A near-normal distribution of child IQ occurs around the midpoint parental IQ (i.e., the average of the two parents' IQs) based on the number of possible ways one can receive from one to ten alleles.

The theoretical distribution of intelligence generated by the polygenic model is the standard Gaussian or bell-shaped curve (see Figure 3.1). The model can be tested directly by comparing this theoretical curve with the actual distribution of intelligence found in our society (shown in Figure 4.1). Even a brief glance reveals that the theoretical polygenic distribution is not a good approximation of the empirically discovered range of intelligence. The most striking disparity is the failure of Gottesman's polygenic model to account for individuals with IQs below 50. (For the problem of IQs above 150, see Jensen, 1969.) Another important deviation is that the theoretical distribution is bisymmetrical, as it is essentially a "normal curve" (with $SD = 15$) from IQ 0 to IQ 200. As many authorities have noted (Jensen, 1969; MacMillan, 1977; Penrose, 1963), empirical findings show that there are many more people with IQs below 50 than would be expected from theoretical predictions.

Workers have tended to agree on an explanation of this excess of very low IQ scores. The explanation was first proposed by E. Lewis (1933),

Table 4.1. *Probabilities of offspring having particular IQs, given particular parental IQs (as predicted by Gottesman, 1968)*

Parents' IQs		Offspring IQs							
Mother	Father	50	60	70	80	90	100	110	120
50	50	1.	—	—	—	—	—	—	—
60	60	.25	.50	.25	—	—	—	—	—
70	70	.04	.24	.44	.24	.04	—	—	—
80	80	.007	.069	.243	.361	.243	.069	.008	—
90	90	.00056	.011	.079	.238	.341	.238	.079	.011
100	100	.000016	.0008	.013	.082	.237	.335	.237	.082

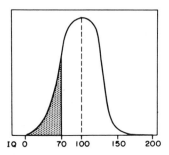

IQ 0   70 100   150   200

Figure 4.1. The actual distribution of intelligence. Notice that there is a larger proportion of scores below IQ 70 than would be predicted by the normal distribution (see Fig. 3.1).

who argued that there are really two separate distributions of intelligence: one for those whose intelligence is the product of some interaction between hereditary and environmental components; and the other for those whose intellectual apparatus has been physically damaged, thus altering the biological side of the formula. Pictorially, the first distribution would approximate the normal curve, while the one for organically damaged persons would overlap the first but have different features. This second distribution begins at IQ 0 (e.g., the case of an anencephalic individual), peaks at approximately IQ 30, and has a very long tail extending into the high IQ range (see Figure 4.2). This long tail is necessary to encompass those cases of brain-damaged individuals who do not display intellectual retardation (e.g., the occasional cerebral-palsied person with an average or above-average IQ). Interestingly, if one combines the two curves in Figure 4.2, the resulting distribution is a relatively good fit to the actual distribution of intelligence (see Dingman & Tarjan, 1960; Penrose, 1963). Such congruence between a theoretical formulation and empirical results is the goal of all scientific inquiry and supports the validity of the two-group approach.

Genetic contributions

Note that this discussion is based on the premise that genetic inheritance has some role in determining individual differences in intelligence. We will carry this a step further and assert that that role is substantial. Although some theorists (e.g., Kamin, 1974) have argued that genes have little responsibility for variations in intelligence (i.e., the heritability index for intelligence is essentially zero), many view such a position as untenable. Drawing from the results of various twin studies, adoption studies, and environmental enrichment studies (see reviews of these studies by Plomin

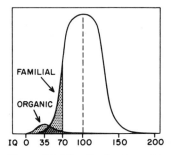

Figure 4.2. The distributions of intelligence of the two groups of retarded people. Notice that the familial group forms the lower tail of the normal distribution, whereas the organic group forms its own, overlapping distribution.

& DeFries, 1980; Scarr & Carter-Saltzman, 1982; Thiessen, 1972; Vernon, 1979; Willerman, 1979), most researchers consider the heritability of intelligence to be somewhere between .45 and .80. This indicates that from 45% to 80% of the variation in IQ scores is due to genetic variability, allowing the remaining percentage to environmental influences. Since the nature–nurture debate has been such a long and heated one, readers have a right to view for themselves the sort of evidence that led us to our unequivocal stance. As one example, Table 4.2 presents heritability ratios of intelligence (as measured by IQ scores) derived in several studies of fraternal and genetically identical twins. Willerman (1979) also offers support for the argument that there is an important genetic component underlying variations in intelligence.

Polygenic predictions

It should be noted that Gottesman's five-gene model is but one possible example of polygenic inheritance of intelligence. A model with four, six, or more genes would produce similar results. The important point is that a number of genes added together produce a specific value of intellectual potential. And while the selection of a five-gene model starting at IQ–50 to account for normal variations in intelligence is arbitrary, this proposal does fit empirical findings that individuals with IQs below 50 almost always show evidence of organic involvement (e.g., Slater & Cowie, 1971; Vernon, 1979). Thus, such a distribution might be close to that expected in a population that permits mating between individuals with different family backgrounds, educations, and IQs.

Using Gottesman's model for the sake of simplicity, let us examine the expected intelligence levels of the offspring of parents with various IQs.

Table 4.2. *Correlations (r) and heritability ratios (H) from studies of identical (monozygotic, MZ) and fraternal (dizygotic, DZ) twins*

Country	Year	MZ r	DZ r	H
England	1958	.97	.55	.93
U.S.A.	1932	.92	.61	.80
France	1960	.90	.60	.75
U.S.A.	1937	.90	.62	.74
Sweden	1953	.90	.70	.67
U.S.A.	1965	.87	.63	.65
U.S.A.	1968	.80	.48	.62
Sweden	1952	.89	.72	.61
England	1954	.76	.44	.57
England	1933	.84	.65	.54
Finland	1966	.69	.42	.51
England	1966	.83	.66	.50

Source: From Zigler, Balla, and Hodapp (1984), with permission. Originally adapted from Vandenberg (1971).

As can be seen in Table 4.1, parents who are themselves retarded (IQs below 70) will often have children with IQs higher than their own. Analogously, nonretarded parents (IQs above 70) will frequently have children with IQs lower than their own. This happens because, simply by the laws of chance, two retarded parents will occasionally pass on enough genes for average intelligence, and nonretarded parents will occasionally pass on few "+" genes and produce a retarded child. In the Gottesman model, two parents with IQs of 70 (meaning each parent has two alleles for higher intelligence) have a chance of producing a child of IQ 90 (receiving all four alleles for higher intelligence). Similarly, two parents with IQs of 100 (five alleles per parent) will, on rare occasions, produce a child of IQ 50 with none of these alleles. But since there are many more parents with IQs of 100 than with IQs of 70, these rare instances will account for a fair percentage of the retarded population.

Once again, we must be concerned with how congruent the model is with empirical findings. We turn to the classic study by Reed and Reed (1965), who followed the family histories of 289 retarded persons in the Faribault Minnesota State School. Relying on previously collected family histories of the parents of the residents in that school from 1911 to 1918, Reed and Reed traced the offspring of retarded and nonretarded family members. Approximately 80,000 persons were included in the study. The care and thoroughness of data collection by two sets of researchers 30 years apart have provided workers with an invaluable resource.

Two tables from the Reeds' study are presented to compare their empirical findings with the expectations derived from the polygenic model. Table 4.3 presents the IQ scores of children with one or two retarded parents, while Table 4.4 shows the IQ scores of children of gifted parents. In both cases, regression to the mean (Eysenck, 1971; Li, 1971) occurs: Gifted parents have children less intelligent than themselves, while retarded parents have children who are brighter. Indeed most offspring of one retarded and one nonretarded parent are not retarded, some have average intelligence, and a few even possess above-average intelligence. These average and above IQs occur in spite of low SES levels (especially likely if the father's IQ is below 70), the alleged cause of "sociocultural retardation."

The phenomenon of regression to the mean appears mostly at the intellectual extremes. In the majority of cases, a good prediction of a child's IQ is the midpoint of the parents' IQ (see Table 4.1). Around any midpoint parental value, one should find a normal distribution of progeny scores. The principle thus emerges that the lower the midpoint of the parents' IQs, the higher the prevalence of mentally retarded offspring. A note of caution must be sounded, however. Prevalence rates should not be confused with absolute numbers. A small prevalence rate in a large cohort of individuals (e.g., parents having a midpoint IQ of 100) should result in an absolute number of retarded children that is the same as or more than the number of retarded children from a smaller-sized cohort with a larger prevalence rate (e.g., both parents retarded).

This reasoning generates the conclusion that there must be retarded people in our society who are the progeny of nonretarded parents. The question remains as to how large this group might be. Reed and Reed's (1965) data led them to conclude that approximately 64% of retarded people have parents whose intelligence is in the average, or at least in the nonretarded, range (IQ above 70). However, this estimate includes individuals whose retardation is associated with known organic damage. (Such damage supposedly occurs irrespective of parental IQs.) We have no way of knowing what part of this 64% is organically involved. Since less than half of the retarded population has demonstrable organic damage, a very conservative estimate is that half of the 64% is organically involved. This would mean that approximately 32% of retarded people have parents of average intelligence and have retardation associated with polygenic inheritance.

Table 4.3. *IQ ranges of children whose one or both parents have IQs below 70*

	IQ range						Total number of children	Average IQ of children	Percentage retarded (IQ below 70)
	0–49	50–69	70–89	90–110	111–130	131+			
Both parents' IQ 69 or below, $\overline{X}$ = IQ 60 (12)	5	23	12	6	0	0	46	67	61
Father IQ 69 or below, $\overline{X}$ = IQ 62, mother IQ 70 or above, $\overline{X}$ = average IQ 92(26)	3	3	20	43	12	1	82	94	7
Mother IQ 69 or below, $\overline{X}$ = IQ 63, father IQ 70 or above, $\overline{X}$ = average IQ 98(15)	0	9	18	20	2	0	49	86	18
Total (53)	8	35	50	69	14	1	177	82	24

Source: Adapted from Reed and Reed (1965), with permission.

Table 4.4. *IQ ranges of children whose one or both parents have IQs of 131 or above*

	IQ range						Total number of children	Average IQ of children	Percentage gifted (IQ above 131)
	0–49	50–69	70–89	90–110	111–130	131+			
Both parents IQ 131 or above, $\overline{X}$ = IQ 154 (1)	0	0	0	0	0	3	3	138	100
Father IQ 131 or above, $\overline{X}$ = IQ 136, mother under IQ 131, $\overline{X}$ = IQ 106 (16)	0	0	0	15	18	8	41	116	20
Mother IQ 131 or above, $\overline{X}$ = IQ 137, father under IQ 131, $\overline{X}$ = IQ 99 (18)	0	0	4	6	22	4	36	115	11
Total (35)	0	0	4	21	40	15	80	123	19

Source: Adapted from Reed and Reed (1965), with permission.

A similar estimate can be derived from a study of the entire population of a county in Sweden (Hagberg, Hagberg, Lewerth, & Lindberg, 1981a). Of the 50 children who were identified as mildly retarded with no known etiology, about half ($N = 26$) could be classified as familial (i.e., had at least one retarded parent), while 24 had parents of average intelligence. As the accepted view is that up to 75% of all retarded people have no known organic etiology, a reasonable estimate is that half of these (about 37% of all retarded people) are the children of nonretarded parents.

It should be noted that the polygenic approach is a fully accepted and noncontroversial model in the fields of genetics and behavior genetics (Cavalli-Sforza & Bodmer, 1971; Willerman, 1979). A crucial if incriminating question is why this model has so little influence in the field of mental retardation. One means of assessing the magnitude of this influence is by searching the literature for studies that include groups of nonorganically retarded individuals who have parents of average intelligence. In a systematic review of five years of published papers on mental retardation (*American Psychological Association Abstracts*, 1977–1982), we failed to find one study that singled out such groups for investigation. Countless studies focused on familial retardation, that is, on retarded individuals whose own parents are retarded. But in actual numbers, there may be fewer familial retarded people than nonorganically retarded people with nonretarded parents. Regardless of the exact prevalence estimate one concurs with, it can only be concluded that researchers have overlooked a sizable group of retarded individuals.

The question must be faced as to why, with all the high quality and quantity of work that has characterized the mental retardation profession for the past two decades, workers have chosen to ignore all of these retarded people. A strong possibility is that the very existence of this subgroup represents a refutation of the conventional wisdom or ideology of the field. With few exceptions, workers in the discipline appear committed to an environmental approach in explaining the etiology of retardation without known organic causes. This approach is at odds with the polygenic model, which generates the clear expectation that a child can be retarded even though he or she is reared in a middle-SES environment by parents of average intelligence. We will now examine the history and impact of this environmental bias, and attempt to reconcile it with polygenic theory.

The environmental bias

In the field of mental retardation, a Zeitgeist has developed that is characterized by a strong reliance on environmental explanations for human traits and behavior. This bias can be traced to thinking within the general field of psychology. A milestone event that helped to ingrain this view was the publication of Joseph McVicker Hunt's influential book, *Intelligence and Experience*, in 1961. Reacting against fixed-IQ views with a vivid genetic coloration, Hunt argued forcefully that variations in intelligence are due primarily to variations in experience. Under this theoretical rubric, the biological integrity of the individual received little attention. Hunt presented the child as an extremely malleable being whose intellectual functioning could be enhanced through relatively small environmental interventions. As late as the 1970s, he was promulgating the view that brief interventions during infancy could result in IQ changes of 48 and 75 IQ points (Hunt, 1971). In a cogent critique of Hunt's and similar views, Scarr and Weinberg (1978) referred to this sort of thinking as "naive environmentalism." Zigler (1970b) also called such one-sided viewpoints into question in his paper, "The Environmental Mystique."

Simplistic environmentalism represented but one strand of thought in the general field of psychology, essentially defining the nurture pole of the nature–nurture controversy. Yet the field of mental retardation enthusiastically adopted environmental arguments with none of the balanced debate on this issue that could be heard in the intellectual community at large. This uncritical approach towards environmentalism has now permeated the mental retardation literature for well over 15 years. Thus, as late as the mid–1970s, workers with international reputations could conclude: "Most professionals in the field today assign the greatest etiologic role to early experimental factors, giving a lesser value to nonheritable somatic noxae and the least weight to polygenic inheritance" (Valente & Tarjan, 1974, p. 16). Even more explicitly, Tarjan proclaimed "If I were forced today to label, in one word, the most important cause of sociocultural retardation, I would use the term impoverishment or poverty" (1970, p. 755).

Standard intellectual fare for these workers was the Iowa studies of the 1940s (Skodak & Skeels, 1949). In brief, Skeels studied 25 children who as infants had been placed in an orphanage where they received little attention or stimulation. At the age of 18 months, 13 of these children, all below average in intellectual development, were transferred to an institution for retarded women. Here each was "adopted" by a retarded woman and given considerable attention, affection, and stimulation. After two years these children showed an average IQ increase of 28 points. The IQs of children who had remained in the orphanage had dropped an average of 26 points in the same period – a difference of 54 points! The two groups also had quite different patterns of adjustment as adults (Skeels, 1966). Those who had been removed from the orphanage showed normal intellectual functioning and good occupational and social adjustment. The adult lives of the children who had remained in the orphanage were characterized by a retarded or borderline level of intellectual functioning and poor employment and social records.

These studies were generally interpreted to mean that children could be "saved" from retardation caused by "social deprivation." In the 1960s workers embraced this hopeful notion, hardly noticing that from their inception the Iowa studies were shrouded in controversy (see Zigler, 1970c). A key investigator in the Iowa studies, Harold Skeels, was honored with the prestigious research award of the Kennedy Foundation on Mental Retardation.

An example of the environmental bias

An important event helping to spread the environmental bias across the mental retardation terrain was the 1968 Peabody-NIMH Conference on Sociocultural Aspects of Mental Retardation (Haywood, 1970a). This conference was chaired by H. Carl Haywood, one of Hunt's students. At the opening session another of his students, Ina Uzgiris, reviewed the literature concerning environmental influences on cognitive development (Uzgiris, 1970a). These papers and the rest of the conference to follow gave the distinct impression that a depriving environment was the key element in producing mental retardation without known organic etiologies. The first discussant (Zigler, 1970c) disagreed with this conclusion and reminded listeners of the acknowledged importance of genetic factors in the determination of human intelligence. The second discussant was Boyd Mc-Candless (1970), one of the investigators involved in the Iowa studies and a lifelong champion of the importance of the environment in determining intelligence. Since the topic of the conference was social and cultural aspects of mental retardation, it was perhaps appropriate that environmental influences received so much of the attention and genetic influences so little. But the legacy of this conference for the field was to help promulgate the view that the environment was almost solely responsible for retardation without known organic determinants.

An obvious corollary to the view that poor environments result in lowered intelligence is that environmental interventions can ameliorate this condition, lead to higher IQs, and thus "cure" mental retardation. The history of the establishment of institutions for retarded persons in the 19th century, and the ultimate fate of these institutions in the 20th century (Rosen, Clark, & Kivitz, 1976; White & Wolfensberger, 1969; Zigler & Harter, 1969), demonstrate the negative consequences of such overoptimistic views (see Chapter 10). But at the Peabody conference, concern with sociocultural influences on mental retardation quickly generated discussions and papers on how environmental interventions could override the effects of socially depriving environments.

A careful reading of the Peabody conference proceedings indicates that this meeting did not have to result in an environmental prejudice. For example, in his summary statement Haywood offered a fairly balanced conclusion:

The evidence that individual differences in intelligence are very strongly associated with genetic determinants is voluminous and convincing. The most generally acceptable statement in this regard is that, when one deals with group data, increasing degrees of familial relationship are accompanied by increasing intellectual similarity. To accept this general statement does not in any way deny the power of experiential factors to influence the levels of intellectual ability attained by individuals. . . . It has become quite apparent that certain unfavorable combinations of environmental circumstances do serve to depress the kinds of functions which are associated with scores on intelligence tests and with performance in academic and social situations. While the evidence is less plentiful, and in some respects less convincing, there are also quite strong suggestions that favorable combinations of experiences, properly programmed with respect to timing, sequence, quantity, and quality, can serve to elevate the characteristic performance levels of individuals who, without such experiences, would almost certainly have performed at significantly lower levels. . . . Intelligence develops within the individual as a function of structured experience interacting with genetic endowment. (1970b, pp. 763–764)

In the face of this standard interactionist position, what evidence is there that the Peabody conference, and others like it, helped prejudice the mental retardation field toward environmentalism? The most striking support is to be found in the nomenclature used in the profession. In 1961, the official AAMD terminology designated retardation without known organic etiology by one of two classes: "cultural-familial mental retardation" and "psychogenic mental retardation associated with environmental deprivation" (Heber, 1961). The cultural-familial label, at least, implies that etiology is traceable to some unspecified interaction between environmental (cultural) and genetic (familial) factors. By 1973, this label had vanished. In its place came Category VIII, retardation due to "environmental influences," with the two subcategories, "psychosocial disadvantage'" and "sensory deprivation." (See Grossman, 1977, p. 185, for a comparison of the 1961 and 1973 terminologies.) This movement from interactionist to environmental labels constitutes nothing more than theorizing through naming. The 1973 nomenclature (also in Grossman, 1983) gives the clear impression that mental retardation without known organic etiology is the exclusive product of a poor environment.

Further evidence of the pervasiveness of the environmental bias may be seen in the pronouncements of the authoritative President's Committee on Mental Retardation (1969). This was the group that introduced us to the concept of the "six-hour retarded child." The notion here was that a child could be "retarded" while in school, but "normal" upon leaving school, both at the end of the day and after graduation. Thus mild retardation was considered nothing more than a situational trait. Such a view is in direct contrast to that of behavior geneticists, who regard intelligence (and mental retardation) as a quantitative trait that characterizes the individual across situations. As if this scientific viewpoint did not exist, a subsequent review of psychosocial mental retardation (Ramey & Finkelstein, 1981, p. 75) included Kushlick and Blunden's (1974) assertion that "mild subnormality is a temporary incapacity related to educational difficulties in school." This review seems to offer us an easy solution to the problem of mild retardation: Close all schools and the condition would vanish.

The Ramey and Finkelstein review, entitled "A Biological and Social Coalescence," is another clear example of the strength of the environmental attitude in the field today. One looks in vain in this paper for some mention of the biological side of "coalescence." Although a genetic–environmental interaction model is adopted, the discussion of the genetic component is limited to a brief mention of Galton and a brief quote from Burt, vintage 1934. The work of countless contemporary behavior geneticists is totally ignored, and there is not even an allusion to the polygenic model, the cornerstone of all behavior-genetic discussions of intelligence.

A genuine coalescence

Clear and strong emphasis must be placed on the fact that acceptance of a polygenic model, which recognizes the role of genes in human behavior, does not preclude acknowledging the importance of the environment, nor does it lead one to champion the status quo. One dramatic example should suffice to make this point. Phenylketonuria is a disorder that produces mental retardation and is known to be caused by a single gene. Once the relation of the defective gene to the metabolism of the amino acid phenylalanine was discovered, it became possible to screen infants and treat those afflicted with a phenylalanine-free diet. Thus an environmental intervention was found to ameliorate the effects on intelligence of a disorder with a clear genetic basis.

Along with many workers, we too consider ourselves interactionists, fully appreciating that the environment has a significant influence on an individual's intellectual functioning. Yet to assert that human behavior is modifiable is to say a truism. The issue that must be addressed is the perplexing one of just how modifiable intelligence actually is. Drawing from the results of various twin studies, adoption studies, and environmental enrichment and deprivation studies (see reviews by Plomin & DeFries, 1980; Scarr & Carter-Saltzman, 1982; Vernon, 1979; Willerman, 1979), most researchers consider the heritability of intelligence to be somewhere between .45 and .80.

Consistent with many workers, we employ the concept of *reaction ranges* when dealing with the environment. "The concept of reaction range refers to the quantitatively different phenotypes that can develop from the same genotype under varying environmental conditions" (Scarr-Salapatek, 1974, pp. 14–15). Indeed, different genotypes may have different ranges, increasing or lowering their susceptibilities to favorable or unfavorable environments.

The net effect of the reaction range concept on IQ is shown by Figure 4.3. If IQ has a low degree of heritability, then it follows that IQ scores can be influenced greatly by the environment. Those who believe in high heritability would argue that the range of phenotypic expression for IQ is relatively small.

Figure 4.3 illustrates the notion that different genotypes may have different ranges, which can raise or lower their susceptibilities to favorable or unfavorable environments. Several major theorists have argued that for a trait such as IQ, the presumed reaction range, under natural habitat conditions, is probably about ± 12 points for average genotypes (Cronbach, 1975; Gottesman, 1968; Zigler, 1970b). Although this range will not make average intelligence possible in a severely retarded child, it does imply the importance of environmental efforts.

An immediate question raised by this discussion is just what constitutes natural habitat conditions or an average environment. Jensen (1969) addressed this issue by introducing the notion of a *threshold effect*. He argued that at some point an environment becomes so debilitating that it can lower the phenotypic expression of IQ. Above this threshold, however, variations in environment probably make little difference. This probable nonlinearity of environmental effects is illustrated in Figure 4.4.

One of the few empirical investigations in this area was conducted by Scarr and Weinberg (1978). These investigators found that the IQs of children adopted as infants into homes of different SES levels are about

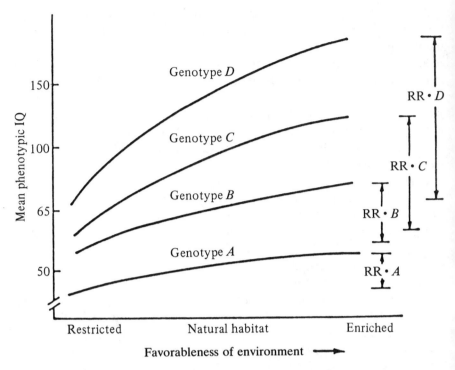

Figure 4.3. The reaction range (RR) of intelligence. Different genotypes will have different reaction ranges. Most theorists (Zigler, Gottesman, etc.) argue that the reaction range for intelligence is approximately ± 12 IQ points, as shown for Genotypes A and B. Others (Hunt) argue that the reaction range is much larger, as shown in Genotypes C and D.

equal when the children are adults. They concluded, "within a range of humane environments, from an SES level of working to upper middle class, there is little evidence for differential (environmental) effects" (p. 688). Thus, although the life experiences of working-class children are very different from those of upper middle-SES children, these differences apparently do not affect IQ scores to any substantial degree.

Another issue is how long a poor environment must be endured in order to have detrimental effects. Negative environmental events during "critical periods" have been considered less potent in recent years. After surveying the many studies of extreme environmental deprivation in the early years, Clarke and Clarke concluded, "the whole of development is important, not merely the early years. There is as yet no indication that a given stage [in development] is clearly more formative than others; in the long-term all may be important" (1976, p. 272). Similar conclusions were drawn from

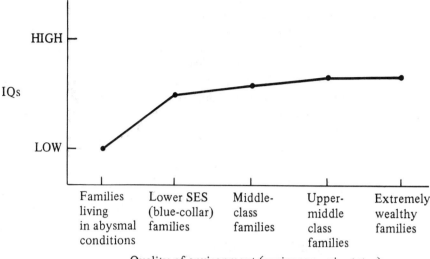

Quality of environment (socioeconomic status)

Figure 4.4. The hypothesized threshold effect of the environment. Whereas extremely poor environments depress one's IQ, environments ranging from lower SES to extremely wealthy do not substantially affect IQ scores.

studies of deprivation as a result of cultural practices (e.g., Kagan & Klein, 1973), maternal deprivation (Rutter, 1979), and disruptions due to short-term hospitalizations during early childhood (Hodapp, 1982). Thus, there is little support for the notion that relatively short-term contact with adverse experiences can hinder intellectual development.

There is some evidence, however, that prolonged exposure to a poor environment can cause some decrements in IQ scores. Jensen (1977) tested some 1,300 white and black children in a rural town in southeastern Georgia. The black children came from a very low socioeconomic position, while the white children were from low and lower-middle SES. (The confounding of race and living standards in this design does pose problems of interpretation.) Jensen found that older black children performed worse on IQ tests than did their younger siblings. He computed this decrement to be about 1.42 points of IQ per year; "that is, for every year's difference in age, over the age range 6–16, . . . total IQ decreases 1.42 points per year" (p. 187). For the white children from slightly higher social classes, no such decrements were observed. Thus, as may be surmised from Sameroff's (1975) transactional model of development (Chapter 2), only a long and continuous history of poor environment–child interactions may lead to a lowering of IQ as development progresses.

Why then do so many low-IQ children come from low-SES homes? Putting genetic reasons aside, let us concentrate on how the daily experiences of the child influence psychological subsystems other than formal cognition. Children growing up in lower-class rather than middle-class environments may have different experiences in regard to parental availability, personal attention at home and in school, expectations of the future, and society's evaluation of their personal worth. One can assume that the heritability indices for such traits as "expectancy of success" and self-image are markedly lower than those obtained for intelligence. Thus a poor environment may depress these traits, which in turn will hamper intellectual performance, making it appear that environment affected intelligence. Of course we do recognize that sometimes the environment in low-SES homes is not an optimal one for intellectual development. There is evidence that long-term, intensive intervention programs can lead to IQ increases in low-SES children (Garber & Heber, 1977). Yet motivational factors may be more malleable (Scarr & Yee, 1980) and more important for school and life success (Zigler, 1970a). Thus, while most environments do not depress IQ, bettering the environment can have some impact on IQ and can certainly improve adaptability.

A classification system for mental retardation

If there exists a relatively sizable group of retarded people without organic etiology who have parents of average intellect, how should these people be classified? In the classification system proposed in Chapter 3, IQ is the ultimate defining feature of mental retardation, while etiology is used as a classificatory principle. This allows us to distinguish three groups of retarded individuals: those with known organic etiologies; those with no known organic etiology and with low-IQ parents (familial retardation); and an undifferentiated group, or those who cannot reliably be placed in the other two categories. The arguments advanced in this chapter now allow us to offer a more differentiated classification of mental retardation and to offer some estimates of the percentage each group contributes to the total retarded population. We have defined as retarded all persons who score below 70 on standard IQ tests. The classification system we propose is:

I. *Mental retardation with known organic etiology.* Individuals in this group generally have IQ between 0 and 60 and comprise approximately 25% of the retarded population.

II. *Familial retardation.* These individuals have IQs between approximately 40 and 70 and have at least one parent whose IQ is below 70. This group comprises around 35% of the retarded population.

III. *Polygenic isolates*. These are the polygenically retarded offspring of parents who are not themselves retarded. Even though the field has paid virtually no attention to this group, the evidence presented above leads us to believe that they form approximately 35% of the retarded population. People in this class have received a "poor genetic draw" (MacMillan, 1977) in ways encompassed by the Gottesman and other polygenic models.

IV. *Environmentally deprived*. Children who suffer from extreme and prolonged neglect or abuse make up a fourth category of mental retardation. Two cases are Victor, the wild boy of Aveyron (Lane, 1976), and Genie, the child discovered in 1971 who had been locked in a closet for the first 12 years of life (Curtiss, 1977). Many other cases undoubtedly exist. We would emphasize, however, that environmental deprivation must be extreme and prolonged in order for it to affect IQ markedly. We have neither a theoretical model nor a data base from which to estimate how many individuals are mentally retarded due to environmental deprivation. However, we assume that truly deprived environments are rare and produce less than 5% of all retarded persons.

We acknowledge that our prevalence estimates for the four categories are but our best guesses at this time. In particular, we realize that there may be more individuals who actually are organically retarded (i.e., persons who should be placed in Category I), but for whom the technology is not yet available to diagnose their etiologies. The relative size of the organic group can thus be expected to rise in the future, but by how much is unknown.

A recent example of organic retardation that was previously classified as of unknown etiology is the Fragile X syndrome, first discovered in 1969 (Lubbs, 1969). In this syndrome, the tips of the long arm of the X chromosome appear pinched, especially when chromosomes are cultured in a medium deficient in folate. The prevalence of this syndrome is unknown at the present time, but some researchers (e.g., Turner & Turner, 1974) estimate that X-linked disorders may be responsible for as much as 20% of retardation among males. Besides accounting for much of the overabundance of males in the retarded population, X-linked retardation may be second in prevalence only to Down syndrome among single-gene disorders.

A second example of an unrecognized (or underappreciated) organic disorder may be lead poisoning. While long acknowledged as causing organic insult (Zigler, 1967), the incidence of lead poisoning may be higher than previously believed. Experts now estimate that "one in five inner-city black children under five years old is carrying a body burden of lead that could affect his or her intellectual development" (Raloff, 1982). The amount of lead intake necessary to depress intellectual functioning and the effects of subclinical levels of lead in the body are yet to be determined.

There is obviously no way of ascertaining the exact percentage of un-diagnosed organic retardation. The ultimate effect of this factor should be to raise slightly the percentage of retarded people accounted for by organic etiologies, while leaving substantially intact the familial, polygenic isolate, and environmentally deprived groups. But we do not believe that the entire retarded population will ever be classified as organic, no matter how ad-vanced tomorrow's technology may become.

Service and treatment implications

We have argued that there is a large group of retarded people in our society for whom there is no category in our current classification system, namely, retarded people without organic involvement who are the progeny of non-retarded parents. If such individuals exist, conceptual rigor demands that a complete taxonomy be able to encompass them.

In assessing the value of a classification system, however, a distinction should be made between the conceptual utility of the system and its use in directing service and clinical activities (see Zigler & Phillips, 1961a & 1961b). The question remains whether we should proceed from the con-struction of a class of polygenic isolates to the clinical and/or social practice of formally labeling members of this class as mentally retarded. While definitional rigor suggests that we should do so (i.e., they do have IQs below 70), an argument can be made for our society to forgo labeling in this case.

This discussion raises the intriguing question of exactly how unlabeled persons are treated as they encounter important social institutions (e.g., school, child guidance clinics). Unquestionably, some persons are never identified as retarded and live their entire lives without any indication of deviance, although as children they would have difficulty meeting the ac-ademic demands of school. If their difficulties led to their being tested, they would probably be designated mentally retarded (Berk, Bridges, & Shih, 1981). But, given the current classification system, the retarded child whose parents have IQs in the average range is an enigma that presents professionals with an unpleasant dilemma: whether or not to give recog-nition to this handicap with a label that his or her family and community find offensive. School psychologists and other clinicians may be apt to employ a variety of less stigmatizing labels for such children, like *under-achiever* and *learning-disabled* (see Polloway & Smith, 1983). Of course there is the issue of whether such terms carry their own stigmas.[1]

Let us also consider that middle-class parents often have high aspirations for their children. If this child is mildly retarded but unlabeled, there is a guarantee of a lifetime of frustration and sense of failure for both parents and child. The label could ease this conflict, allowing the parents to set more realistic expectations and the child the opportunity to meet them. We must seriously ponder the following statement by Nicholas Hobbs:

> Classification can profoundly affect what happens to a child. It can open doors to services and experiences the child needs to grow in competence, to become a person sure of his worth and appreciative of the worth of others, to live with zest and know joy. On the other hand, classification, or inappropriate classification, or failure to get needed classification – and the consequences that ensue – can blight the life of a child, reducing opportunity, diminishing his competence and self-esteem, alienating him from others, nurturing a meanness of spirit, and making him less a person than he could become. Nothing less than the futures of children is at stake. (1974, p. 1)

Conclusion

We have proposed in this chapter a new classificatory system to describe the phenomenon of mental retardation. In the process, we have shown how the current system of the AAMD may actually misclassify a significant number of retarded persons under its category VIII ("retardation due to environmental influences"). A new system, based on a truly interactionist perspective, can account for retardation caused by both genetic and environmental factors.

Our goal in proposing such a system is to make progress toward a truly scientific study of mental retardation. For too long, the field has been enamored with pure environmentalism, at the expense of a classification system that best explains the phenomenon under study. Workers in the mental retardation field must now assess the heuristic value of the proposed classification system and determine the numbers of retarded individuals included within each category.

[1] The phenomenon of "wastebasket categories" has not escaped the notice of professional groups who deal with children on an everyday basis. A resolution passed by several national organizations of school psychologists concludes: "The National Association of State Consultants for School Psychologists' Services is concerned about reports that a significantly large number of children who are experiencing difficulty in school are being inappropriately classified as handicapped, particularly learning disabled, and that such occurrences have the potential for serious harm to these children. NASCSPS does not condone inappropriate assessment and placement practices."

5   How many retarded people are there?

In the preceding two chapters we have attempted to define who should be classified as mentally retarded and how these people should be subclassified. Now we will consider just how large a population is involved. As we saw earlier, this depends primarily on the definition of mental retardation employed. Yet even if there was a unanimous definition, there would have to be standard methods of census-taking. Unfortunately, there are not. Prevalence estimates for mental retardation thus range so widely that we cannot truthfully say whether mental retardation is a relatively minor social problem or one that is very widespread. If this state of affairs is confusing to workers in the field, imagine the impact of such ambiguity on decision makers who have the responsibilty for allocating funds and constructing social policy affecting the lives of all our nation's mentally retarded citizens. With the experts themselves divided on the issue, officials can do nothing more than throw up their hands and wish that they knew how large the social problem posed by mental retardation actually is. In this chapter we will examine current prevalence estimates and attempt to reconcile their definitional and methodological incongruities. We hope not only to reach a consensus on the size of the retarded population, but in the process to expose the many factors involved in identifying all retarded persons.

In 1961 the AAMD was defining as retarded all individuals with IQs lower than one standard deviation below the population mean (Heber, 1961). Then there were about 32 million retarded Americans. A decade later the AAMD changed the IQ criterion to two *SDs* below the mean (Grossman, 1973), leaving only 6 million retarded people. It is fair to say that the true prevalence of mental retardation was not reduced by 81% in these few years. This casts doubt on both estimates.

Definitions in practice

The situation today is no better. The current AAMD definition of mental retardation reads as follows: "Mental retardation refers to significantly subaverage general intellectual functioning resulting in or associated with impairments in adaptive behavior and manifested during the developmental period" (Grossman, 1983, p. 11). Ignoring the criterion of age of onset for the time being, the dual criteria of intellectual functioning and social adaptation give considerable flexibility (or imprecision) to the diagnosis of mental retardation. As we pointed out in Chapter 3, social adaptation is not a well-defined construct; it varies across subcultural groups, changing societal expectations for various age groups, and important life changes for each individual (e.g., losing a job). Since this sort of imprecision may spare some individuals from and subject others to the mental retardation label, it creates a poorly defined clinical entity. It also makes the job of describing the characteristics of the mentally retarded population virtually impossible.

In a cogent analysis of the definition question, Silverstein (1973) pointed out that when the definition relies both on IQ and adaptation criteria, the exact prevalence rate for mental retardation depends on: (1) the correlation between the IQ measure and whatever measure of social adaptation is employed, and (2) the cutoff scores used on each measure to define mental retardation. Meeting the problem head-on and doing the arithmetic for us, Silverstein concluded that even with a two-*SD* cutoff on both indices, the nationwide prevalence of mental retardation can range from 104,000 to 4,550,000 depending on the correlation of the measures (see Table 1.1). The field of mental retardation cannot tolerate a possible error factor of 45 in our prevalence rates. In another study (Reschly, 1981), the prevalence figure for retardation among blacks and native Americans dropped dramatically when both IQ and various adaptive behavior criteria were employed, and dropped even further when a composite of all the behavioral measures was used. Excluding errors of measurement, the IQ-alone definition we advocate yields a figure of approximately 5 million retarded citizens. This more stable statistic can at least provide a basis for planning the scope of programs and resources required to meet the needs of retarded Americans.

The argument that IQ be used as the sole defining criterion for mental retardation appears consonant with the everyday procedures of clinicians and research workers in the field. Adams (1973) examined the diagnostic procedures used to evaluate 5- and 6-year-old children and concluded that "clinicians continued to use IQ as the prime determinant in classification" (p. 80). A similar conclusion can be drawn from a survey of articles in the *American Journal of Mental Deficiency* from 1974 through 1978 (Smith & Polloway, 1979). In 72.7% of all studies, investigators selected research samples solely on the basis of IQ-related indices, while only 5.3% included measures of both intellectual and adaptive functioning. Thus, in their daily practices neither clinicians nor researchers employ social adaptation as a criterion of mental retardation, even if both factors are present in the official definition. A reliance on IQ scores as the major criterion for diagnosis of retardation probably occurs in school settings as well (Berk et al., 1981; Junkala, 1977).

The question of IQ consistency

While experts may generally ignore social adaptation in their identification of mental retardation, the consruct may help to explain the change in prevalence rates with age. There is general agreement that the number of people diagnosed as retarded climbs once children enter school, peaks in the early teen years, and declines thereafter. This fact has led several researchers (e.g., MacMillan, 1982; Tarjan, Wright, Eyman, & Keeran, 1973) to conclude that the prevalance of mental retardation decreases once adulthood is reached. In fact, a commonly heard cliché in the field is that 50% of the cases of retardation vanish after the school years. Whether true or not, age-related changes in prevalence levels are an inherent assumption in the phenomenon of *decertification* (the removal from the mentally retarded classification of someone once so classified).

The shift in prevalence rates is related to a central issue in the field of psychology, namely, whether intelligence is a relatively stable human trait or varies with the situational demands inherent in any person–environment interaction. Those championing the stable-trait position view intelligence as operative across situations (see Chapter 1). They would thus expect true prevalence rates of mental retardation to be roughly constant across ages. An opposing viewpoint is that mental retardation does not inhere within the person, but is situationally determined by the ever-changing demands of person–environment interactions (e.g., Mercer, 1973a, 1973b). Within this formulation, the individual would shift from situation to situation. Since the situations encountered in everyday life differ greatly from age to age, situationists could accept the view that the prevalence rates for mental retardation change dramatically over the life span.

The documented age changes in the number of people diagnosed as retarded give more credence than is merited to the view that the true prevalence of retardation changes with CA. The error lies in equating diagnosed cases with actual prevalence. The true prevalence of a disorder is the number of diagnosed cases (minus false positives due to errors of measurement) plus the number of undiagnosed cases. For any disorder, at any age, there is always a ratio of diagnosed to undiagnosed cases. Thus, the changing prevalence rates of mental retardation that have been reported for different ages may have much more to do with the diagnosed:undiagnosed ratio than with changes in the true occurrence of the disorder. Workers must clearly differentiate between detection rates and prevalence rates, for confusing the two results in the nonsensical conclusion that many children *become* retarded upon school entry, and are somehow "cured" upon graduation.

Changes in definition or detection?

It is not surprising to discover that the detection rates are relatively low in both the preschool and postschool periods. For one reason, there is little incentive for engaging in the detection process in the early years. Even if there were, as in the case of high-risk children, we have no very satisfactory way to assess the intelligence of very young children. These two factors (discussed in more detail below) could easily account for underdetection of all but the most severely retarded children under 5 years of age.

Why then the great increase in the detection of mental retardation during the school years? The most obvious explanation is that school places increasing cognitive demands on children, demands that many children with low IQs cannot meet. Further insights come from realizing that the IQ reflects two cognitive developmental phenomena: (1) the rate of cognitive development (the lower the IQ, the longer the individual will take to reach any given level of development), and (2) the level of cognitive development achieved (compared to the child's age). Thus nonretarded children are not only at a higher cognitive level than their retarded classmates at each and every grade in school, but their cognitive abilities are increasing at a faster rate. Hence the disparity in cognitive level (as assessed by differences between the two groups in MA) increases over the school years. As the retarded child falls further and further behind, there is an ever greater likelihood that his or her intellectual deviance will be noted and an effort made to detect the nature of the child's problems.

This line of reasoning may help to explain the peak in prevalence levels in the early teen years. Between the ages of 10 and 14 most children of average intellect reach Piaget's stage of formal operations. From this time on, the school curriculum presents intellectual tasks that require logical operations. However, the retarded child of this CA has not yet attained this level of intellectual functioning. During this period of schooling we would therefore expect the problem of nonlearning to become most noticeable and for school personnel to engage in increased detection efforts.

This explanation also helps us to understand why the detection rates for mental retardation drop precipitously during the postschool years. Everyday social competence during the school years is largely defined by degree of academic success, which in turn is highly correlated with IQ (Zigler & Trickett, 1978). (Indeed, intelligence tests were originally created to predict school performance.) Successful adaptation to the nonschool environment, however, is relatively more dependent on nonintellective attributes, such as persistence, acceptance of social responsibilities, and compliance with society's social and moral codes (Granat & Granat, 1978). Evidence on this point may be seen in a review by Windle (1962), who found that the relation between IQ (range 40–80) and functioning in the community-nonschool environment is essentially zero. Once the demands of school are behind, the level of cognitive functioning achieved by most retarded persons is adequate for at least a marginally self-sufficient existence in our society. We thus see in the postschool years a weakening incentive for detection. But this does not mean that retardation is a "childhood disease." Those who emphasize the 50% of retarded people who vanish ignore the 50% who continue to be a concern to society. It is also likely that many of those who have become less visible are still in need of supportive services.

To summarize our argument, if a reliable and conceptually-based definition of mental retardation (e.g., IQ below 70) is employed, the diagnosis, and therefore the prevalence, of mental retardation should remain constant throughout the life span. What have been reported as differences in prevalence rates among age groups are actually differences in detection rates. In the next section we examine the empirical evidence relevant to this assertion.

The 3% versus 1% argument

What percentage of our population is mentally retarded? Through convention and sheer repetition, the figure most frequently quoted is 3%. To understand where this estimate comes from, we turn to the fact that there are two distinct types of retardation, one with known organic etiologies and the other without known organic involvement. This two-group approach has two commonly accepted corollaries: (1) A much smaller percentage of retarded people are in the organic as compared to the nonorganic group (the most common estimate being 25% vs. 75%), and (2) the average IQ of the organic group is markedly lower than that of the nonorganic group.

As discussed in Chapter 4, retarded people with no known organic involvement probably represent the lowest segment of the normal or Gaussian distribution of intelligence. Using a below-70 IQ definition of mental retardation (approximately two *SDs* below the mean of 100), 2.28% of the general population should be placed in the retarded range. To estimate the true prevalence, we would have to add to this figure the percentage of people whose retardation stems from organic damage (a cause not thought to reflect normal variations in intelligence). While the size of this group has been disputed, the literature over the past quarter of a century suggests that the ratio of organic to nonorganic cases should be no greater than 1:3. Thus, the prevalence of mental retardation in our population may be calculated as 2.28% + .76% (organic) = 3.04%. Even this brief exposition should make clear that the 3% estimate is a guess based on a number of questionable assumptions.

Deriving the 1% estimate

A decade or so ago, a group of leading figures in the MR field (Tarjan, Wright, Eyman, & Keeran, 1973) did indeed challenge the assumptions underlying the 3% estimate. They espoused instead the view that the prevalence rate for mental retardation is approximately 1%, or 2 million people rather than the frequently cited 6 million. The 1% estimate was thought to be supported by an epidemiological study by Mercer (1973a, 1973b). This reduction in the prevalence estimate was based primarily on two assumptions: that individuals enter and exit from the state of mental retardation, and that a single IQ-below-70 criterion for mental retardation is indefensible. To connect the two estimates, the Pacific State group argued that 3% of the population will be considered retarded at some point in their lives, but at any given time only 1% of our population is retarded.

Let us briefly examine these two assumptions. Whether the prevalence rates for mental retardation change over the life span is essentially an empirical issue. The most logical place to look for evidence is in the carefully collected standardization data of our major IQ tests. If there are indeed different prevalence figures at different ages, then the means and/ or standard deviations of IQ distributions should change with CA. For example, if the true prevalence of mental retardation is less in the postschool years, the mean during this age period should be higher and the *SD* lower. In point of fact, the standardization data for the Stanford-Binet (Terman & Merrill, 1973) reveals no such variations with age, leading the test constructors to conclude that "fluctuations from one age level to the adjacent age level were probably primarily a matter of sampling and measurement error" (p. 358).

Even more compelling evidence concerning the incidence of mental retardation may be found in several longitudinal studies of changes in IQ over the life span. If there are indeed changes in the prevalence rates of mental retardation, then we would expect the IQs of all individuals, whether low or high, to fluctuate considerably with age. After examining data from several of the major longitudinal studies of intelligence, we conclude that levels of intelligence are essentially stable throughout the life span (for a review of these studies, see MacMillan, 1982; also, see Silverstein, 1982, for a study of IQ stability in EMR children).

The central issue in the controversy between the 1% and 3% prevalence figures hinges on the definition of mental retardation that one accepts. In Chapter 3 we presented a case in favor of the single criterion, below-70 IQ, as the most appropriate definition for mental retardation. The Pacific State group argued that to be included within the prevalence figures for mental retardation, the individual must show both a low IQ and social maladaptation. The difference in the two prevalence estimates, as well as between the two schools of thought they represent, reduces finally to the percentage of people with IQs below 70 who do and do not make successful adaptation to society following the school years. If no one adapts success- fully, the single-criterion and dual-criteria definitions become identical and both result in a prevalence estimate of about 3%. If one assumes that the prevalence peaks at about 3% during the late school years and that two thirds of persons labeled retarded by the schools make a successful social adaptation in the postschool years, then the prevalence rate using the two- variable criterion is slightly above 1% (the smaller number of school-age individuals multiplied by 3% plus the larger adult population multiplied by 1%). Thus the Pacific State group has not proposed that persons labeled retarded during the school years achieve higher IQs (i.e., become more intelligent) upon leaving school, but rather that more of them are able to adapt to the new demands society makes on them.

Regardless of whether one agrees with the two-factor definition, it is clear that using it must inevitably lead to an impasse concerning the accurate assessment of the prevalence of mental retardation in our society. No real consensus has developed as to what constitutes successful adjustment dur- ing the adult years. And we simply do not know how many people with IQs below 70 function effectively (employing any definition) in the posts- chool years. We can see how one's stand on the 3%–1% controversy can color the answer to this question. Those who favor the 1% figure emphasize how well retarded people do in the postschool years. Supporters of the 3% figure tend to emphasize how poorly those labeled as retarded during the school years do later. The proportion of individuals with below-70 IQs who are deemed satisfactorily adjusted ultimately depends on the intensity of the detection effort (i.e., the closer the surveillance of the retarded individual, the more likely social inadequacies will be discovered) and the criteria chosen for successful adaptation in society. It is inherently unsatisfying to have the determination of the prevalence of a disorder rest so heavily on the intensity of detection efforts based on such variable criteria.

The decision to subscribe to either the 3% or 1% school of thought is more than a theoretical matter. It has real, pragmatic consequences in regard to the daily lives of retarded persons. The benefits of the 1% view lie in allowing adults with IQs below 70 to avoid any negative consequences of being labeled mentally retarded. The benefits of the 3% view are that special services and opportunities might be available, including indirect ones, such as the offer of tax incentives to employers who hire handicapped persons.

A compromise estimate

Even though we reject the two-factor definition of mental retardation, certain sound points made by the Pacific State group have convinced us that the prevalence of retardation in our society must be less than 3%. These points relate to (a) the difficulty of detecting mental retardation in infancy, and (b) differential mortality rates at different IQ levels. Any final estimate of the prevalence of mental retardation must allow for these two phenomena.

Concerning the first point, the only children identified as retarded in the first few years after birth are those with severe retardation and/or obvious physical impairments or genetic syndromes that are easily diagnosed. The number of other retarded children in this age group is undoubtedly underestimated, because of several factors. For one, societal expectations of infants and toddlers are minimal compared to the school years. Since young children develop at such different rates in different behavioral areas, few parents would notice delays until at least the onset of spoken language (18–24 months). Another factor leading to lower rates of identified retardation in young children is the inability of infant intelligence tests to predict later IQs (Bayley, 1949; Lewis, 1976; McCall, 1979). While extremely low scores on infant tests may be somewhat more predictive of lower intelligence at later ages (Bayley, 1949; McCall, 1979), we are currently unable to diagnose most children who are mildly or moderately retarded before at least 3 or 4 years of age. Even if we could, few children ever experience an IQ test until well beyond that age period.

Given the factors that militate against early diagnosis, the 3% prevalence estimate of mental retardation must be lowered slightly. That is, even if 3% of the children will be diagnosed as mentally retarded at later ages, only a small fraction of these will be identified in the earliest years. But how much should a lowered detection rate in the first five years of life lower the overall prevalence figure? U.S. Census data (1980) indicate that approximately 7% of the U.S. population is below 5 years of age. Given our assumptions that intelligence is a stable trait and that there is a uniform percentage of retardation at every age, 7% of the retarded population should also be aged 0–5. Even if none of these children was to be identified, 93% of all retarded people would reman, yielding a smallest possible prevalence rate of 2.79% (.93 × 3%).

At present, most of the approximately .4% of children suffering from severe retardation (below IQ 50) are identified in the 0–5-year age range (Abramowicz & Richardson, 1975). As improvements in early screening for retardation are made, we can expect that increasing numbers of less severely retarded children will be identified at early ages.

For example, Lemkau and Imre (1969) have shown that when one actually tests all of the preschool children suspected of being retarded in a particular city or county, the rates of retardation for this group are higher than originally supposed. In their study, 5.3% of 1- to 5-year-old children received IQ scores in the retarded range (below 69), as compared to 6.6% of 5- to 9-year-olds and 8.9% of 10- to 14-year-olds. Thus, even though the early scores may not be particularly trustworthy, intelligence tests reveal rates of retardation in preschool children not too far off from those obtained with older children.

The 3% estimate must be reduced further to account for the differential death rates between retarded and nonretarded groups. Surveys of retarded persons living in institutions (Tarjan, Wright, Kramer, Person, & Morgan, 1958) and in the community (McCurly, Mackay, & Scally, 1972; Eyman & Miller, 1978) have shown that retarded persons in general die at earlier ages. This is particularly true of persons who are profoundly and severely retarded, and for those who are nonambulatory (Edgerton, Eyman, & Silverstein, 1975; Eyman & Miller, 1978). While no life expectancy data are available, the mean age of death is somewhere in the late teens or early 20s for profoundly retarded persons, in the 40s for severely retarded persons, and in the 50s for persons who are mildly or moderately retarded. (As medical knowledge increases, life spans for all levels of retardation will probably increase.)

As the earliest deaths occur in the most impaired individuals, who are few in number, the prevalence estimate is not much affected by the radically higher death rates of this group. The difference in mean age at death between mildly retarded persons and the population at large (approximately 20–25 years) is noteworthy, however, especially since there may be

12 times as many mildly retarded individuals as there are retarded persons in all other levels combined (Haywood, 1979). The shorter life span of mildly retarded persons leaves fewer of them in the 55–80 age group, a group that currently comprises 20.8% of the U.S. population (U.S. Census, 1980). While it is not quite clear how much the 3% prevalence rate should be lowered to take into account these differential death rates, a lowering of 10–15% of those included in the 3% figure seems reasonable.

This analysis leads us to conclude that the 3% prevalence rate for mental retardation is somewhat higher, just as a 1% figure is much too low. A defensible estimate for the prevalence of mental retardation in our society would appear to fall between 2% and 2.5% (i.e., adjusting the 3% figure on the basis of differential death rates and our inability to diagnose mild retardation in the early childhood years). We shall now turn to population studies to assess the accuracy of this estimate.

Prevalence studies

Studies of the prevalence of mental retardation differ in a variety of ways. Some examine only those children and adults with severe (i.e., below IQ 50) levels of retardation while others include individuals of all levels; a few even include borderline individuals, with IQs up to 85. Some researchers rely on IQ tests in making diagnoses, others use tests of social adaptation or achievement, and still others use no tests at all. Many investigators calculate prevalence on the basis of the number of persons who use social services, while others attempt to identify all persons who score below two standard deviations from the mean, regardless of whether they are known to local agencies.

In this section, studies that include at least the following elements will be used to ascertain the prevalence of mental retardation:

1. Each study must examine the prevalence of retarded persons in the population at large, not just among individuals in institutions, hospitals, special schools, or clinics, or those known to local authorities.
2. The design must include a strong attempt to identify previously unidentified cases of mental retardation.
3. Investigators must directly employ standard intelligence tests in deriving their prevalence estimates.

Table 5.1 provides a summary of all population studies performed since 1960 that meet our criteria.[1] (For reviews of earlier surveys see Gruenberg,

---

[1] Two points must be made in regard to the studies chosen. First, many of the "classic" prevalence studies are omitted because each person was not individually tested. Second, the date at which a test was standardized relative to when it was used in the prevalence study is of interest, as there might be a trend toward a higher population mean on IQ tests not recently standardized. (See President's Commission on Mental Retardation, note 3; and Robinson, 1980, note 4, for a discussion of this issue.)

Table 5.1. *Prevalence studies*

Study	Location	Ages	Tests employed	Case-finding procedures	Estimate of MR prevalence
Birch, Richardson, Baird, Horobin, & Illsley (1970)	Aberdeen, Scotland	8–10	Moray House Picture Test of Intelligence	Moray House test given to 95% of Aberdeen 7-year-olds	2.74%
Mercer (1973a, 1973b)	Riverside, Calif.		Stanford-Binet LM & Kuhlman-Binet	"Disproportionate random sampling" + weighting 644 persons.	2.14%
Rutter, Tizard, & Whitmore (1970)	Isle of Wight, England	9–11	WISC (1949 – restandardized on Isle of Wight population)	All 9- to 11-year-olds living on island: 2,344 children.	2.53% (Isle of Wight norms)
Reschly & Jipson (1976)	Pima county, Ariz.	1st, 3rd, 5th, 7th, in reg. & special schools	WISC-R	Stratified random sample of 950.	3.53%
Granat & Granat (1973, 1978)	Sweden	19-year-old males	Ullerkas Sjukhus battery (a Swedish IQ test) & Stanford-Binet	Random sample of 5,605 Swedish male 19-year-olds.	2.21%
Drillien, Jameson, & Wilkinson (1966)	Edinburgh, Scotland	7½–14½	Stanford-Binet (T-M revision) & WISC	Public health registers and other institutions for physically & mentally handicapped children throughout Scotland, group IQ tests given to all Edinburgh children at age 7½.	1.13%
Åkesson (1961)	Malmohus county, southern Sweden	All	Stanford-Binet L	Official sources and key inform-ants from 10 randomly chosen	1.75%

parishes in a southern Swedish county (MR defined as two SDs from mean = IQ < 68).

Study	Location	Age	Test	Description	Rate
Lemkau & Imre (1969)	"Rose County"	1–19	Stanford-Binet (unclear which tests used for preschoolers)	Preschoolers: household survey to identify all children scoring less than Social Quotient 81. School-aged children: all receiving a Lorge-Thorndike IQ < 79 or a PPVT IQ < 79 were given individual Stanford-Binet tests. 7,383 children screened.	7.44%
Hagberg, Hagberg, Lewerth, & Lindberg (1981a and 1981b)	Gothenburg, Sweden	8–12	Swedish WISC & Terman-Merrill	Registers of National Bureau for Provision of Services (BPSMR). Contacts of schools for MR & physically handicapped, hospitals. All school nurses and school psychologists contacted.	0.67%
Jonsson & Kalveston (1964)	Stockholm, Sweden	8- to 17-year-old boys		Randomized, systematic sample of 222 Stockholm boys (MR = 2 SDs below mean).	2.3%

1966; Wallin, 1958.) The median estimate of the prevalence of mental retardation from the 10 studies in Table 5.1 is 2.25%. Studies that test the entire population (Birch, Richardson, Baird, Horobin & Illsley, 1970; Rutter, Tizard, & Whitmore, 1970) and those that undertake random (and weighted) sampling (Granat & Granat, 1973; Jonsson & Kalveston, 1964; Mercer, 1973a, 1973b; Reschly & Jipson, 1976) closely appproximate the estimate that the prevalence of mental retardation is somewhere between 2% and 2.5%. Studies that test only persons suspected of being retarded by clinic, key informant, or survey report (Åkesson, 1961; Drillien, Jameson, & Wilkinson, 1966; Hagberg, et al., 1981a, 1981b; Lemkau & Imre, 1969) provide the extreme values (0.67% to 7.44%) of the distribution.

Let us examine for a moment the case-finding procedures of the three studies that are furthest from the hypothesized 2-2.5% figure. Investigators in the two studies reporting the lowest prevalence rates (Drillien et al., 1966; Hagberg et al., 1981a, 1981b) began with medical or state records, then examined children in schools for the physically handicapped, and then sought referrals from school personnel or from the results of group tests. The orientation of both sets of researchers was essentially medical, and the lower prevalence rates are most probably the result of this orientation. It seems probable that both these studies overlooked large numbers of retarded children, especially those with retardation in the mild range and/ or of unknown etiology. There was simply no reason why many of these children would have come to the attention of the medical authorities.

The study of Lemkau and Imre (1969), on the opposite end of the prevalence range (7.44%), employed a radically different case-finding approach. The researchers first mailed census forms to every household in the county. A trained observer then visited each home, and screened children (i.e., those suspected of being retarded) were identified by the use of specific criteria. All screened children were then given intelligence tests. Among 2,266 preschoolers, for example, 592 were identified for further examination, and of these, 116 scored 69 or below on standard intelligence tests. Thus, information was collected on all children, some were designated for further testing, and, of these, only about one fourth actually tested in the retarded range. The prevalence rates obtained in this study are well above the others, providing a clear example of our dictum that the more intensive the detection effort, the higher the prevalence rates obtained.

The studies reported here are unfortunately few in number, and they are not as nationally or internationally representative as one might like. Prevalence rates will of course be affected by demographic factors such as in- and out-migration and the age, sexual, and racial composition of the particular region under study (see MacMillan 1982; Robinson & Robinson, 1976). The studies reported here differ in all these regards. Nonetheless they furnish the best available data. The median overall prevalence rate of 2% to 2.5% seems the most reasonable conclusion to be drawn from these surveys. This rate translated into numbers means that there are currently 4.6 to 5.75 million retarded people in the United States.

Retardation due to organic versus unknown etiologies

An issue related to the prevalence question concerns what percentage of retarded people have mental retardation due to known organic etiologies, and what number display mental retardation in the absence of known organic involvement. As in the case of the overall estimates in general, this more fine-grained question is usually answered on the basis of convention or appeals to authority rather than by means of carefully conducted empirical investigations. Thus, it is an article of faith within the mental retardation field that 75% of retarded people show no organic pathology, and 25% show damage due to prenatal, perinatal, or postnatal insult (Tarjan, 1970; Zigler, 1967). However, few if any studies have attempted to document this estimate in recent years, despite the fact that the two groups differ dramatically in physical and intellectual terms as well as in care and training needs.

A survey of the current literature revealed only seven studies that empirically investigated the ratio of organic to etiology-unknown cases in the retarded population. Their results are summarized in Table 5.2. These findings lead to the heretical but fairly safe assertion that the percentage of organic cases of mental retardation is markedly higher than the 25% typically assumed. The studies indicate, when the median values in Table 5.2 are taken, that 55% of cases of retardation involve known organic etiologies, whereas the remaining 45% are linked to unknown causes. This ratio of course must be qualified by the fact that there is a much greater likelihood that cases involving organic damage will be detected. Our best estimate at this time is that the ratio of organic to etiology-unknown cases is much closer to 50 : 50 than to the widely accepted 25 : 75. We also acknowledge that our own estimates of the percentages of retarded people in each of the various categories of mental retardation (Chapter 4) may also need to be modified. If this higher proportion of organically retarded relative to nonorganically retarded persons is substantiated by future research, each of our categories of nonorganic retardation (familial, polygenic

Table 5.2. *Percentages of individuals with organic and unknown etiologies*

Study	Total number of retarded cases	Organic etiology	Unknown etiology
Drillien, Jameson, & Wilkinson (1966)	406	61.8%	38.2%
Hagberg, Hagberg, Lewerth, & Lindberg (1981a, 1981b)	164	55.5%	44.5%
Blomquist, Gustavson, & Holmgren (1981); Gustavson, Holmgren, Jonsell, & Blomquist (1977)[a]	332	67.2%	32.8%
Åkesson (1961)	132	6.8%	93.2%
Rutter, Tizard, & Whitmore (1970)[b]	58	53.4%	46.6%
Smith & Simons, 1975	98	60%	40%
Czeizel, Lanyi-Engelmayer, Klujber, Metnéki, & Tusnády (1980)[c]	1276	44.2%	55.8%
	Median values	55.5%	44.5%

[a]These studies are actually an examination of severe (i.e., below IQ 50) and moderate retardation in the same population by the same researchers.

[b]Percentages of below 70 IQ children from restandardized WISC (i.e., restandardized on Isle of Wight population).

[c]From Table 1 of this study – children with "familial-cultural" retardation and those with "unknown" etiologies, from both special schools and institutions for retarded persons, are compared to the number of organically retarded children from both of these institutions.

isolate, and environmentally deprived) will contain smaller percentages of retarded individuals.

IQ differences

Another unresolved demographic issue concerns the range of intelligence associated with the two major classes of mental retardation. The organic and etiology-unknown classes form one axis in any comprehensive taxonomy of mental retardation. A second axis is defined by the magnitude of the retardation as indicated by IQ. Along this axis, we find such terms as mild (IQ 50–69), moderate (IQ 40–54), severe (IQ 25–39), and profound (IQ below 25) retardation. There is some consensus in the field that a systematic relation obtains between these two axes. Those with known organic etiologies are assumed to have lower IQs (although there are some exceptions), whereas those with unknown etiologies are assumed to have higher IQs (see Figure 4.2). Again, however, assertions concerning the exact nature of the relation between etiology and IQ appear to be based on convention rather than actual data.

In approaching this issue, we must begin with the clear understanding that mental retardation is not a homogeneous entity and that individuals labeled mentally retarded (IQs between 0 and 70) are extremely heterogeneous in regard to the cause of their retardation, their levels of cognitive ability, and the adjustments they make to society. The only common element displayed by all retarded persons (by any definition of mental retardation) is that at some point in their lives they display a level of cognitive functioning below that of the average individual of the same age in our society.

As is typical in most taxonomic enterprises, workers have attempted to construct subclasses of mental retardation characterized by greater homogeneity. For example, grouping individuals within rather narrow IQ ranges is straightforward and results in considerable homogeneity within each subclass. For example, those with IQs below 20 are more likely to be bedridden, and those above 60 can generally attend public schools. This is not true of the etiologic axis, however. Consider those with the organic classification. There are now over 200 known etiologies for organic retardation (Lubs & Maes, 1977), with more being discovered as time goes on.

The IQs of those in the organic group are also extremely heterogeneous, ranging from 0 to 70. Indeed one could suffer brain damage and still function and test within the average or gifted range. This possibility leads to the intriguing question of how much an individual's polygenic inheritance continues to influence the expression of intelligence even though he or she might have suffered organic insult. Do organically damaged individuals with better genetic endowment have higher IQs than similarly damaged individuals with poorer genetic endowment (assessed perhaps by the midpoint of the parents' IQs)? There is some evidence that such may be the case with some circumscribed types of organic impairment (e.g., Down syndrome; see Hodapp & Zigler, in press). More research on this issue would greatly increase our understanding of organic retardation.

The class of unknown etiologies also encompasses a very heterogeneous group of individuals. As we indicated in Chapter 4, this grouping comprises three subclasses: familial retarded individuals (whose etiology is traceable to at least one parent with an IQ below 70), polygenic isolates (whose etiologies primarily reflect polygenic factors), and a small number of persons who have suffered extreme and prolonged environmental deprivation. The behavioral characteristics of each of these groups is unknown at this time.

In terms of IQ, however, those with unknown etiologies are not as heterogeneous as those with organic etiologies. The conventional estimate is that nonorganic retardation is characterized by IQs between 50 and 70. This estimate derives from the polygenic model for the distribution of intelligence; its popularity can be traced to Gottesman's (1963) seminal paper (see Chapter 4). In the process of constructing a five-gene model for the distribution of intelligence, Gottesman placed the lowest point of the IQ range at 50. (He could, for example, have picked a six-gene mode, with each " + " allele worth 10 points, covering the IQ range from 40 to 160.)

In any event, the acceptance of 50 as the lower IQ limit for the unknown-etiology group is now evident among many renowned workers in the field. For example, Tarjan (1975) asserted that the degree of retardation of persons of unknown etiology is "usually mild," and Heber (1970) noted that "most of this group fall in the range of IQ 50–70" (p. 5). Similarly, Robinson and Robinson (1965) stated that "by far the majority of such children [of unknown etiology] fall within the mild range of subnormality" (p. 213). While all of these workers acknowledge that some individuals of unknown etiology may fall in the moderate, severe, and even the profound ranges of mental retardation, all agree that most of these cases are mildly retarded.

This entire issue of IQ levels of retarded persons of organic and unknown etiologies has recently come under new scrutiny. Employing questionnaire responses from 18 U.S. institutions for the retarded, Cleland, Case, and Manaster (1980) found that individuals of "familial" and "unknown" etiologies are numerous at all retarded levels, even among the profound and severe groups. Further, these investigators discovered that organically retarded people constitute the majority of cases at each level of retardation (even among the mildly retarded). Both of these conclusions are at variance with the consensus views of retardation due to organic and unknown etiologies as described above.

Some understanding of the Cleland et al. (1980) findings can be gained by noting that this particular study was performed by examining institutionalized populations. It is extremely likely that individuals with very low IQs and/or organic damage will be overrepresented in such samples. In point of fact, of the approximately 20,000 cases examined by these workers, only 29% were from combined familial and etiology-unknown classes, while 71% were organically retarded. This 29 : 71 ratio contrasts sharply with the rough 50 : 50 estimate derived from the population studies in Table 5.2. Furthermore, over three fourths of the Cleland et al. sample had IQ scores below 40. When compared to Haywood's (1979) estimate that "there

Table 5.3a. *Percentage of retarded persons of unknown etiology at each IQ level*

	0	10	20	30	40	50	60	70	
Hagberg, Hagberg, Lewerth, & Lindberg (1981a, 1981b)			24.6%				75.4%		N = 73
Blomquist, Gustavson, & Holmgren (1981); Gustavson, Holmgren, Jonsell, & Blomquist (1977)			32.1%				67.9%		N = 109
Åkesson (1961)			30.9%				69.1%		N = 123
Drillien, Jameson, & Wilkinson (1966)		.6%	1.9%		7.7%	13.5%	76.1%		N = 155

Table 5.3b. *Percentage of organically retarded persons at each IQ level*

	0	10	20	30	40	50	60	70	
Hagberg, Hagberg, Lewerth, & Lindberg (1981a, 1981b)			60.4%				39.6%		N = 91
Blomquist, Gustavson, & Holmgren (1981); Gustavson, Holmgren, Jonsell, & Blomquist (1977)			56.5%				43.5%		N = 223
Åkesson (1961)			66.7%				33.3%		N = 9
Drillien, Jameson, & Wilkinson (1966)		19.1%	7.6%		28.7%	16.7%	27.9%		N = 251

Note: Studies by Drillien, Jameson, and Wilkinson, 1966, and by Åkesson, 1961, both employ IQ 55 as the dividing line between severe and mild levels of mental retardation; all other studies use IQ 50.

Table 5.4. *Percentage of retarded persons of organic and unknown etiologies at each IQ level*

		0	10	20	30	40	50	60	70
Hagberg, Hagberg, Lewerth, & Lindberg (1981a, 1981b)	% U		24.7%					60.4%	
	% O		75.3%					39.6%	
	N =		N = 73					N = 91	
Gustavson, Hagberg, Hagberg, & Sars (1977)	% U		11.5%				No mildly retarded subjects in this study		
	% O		88.5%						
	N =		N = 122						
Åkesson (1967)	% U		80%				No mildly retarded subjects in this study		
	% O		20%						
	N =		N = 105						
Gustavson, Holmgren, Jonsell, & Blomquist (1977) Blomquist, Gustavson, & Holmgren (1981)	% U		21.7%					43.3%	
	% O		78.3%					56.7%	
	N =		N = 161					N = 171	
Åkesson (1961)	% U		86.4%	14.3%	33.3%			96.6%	
	% O		13.6%	85.7%	66.7%			3.4%	
	N =		N = 44	N = 84	N = 63			N = 88	
Drillien, Jameson, & Wilkinson (1966)	% U	2%	13.6%					62.8%	
	% O	98%	86.4%					37.2%	
	N =	N = 49	N = 22					N = 188	

U = % etiology unknown
O = % organic

Mean for etiology unknown	= 40.2%*
Mean for organic	= 59.8%*
Median for etiology unknown	= 23.2%*
Median for organic	= 76.8%*

*These numbers represent subjects with IQ 0–50 or 55, depending on each study

Mean for etiology unknown	= 65%
Mean for organic	= 34%
Median for etiology unknown	= 61%
Median for organic	= 38%

These numbers represent subjects with IQ above 50 or 55 depending on each study are 12 times as many mentally retarded persons in the IQ 50 to IQ 70 range as there will be IQs less than 50" (p. 431), we see that, in this respect as well, institutionalized samples are not representative of the entire retarded population.

Tables 5.3 and 5.4 summarize the findings of several studies examining percentages of organic and unknown etiologies among severely (below 50 IQ) and mildly (IQ 50–70) retarded persons. The large majority (median = 76.8%) of severely retarded persons show clear organicity; only 23% are of unknown etiology. Mildly retarded people display an opposite pattern. The median ratio of unknown to organic etiologies among the mildly retarded cases is 63 : 37. The tables further show that of all the organically retarded persons studied, 60% have IQs below 50, while 40% are mildly retarded (IQ 50–70). Conversely, of all cases of unknown etiology, 25% are severely retarded, whereas 75% fall in the mild range of retardation.

We see then how a different picture of mental retardation is gained by examinations of general populations as opposed to institutionalized residents or diagnostic clinic patients. The Cleland et al. (1980) findings – that there are sizable numbers of familial and undifferentiated retarded people at all levels of retardation and that many organically retarded people are found at all IQ levels – seem true only for residential institutions. Various population studies support the traditional view of the intellectual levels of those with organic and unknown etiologies. Individuals with unknown etiology are predominantly mildly retarded (and constitute the majority at the mild level of retardation), while organically retarded persons are more likely to be severely retarded (and constitute the majority at the severe level of retardation).

Conclusion

We have attempted in this chapter to clarify several issues related to the prevalence of mental retardation. After carefully considering the arguments in the 3% versus 1% debate, and the data from several population studies, we conclude that approximately 2% to 2.5% of the population is retarded (as defined by an IQ below 70). This estimate translates to a national prevalence rate of 4.6 to 5.75 million people.

In further examining these population studies, we found that the oft-cited 75% : 25% ratio of nonorganic to organic retardation may not be accurate. Our review leads us to conclude that the ratio may be closer to 50 : 50, there being about equal numbers of nonorganically and organically retarded persons in the relevant prevalence studies. However, we did find support for another widely held position, that organically retarded people are more likely to be severely and profoundly retarded, and that those retarded people who show no organic etiology are predominantly found in the mild-to-moderate ranges of retardation.

Part III

Motivation and personality development of retarded persons

6   The retarded child as a whole person

In the preceding chapters we have dealt with the difficult issues involved in determining who is retarded and who is not, in categorizing retarded people into meaningful subgroups, and in estimating the size of the retarded population. This extended focus on definitions and data can lead to a common but unforgivable oversight: There are human beings behind those numbers. Hidden within the theories and statistical charts are real people who think, laugh, cry, hope, dream, and have more than their fair share of disappointments. In this chapter we attempt to right this wrong by turning our attention from the group to the individual retarded person.

There are several reasons why the words "person" and "personality" do not seem to be part of the jargon in the field of mental retardation. One is that subnormal intellectual functioning is such a striking phenomenon; it is the first thing noticed and retains our attention. While this is understandable, professionals and laypeople can become guilty of treating the retarded person as nothing but a low IQ score. Once we know a child is retarded, we act as if we know all there is to know. When the child performs a task poorly, for example, we are quick to blame a lack of intelligence and do not think to wonder if he or she might be afraid of us and unwilling to try.

This tendency can clearly be seen in a common research design that compares institutionalized retarded children, many of whom spend their lives in the very lowest segment of the lowest socioeconomic class, with middle-class children who live at home. Such groups differ not only with respect to their IQ scores but also in their total life histories and the nature of their current socioemotional environment. One wonders how many differences discovered in such comparisons reflect the effects of institutionalization, or the circumstances that led to the child's placement, rather than some cognitive aspect of mental retardation. These facts lead us to underscore a logical point that must be kept in mind when interpreting research involving retarded persons: You cannot safely attribute performance differences between retarded and nonretarded groups to a difference in a trait such as IQ if the groups also differ in other ways that could reasonably be expected to affect their behavior.

The overly cognitive approach to mental retardation also stems from the paucity of empirical work dealing with personality functioning in retarded individuals (see Gardner, 1968; Heber, 1964). Had such a body of work developed over the years, it may have moderated the cognitive emphasis that colors explanations of retarded persons' behavior. And not only has there been surprisingly little work done on personality development in mental retardation, but many of the views advanced have been at best inadequate, and at worst patently ridiculous. Zigler and Harter (1969) pointed out that in the early years of this century, the prevailing viewpoint was that retarded people are essentially immoral, degenerate, and depraved (see Chapter 10). Despite some progress, the intervening years have not brought a very great change in such stereotypic thinking about retarded persons (see, for example, Mautner, 1959). The persistence of this view was pointed out by Gardner (1968), who quoted a number of later workers guilty of stereotypic thinking. Others have observed how this attitude has even been extended to the view that mental retardation represents some sort of subspecies or group of less than human organisms (Wolfensberger & Menolascino, 1968; Zigler, 1966a). Nowhere are such condescending beliefs seen more clearly than in mandatory sterilization laws. Passed in many states so that retarded persons could not propagate their "defects," these laws denied them an integral aspect of their humanity.

Some of this slander can be traced to a common, but unnecessary, outcome of categorizing and labeling. Individuals can be fairly easily differentiated with respect to their levels of intelligence. This ease of differentiation leads to the practice of categorizing people along some dimension of intellectual adequacy. For example, a line can be arbitrarily drawn at IQ 70 to distinguish the retarded and nonretarded populations. This both figuratively and literally separates retarded individuals from everyone else. Since the conceptual distance between *subnormal* and *abnormal* is minimal, it is an easy step to regard retarded people as a homogeneous group, defective in all areas and different by their very nature from those possessing higher IQs. We submit that too often such is the practice in the field of mental retardation.

Thus far we have painted a rather unflattering picture of the disposition of the mental retardation field – one characterized by a narrow-minded cognitive emphasis that belittles or downgrades personality factors. Yet cognitive and personality factors can be integrated to form a much clearer understanding of why retarded people behave as they do. As we have emphasized repeatedly in this book, the behavior of retarded people, as of all human beings, is complex and multidetermined. Intelligence certainly has a powerful influence on daily functioning. But so do emotional and motivational factors that underlie each person's manner of response to daily events. Take the requirements of the typical school day. One of course needs the intellectual wherewithal to complete the required tasks. But one also needs to be motivated to complete them. The child who views them as unimportant, is afraid of failure, or is worried about what is going to happen on the playground that afternoon is not likely to do well even if the work is well within his or her capabilities.

Retarded children may be more prone to such motivational handicaps than their nonretarded classmates. Familial retarded children in particular are more likely to come from lower-SES homes where certain values and lifestyles are not always harmonious with school expectations. The retarded child has also experienced frequent failure, which can lead to low or non-existent goal-setting, learned helplessness, negative self-image, and an unwillingness to try. Low-IQ children may also be subjected to the stigma associated with the retardation label or with placement in special classes. These and related experiences can only convince the retarded child that he or she is not as good as others, an attitude that further lowers performance.

Research on motivational variables in the performance of retarded persons has focused on experiences in the socialization process that give rise to these and other motives, attitudes, and response styles often associated with mental retardation. In many cases this work has demonstrated a motivational cause underlying behavior previously attributed to cognitive shortcomings. The remainder of this chapter will present an overview of studies of several of these noncognitive determinants of performance. The effects of institutionalization, which causes a dramatic change in lifestyle and confounds much research comparing institutionalized retarded children with nonretarded children who live at home, will receive separate coverage in Chapter 10.

Two important points must be discussed before we survey the research. The first is that we are speaking in general terms. Differences among individuals can be expected not only because people are different, but because of variations in their socialization histories. Personality differences among retarded individuals should also be expected, given that they have had different home backgrounds, school experiences, and social encounters. All of this is to say that retarded persons do not have a universal personality type that accompanies their low IQs, and they do not all live their days in the same way. Findings on how life experiences affect personality thus apply to both retarded and nonretarded *groups*, but do not necessarily apply to any given child.

The second caution is that our extended focus on personality factors does not imply that the cause of mental retardation is motivational. There are many causes of mental retardation, but its essential feature remains attenuated cognitive functioning. However, there have been repeated demonstrations that the performance of many retarded persons on a variety of tasks is poorer than would be predicted from their general level of cognitive ability. Much of this performance deficit is due to the attenuating effects of motivational factors (Zigler, 1973). If these hindrances were removed and the individual functioned in a manner commensurate with his or her intellectual ability, that individual would still be intellectually retarded when compared with nonretarded peers. Thus a concern with motivational factors holds no promise of a dramatic cure for mental retardation.

The benefits of the motivational approach are in informing us how to help retarded persons realize their full intellectual capacity. This goal is not only realistic, but is of tremendous social value. Well-documented evidence shows that the everyday adjustment of human beings, retarded or nonretarded, depends as much if not more on personality features as on cognitive ability (e.g., Granat & Granat, 1978; Windle, 1962). While we cannot change the IQ a great amount, changes in motivational structure can make the difference between successful and unsuccessful social adaptation. This line of thought bolsters a recurring theme in this volume, namely, that as important as the formal cognitive processes are, their role has been overestimated, especially with respect to meeting the daily demands of society or the individual's overall social competence.

Early research on motivational factors

Much of the early work on the behavior of retarded people stems from the Lewin-Kounin rigidity formulation. This theory had little to do with motivation. It took the opposite course of explaining all differences in the behaviors of retarded and nonretarded people on the basis of cognitive factors. In brief, Lewin (1936) described an individual's sphere of cognition as being divided into different subspheres called *regions*. An aspect of this cognitive system is degree of differentiation, or the number of cognitive regions. Lewin also described the so-called firmness–weakness dimension of the boundaries between these regions, which determines the degree of ease with which a person can move from one region to another. Lewin viewed the retarded child as cognitively less differentiated, that is, as having fewer cognitive regions, than a nonretarded child of the same chronological age. He also argued that the physical boundaries separating a retarded person's cognitive regions are firmer and relatively impermeable, making retarded people more rigid in their thinking.

Building upon Lewin's work, Kounin (1941a) offered the findings of five experiments in which he employed older and younger retarded individuals, and individuals of normal intelligence. The degree-of-differentiation variable was controlled by equating the groups on MA. As predicted, the performance of the three groups differed on certain tasks in all five of these experiments, the differences being attributed to differences in the permeability of the cognitive boundaries.

In Kounin's concept-switching task, for example, the child was given a deck of cards and asked to sort them first on the basis of one principle (shape) and then another (color). Nonretarded children evidenced the least difficulty, and the older retarded persons the most difficulty in shifting from one sorting principle to another, while the younger retarded children fell between these two groups. Kounin argued that less permeable boundaries between regions made it more difficult for the older retarded individual to switch from one concept to another.

In a study designed to test the Lewin-Kounin rigidity formulation, Stevenson and Zigler (1957) investigated the ability of retarded and nonretarded children to acquire one response and then to switch to a new response in a situation that required making a discrimination. The solution of the reversal problem was thought to require movement to a new cognitive region, making it more difficult for the retarded groups because of their more rigid cognitive boundaries. As in the Kounin study, nonretarded and older and younger retarded groups, matched on MA, were employed. Surprisingly, the results showed a striking similarity in performance among groups. Groups did not differ significantly in how long it took to learn the initial problem, in the number of subjects from each group who learned the reversal problem, or on a direct measure of rigidity (the frequency of responses on the reversal problem that would have been correct on the initial discrimination problem). Other studies in this area (Balla & Zigler, 1964; Plenderleith, 1956; Stevenson & Zigler, 1958; Zigler & Balla, 1982d) also failed to support the hypothesized cognitive rigidity of mentally retarded individuals.

The different results of Lewin and Kounin versus Stevenson and Zigler led to a new line of research. Zigler and his colleagues began to ascribe the performance on rigidity tasks in part to the social deprivation experienced by institutionalized retarded persons. Stevenson and Zigler noted that in their studies there was minimal interaction between the children and the experimenter, while in Kounin's tasks personal instructions were used. Thus differences in rigid behaviors between nonretarded and retarded groups in the instruction-initiated tasks may have been related to differences in the children's motivation to comply with the instructions rather than to cognitive rigidity. This hypothesis was based on the assumption that institutionalized retarded children tend to be relatively deprived of adult contact and approval and hence have an increased desire to interact with adult figures.

In an effort to employ tasks comparable to those used in Kounin's earlier study, Zigler, Hodgden, and Stevenson (1958) constructed three simple motor tasks, each having two parts. The study deviated from Kounin's procedure in that two conditions of reinforcement were used. The experimenter maintained a nonsupportive role in one condition and reinforced the child's performance in the other. Not only did the retarded children spend more time on the games than their nonretarded peers in both conditions, but they spent a significantly greater amount of time playing the games when they received support. The nonretarded children were not much affected by reinforcement condition.

The marked sensitivity of the retarded groups to degree of social reinforcement lent a certain amount of support to the social deprivation hypothesis. However, certain of the Zigler, Hodgden, and Stevenson (1958) findings were reminiscent of those found by Kounin. For example, more retarded than nonretarded children stopped the games when the examiner asked if they wanted to play other games, suggesting their desire to comply with instructions. Retarded children also performed an inordinately long time on the boring and monotonous tasks, and they played the second part of a two-part task longer than they did the first part, even though both parts were highly similar. In light of this, the Zigler, Hodgden, and Stevenson findings hardly constituted any death blow to the Lewin-Kounin ridigity formulation. At most they indicated that the production of rigid behaviors is also influenced by motivational effects, a view not very much at variance with Lewin and Kounin's own stance concerning motivational factors.

A more definitive test of the cause of the Lewin-Kounin findings was attempted by examining whether more socially deprived retarded children were indeed more rigid (Zigler, 1958, 1961). The specific hypothesis was that the greater the amount of preinstitutional social deprivation experienced by the retarded child, the greater would be his or her motivation to interact with an adult, making such interaction (and any adult approval or support that accompanies it) more reinforcing than for a retarded child who experienced a lesser amount of social deprivation. Interestingly, in testing such a hypothesis, interest shifts from differences between the retarded and nonretarded groups to differences within a retarded group.

In order to examine the social deprivation experienced by retarded children, a measure of the construct was required. Since the events that constitute social deprivation had never been adequately delineated, this study employed raters to evaluate the preinstitutional histories of the children in terms of what they felt to be the degree of social deprivation. On the basis of these ratings, 60 retarded children were categorized as high or low socially deprived. The groups were equated on MA, CA, and length of institutionalization. The study employed a socially reinforced, instruction-initiated, two-part satiation game similar to those used previously. Results showed that the more socially deprived children spent a greater amount of time on the game, and again played the second part of the task longer than the first.

These findings cast strong doubt on the Lewin-Kounin rigidity formulation, since this formulation could not explain differences in rigid behaviors between groups of retarded children equated on both CA and MA. Instead, the rigidity observed in retarded individuals was linked to a high motivation to maintain interaction with an adult and to secure approval from him or her through compliance and persistence. These results also offered evidence that the institutionalized retarded child's desire to interact with an adult increased with the degree of preinstitutional social deprivation experienced. Thus behavior previously attributed to rigidity was now related to motivational determinants – and mental retardation research took a new motivational and personality-oriented direction.

Social deprivation and desire for social reinforcement

Few constructs in psychology have been more frequently employed, yet more inadequately defined, than social deprivation. Length of institutionalization, though frequently utilized as an operational measure, is not an appropriate measurement, although conditions of institutionalization are certainly a determinant of the child's current behavior. Institutionalization is not even a psychological variable. Generally, it refers to some vague social status of the individual. To be clear about its relation to social deprivation, one must designate specific social interactions in the institution that give rise to particular behaviors. Further, children are not born in the institution they often call home. They enter institutions fully endowed with family and social histories that are not left behind when they pass the

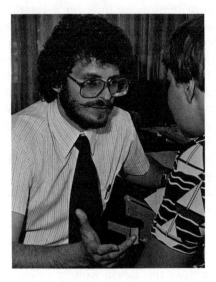

'Photo 3. Individual counseling. (Photograph courtesy of Elwyn Institutes, Elwyn, Pennsylvania)

institution gates. This is true of noninstitutionalized retarded children as well, whose unique backgrounds can influence their responses in school and testing situtation.

These considerations led to the construction of a standard, objective measure of preinstitutional social deprivation (the Pre-Institutional Social Deprivation scale, or PISD). This instrument has been continuously refined over the years (Butterfield & Zigler, 1970; Zigler, Butterfield, & Goff, 1966). The scale now includes factors such as a lack of continuity of care by parents or other caretakers, an excessive desire by the parents to institutionalize their child, impoverished economic circumstances, and a family history of marital discord, mental illness, and child abuse or neglect. Each of these factors has now been found to affect a wide variety of behaviors.

The positive-reaction tendency

The early work of Zigler and his colleagues led to a large and important body of research that has proven that social deprivation does indeed result in a heightened motivation to interact with a supportive adult – an increased responsiveness to social reinforcement that has been called the positive-reaction tendency (Balla & Zigler, 1975; Balla et al., 1974; Zigler, 1961; Zigler & Balla, 1972; Zigler, Balla, & Butterfield, 1968). The standard instrument developed to assess this responsiveness is the marble-in-the-hole game. The person is instructed to drop marbles of one color into one hole of a large box and marbles of a second color into a second hole. He or she is allowed to persist at the task until satiated. The correct holes for the colored marbles are then reversed and the child again drops marbles until satiated. The measure of responsiveness to social reinforcement is the total time that the person persists on both parts of the task. The child is periodically reinforced by the examiner through smiles and verbal praise. Study after study has shown that socially deprived children are more responsive to the attention and support of the adult than nondeprived children, and consequently persist at this boring task longer. This heightened motivation to interact with a supportive adult, stemming from a history of social deprivation, certainly seems congruent with the sort of attention- and affection-seeking behavior often seen in retarded individuals.

A quick survey of some of these studies gives an indication of how broad the effects of social deprivation can be. For example, Harter and Zigler (1968) found that an adult experimenter was a more effective social reinforcer than a peer experimenter for institutionalized retarded children, but not for those who lived at home. Thus, the institutionalized retarded child's motivation to obtain social reinforcement appears to be based on a need for attention and praise dispensed by an adult, rather than on a more generalized desire for reinforcement dispensed by any social agent (e.g., a peer). In another study (Harter, 1967), institutionalized retarded individuals took significantly longer to solve a concept formation problem in a social condition where they were face-to-face with a warm supportive experimenter who praised their performance than in a standard condition where the experimenter was silent and out of view. The retarded children in the social condition appeared highly motivated to interact with an approving adult, so much so that it seemed to compete with their attention to the learning task. Balla (1967) observed that institutionalized retarded children in a schoolroom setting may employ school as a place to interact with adults in an effort to compensate for the lack of such interactions elsewhere. These children utilized the school setting to satisfy their motivation for social interaction, rather than to learn.

Balla's observational study constitutes an important link in the chain of evidence we have been attempting to forge. Balla conducted observations in the homes of nonretarded and retarded children and in several institutions that housed children of both intelligence levels. His findings provide direct observational support for the importance of an adult social reinforcement factor. The quantity and quality of adult social interactions were very similar for the institutionalized children, regardless of whether or not they were retarded; the same was true for the noninstitutionalized groups. This helps to explain many findings of performance differences between retarded and nonretarded children who are matched on MA and therefore should perform similarly. When institutionalized retarded children are placed in a situation where social interaction is readily available, they choose to remain in the situation longer than nonretarded children who live at home and typically receive an appropriate amount of social reinforcement.

We have talked about the socially deprived child's craving for social reinforcement. This heightened motivation has also been viewed as an indicator of an important phenomenon discussed in the general child development literature, namely, dependency. Thus, with a slight shift in terminology, we might conclude that a general consequence of social deprivation is overdependency. We cannot place enough emphasis on the role of such overdependency in the behavior of retarded persons. Given some minimal intellectual level, the shift from dependence to independence is perhaps the single most important factor enabling retarded persons to become self-sustaining members of society (e.g., Zigler & Harter, 1969).

Some indication of the pervasiveness of the atypical dependency of institutionalized retarded persons may be found in a study by Zigler and Balla (1972). Retarded and nonretarded children of three MA levels, approximately 7, 9, and 12, were compared in terms of their performance on the marble-in-the-hole task. In keeping with the general developmental progression from helplessness and dependence to autonomy and independence, both retarded and intellectually average children of higher MAs were found to be less motivated for social reinforcement than children of lower MAs. However, at each MA level, the retarded children were more dependent than the nonretarded children. This disparity in dependent behavior was just as marked at the highest as at the lowest MA level. Indeed, the oldest retarded group persisted at the marble-in-the-hole task almost twice as long as the youngest nonretarded group.

The relation between preinstitutional social deprivation and need for social reinforcement was strongest for the youngest group, suggesting that the younger the child, the more his or her behavior depends on life experiences within the family context. Perhaps as children grow older and interact with a broader spectrum of socializing agents, their motivation for social reinforcement becomes less determined by the quality of social interaction they have experienced within the confines of family life. Such a view is certainly consistent with the observation that as a child grows older, his or her personality structure is more influenced by peers, teachers, and other outside socializing agents.

The negative-reaction tendency

A phenomenon that appears to be at variance with retarded children's increased desire for social reinforcement is their reluctance and wariness to interact with adults. This apparent inconsistency has been a part of a controversy over whether social deprivation leads to an increase in the desire for affection or to apathy and withdrawal. Experimental work to date has suggested that social deprivation results both in a heightened motivation to interact with supportive adults (positive-reaction tendency) and in a reluctance and wariness to do so (negative-reaction tendency).

The negative-reaction construct has been employed to explain some of the performance differences between retarded and nonretarded individuals originally reported by Kounin (1941a, 1941b). Recall that Kounin presented retarded children with two nearly identical, monotonous tasks and asked them to play each part of the game until they wished to stop. These children played part one of the game longer than did nonretarded children, a finding that seemed consistent with Kounin's rigidity formulation. But the retarded children played the second part of the game even longer than they did the first. Zigler (1958) suggested that the institutionalized children learned during part one that the experimenter was not like other strange adults they had encountered who initiated painful experiences (physical examinations, shots, etc.) while making supportive comments. This results in a reduction of the negative-reaction tendency. Part two is then met with a positive-reaction tendency unattenuated by the negative-reaction tendency; they can now enjoy the reinforcement and so play longer on part two than they did on part one.

A study by Zigler, Balla, and Butterfield (1968) threw some light on the particular experiences that might make retarded children fear and mistrust adults. These investigators found that the parents' marital harmony factor in the PISD scale was most related to the manifestation of the negative-reaction tendency. The items in this factor include the nature of the parents' marital relationship, the father's and mother's mental health, and their general attitude toward the child. To further investigate the role of specific factors in the manifestation of wariness, Harter and Zigler (1968) employed both adult and peer examiners (children of normal intellect). Regardless of the examiner's age, institutionalized retarded children had a higher negative-reaction tendency than did retarded children who lived at home.

Thus institutionalized retarded children exhibit a generalized wariness of strangers, regardless of whether the strangers are adults or children.

We generally think of social deprivation as a relatively long-term condition. But there is evidence that even short-term experiences can have detrimental effects. In an early study (Shallenberger & Zigler, 1961), intellectually average and institutionalized retarded children experienced either a positive or negative interaction with an adult prior to playing the marble-in-the-hole game. In the positive condition, all of the child's responses met with success and were praised. In the negative condition, all the child's responses met with failure and expressions of disapproval. For both the retarded and nonretarded groups, greater wariness was demonstrated following the negative condition. In addition, the retarded children were more strongly affected by the negative interaction than were the nonretarded children. (Similar results, using a slightly different methodology, were found by Weaver, 1966, and Weaver, Balla, & Zigler, 1971.)

If such brief negative encounters can make children wary, imagine the effects of a lifetime of social deprivation. Balla et al. (1980) found that after approximately eight years of institutional experience, retarded individuals with a history of high preinstitutional social deprivation were still more wary than less deprived individuals. Balla, McCarthy, and Zigler (1971) found that retarded individuals institutionalized at a younger age were less wary than those institutionalized when older, perhaps because they were not exposed to depriving home experiences for as long.

A logical conclusion of all this research is that wariness of adults and of the tasks they present leads to a general attenuation in the retarded child's social effectiveness. Retarded children's poor performance on tasks presented by adults is therefore not to be attributed entirely to intellectual factors, but must be interpreted in light of their atypically high negative-reaction tendency. This tendency motivates them toward behaviors (e.g., withdrawal) that reduce the quality of their performance to a level lower than that dictated by their intellectual capacity.

The reinforcer hierarchy

Due to a variety of experiential factors, the retarded individual's responses to various types of incentives may be quite different from the responses of nonretarded individuals of the same mental age. Stated somewhat differently, the position of various reinforcers in the reinforcer hierarchies may differ in retarded and nonretarded children. Consider Kounin's concept-switching study discussed earlier in this chapter. The only reinforcer dispensed for switching concepts was the reinforcement inherent in being correct. Being correct may be more reinforcing for nonretarded than for retarded children, who may value the positive attention of the examiner much more than the satisfaction derived from performing the task correctly.

Much of the experimental work on the reinforcer hierarchy has focused on differences in response to tangible and intangible reinforcement (see Havighurst, 1970). This work is of special importance, since intangible reinforcement (information that a response is correct) is the most immediate and frequently dispensed reinforcement in real life (and in the typical test situation). The general conclusion of this research is that with a few exceptions, retarded children are less responsive to intangible reinforcement than are nonretarded children of equivalent MA. In addition, lower-SES children appear less motivated to be correct for its own sake than middle-SES children (e.g., Cameron & Storm, 1965; Zigler & Kanzer, 1962). These findings point out a fatal flaw in the typical research design, which compares middle-SES, nonretarded children with familial retarded children who are generally from the lower SES. Such a match gives double insurance that group differences will be found, not because of something inherent in mental retardation but because of differing reinforcer hierarchies.

The importance of the type of reinforcer dispensed was highlighted in Stevenson and Zigler's study (1957). When tangible reinforcers were given, institutionalized familial retarded children were no more rigid than nonretarded children on a discrimination reversal-learning task. Interestingly, on a concept-switching task both retarded and upper-class nonretarded children switched more readily in a tangible than an intangible reinforcement condition (Zigler & Unell, 1962). Clearest evidence for differences in motivation to be correct for its own sake is contained in a study by Zigler and deLabry (1962). These investigators tested MA-matched nonretarded middle-SES, nonretarded lower-SES, and retarded children on a concept-switching task. In one condition, the only reinforcement dispensed was the information that the child was correct. In the second condition, the child was rewarded with a toy of his or her choice for switching concepts. In the "correct" condition, both the retarded and the nonretarded lower-SES groups had poorer performance than the nonretarded middle-SES children. However, no differences were found among the three groups when they received tangible reinforcers. Furthermore, no differences in the ability to switch concepts were found among the three groups receiving what was assumed to be their optimal reinforcer (tangible for the retarded and the nonretarded lower-SES, and intangible for the nonretarded middle-SES).

We must caution that although retarded children as a group may value being correct less than do middle-SES children as a group, this may not hold true for any particular child. The crucial factor is not IQ or membership in a particular social class, but rather the social learning experienced by the child. This point is aptly underlined in a study by Byck (1968), who examined the performance of institutionalized Down syndrome and familial retarded children on a concept-switching task. Half of the children in each group were reinforced with a tangible reward (a small toy), and the other half with social reinforcers, including the information that they were correct. Superior concept-switching was displayed by the Down syndrome children in the intangible as compared to the tangible condition, whereas the reverse was true for the familial groups. This finding is consistent with the literature on social class and reinforcer effectiveness noted earlier, since familial retarded children generally come from lower-SES background, whereas children with Down syndrome come from all social classes.

In related work, attention has shifted to the more general phenomenon of the intrinsic reinforcement that inheres in being correct, regardless of whether an external agent dispenses an additional reinforcer. This shift in orientation owes much to White's (1959) formulation concerning the effectance of mastery motive (the notion that using one's cognitive resources to their utmost is intrinsically gratifying and thus motivating). As with the case of intangible reinforcers, the strength of the effectance motive may be different for retarded and nonretarded children.

Evidence on this point was provided by Harter and Zigler (1974). They presented MA-matched groups of nonretarded children, and retarded children who lived at home or in an institution, with four tasks measuring various aspects of effectance motivation. Consistent with the findings of such studies as Zigler and deLabry (1962), nonretarded children chose a nontangible reward (a "good player" certificate) over a tangible prize more often than did either retarded group. Furthermore, the nonretarded children showed the greatest desire to master a problem for the sake of mastery and to choose the most challenging task, and showed the greatest curiosity and exploratory behavior. The noninstitutionalized children showed less of these elements of effectance motivation, and the institutionalized children, in most cases, demonstrated the least. Thus, not only do retarded children differ from their nonretarded peers, but groups of retarded children, matched on intellectual functioning, differ from one another with respect to a general motive thought to influence a wide variety of behaviors.

Expectancy of success

Another factor frequently noted as a determinant in the performance of retarded persons is their high expectancy of failure. This is thought to be a consequence of frequent encounters with tasks and situations that re-tarded people are intellectually ill-equipped to handle (see Cromwell, 1963). The pervasiveness of these feelings of failure can be seen in a series of studies by MacMillan and his colleagues (MacMillan, 1969; MacMillan & Keogh, 1971; MacMillan & Knopf, 1971). In these studies children were prevented from finishing several tasks that they had begun, and were sub-sequently asked why the tasks were not completed. Retarded children consistently placed the blame on themselves, while nonretarded children did not.

Another line of research has focused on the effects of success and failure expectancies on problem-solving behavior. The task typically employed in these studies is a three-choice discrimination problem in which one stimulus is reinforced only some of the time it is chosen, but the other two stimuli are never reinforced. Children with low expectancies of success, as gauged by aspiration level or need-achievement measures, are more likely to dis-play a maximizing strategy (persistent choice of the partially reinforced stimulus) on this task than children with high expectancies of success (Gruen, Ottinger, & Zigler, 1970; Kier, Styfco, & Zigler, 1977; Ollendick & Gruen, 1971). Apparently children with low aspirations accept less than 100% success as an acceptable outcome, whereas those who expect 100% success, or a level of success greater than that allowed in the situation, try strategies other than maximizing in the hope of being right all the time.

Consistent with the expectancy of success formulation, retarded children have been found to exhibit more maximizing behavior than children of average intelligence (Gruen & Zigler, 1968; Stevenson & Zigler, 1958). However, this tendency could also be interpreted in terms of cognitive rigidity. That is, the inherent rigidity of retarded persons might lead them to persevere in choosing one of the three stimuli, and not to abandon the choice even when it results in nonreinforcement.

One way to test the motivational explanation is to see if nonretarded children who also experience failure likewise maximize more. Stevenson and Zigler (1958) gave nonretarded children either a success or failure precondition prior to performing on the partially reinforced three-choice learning task. Children who experienced prior failure indeed showed a higher incidence of maximizing behaviors than those who experienced suc-cess. However, these brief preconditions hardly constitute an experimental analog to the real-life experiences of retarded children, who experience failure day after day. A more valid test of the effects of failure on ex-pectancy of success is whether maximizing behavior is found in nonretarded children who have also experienced relatively high amounts of failure. Lower-SES children would appear to have such a background. The motivational position would therefore predict similarity in performance by retarded and lower-SES nonretarded children on the partially reinforced three-choice problem. The rigidity position would lead us to expect a dissimilarity in the performance of these two groups, with the lower-SES children behaving more like their middle-SES peers.

Gruen and Zigler (1968) tested middle- and lower-SES nonretarded children, and noninstitutionalized familial retarded children of comparable MAs, on the partially reinforced learning task. Among other experimental manipulations, some of the children in each group were administered a number of pretraining tasks in which they experienced a high degree of success; others experienced a very low level of success; and the rest did not receive any pretraining.

No effects as a result of prior conditions of success and failure were found for the lower-SES and retarded children. However, for middle-class children, the preliminary success condition resulted in less maximization (fewer correct responses) than the other two conditions. Studies by Gruen et al. (1970) and Kier, Styfco, and Zigler (1977) showed that each child's aspiration level, rather than social class per se, influenced his or her maximizing behavior.

This line of reasoning was further confirmed in a study by Ollendick, Balla, and Zigler (1971), who employed more intense and relatively long-term success and failure conditions. They found that for institutionalized familial retarded children, failure experiences did result in a low expectancy of success, while success experiences resulted in a higher expectancy of success. Since all of the children were retarded, these data suggest that degree of maximizing behavior is motivationally-based rather than being indicative of cognitive rigidity.

Gruen, Ottinger, and Ollendick (1974) attempted to determine whether the success-failure findings could be replicated in a more lifelike school setting. They found that retarded children in regular classes (who were presumably exposed to repeated failure) had higher expectancies of failure than retarded children in special classes (exposed to relatively higher levels of success). However, Caparulo (1979), who investigated mildly retarded boys who were either partially or totally mainstreamed, did not find expectancy of success to be systematically affected by the intensity of the mainstreaming experience.

The findings presented in this section generally offer support for the view that motivational factors arising from experiential events are important determinants in a child's problem solving. Perhaps one reason for some of the inconsistent results is that expectancy of success is only one determinant of maximizing behavior. The small number of correct responses made by middle-SES children might reflect not only the amount of success they are willing to settle for, but also the amount of confidence they have in their own cognitive abilities. Children who believe they can succeed would be willing to abandon maximization and undertake a search for a more successful strategy. Children who do not expect much success and also have little confidence in their own resourcefulness are more likely to maintain the maximizing strategy.

Outer-directedness

In addition to a lowered expectancy of success, a history of failure can lead to a style of problem solving characterized by outer-directedness. That is, the child who frequently fails comes to distrust his or her own solutions to problems and therefore seeks guides to action in the immediate environment. Three factors have been advanced as important in determining the child's degree of outer-directedness: the general level of cognitive development, the incidence of success resulting from self-initiated solutions, and the extent of the child's attachment to adults (Balla et al., 1980). Either too little or too much imitation is viewed as a negative psychological indicator. Some intermediate level of imitation is viewed as a positive developmental phenomenon, reflecting the child's healthy attachment to adults and responsivity to the helpful cues that adults emit.

In general, the developmental aspect of the outer-directedness formulation has received experimental support. With nonretarded children, outer-directedness has been found to decrease with increasing MA (MacMillan & Wright, 1974; Ruble & Nakamura, 1973; Yando & Zigler, 1971; Zigler & Yando, 1972). This developmental shift has also been found in institutionalized retarded persons (Turnure, 1970a, 1970b) and in noninstitutionalized mildly retarded children (Balla, Styfco, & Zigler, 1971; Gordon & MacLean, 1977). Apparently with younger children, outer-directedness is more conducive to problem solving than is dependency upon poorly developed cognitive abilities. With growth and development, children should become more inner-directed, since their expanded abilities lessen their need for external cues. Furthermore, as children grow older they receive independence training, as adults gradually reduce their cues in both number and detail. This further decreases the effectiveness of an outer-directed style.

The success-failure aspect of the outer-directedness formulation has generated the prediction that retarded children, because of their histories of failure, are more outer-directed in their problem-solving behavior than are nonretarded children of the same MA, a prediction that has been confirmed in several studies (Achenbach & Zigler, 1968; Balla, Styfco, & Zigler, 1971; Sanders et al., 1968; Turnure & Zigler, 1964; Yando & Zigler, 1971). These studies have also indicated that both nonretarded and retarded children become more outer-directed following failure experiences than success experiences.

There is some evidence that residential care is more likely to foster the retarded child's optimism and self-confidence than is the nonsheltered school in the community setting. Indeed, Rosen, Diggory, and Werlinsky (1966) found that, compared to noninstitutionalized retarded groups, those who lived in institutions set higher goals, predicted better performance for themselves, and actually performed at a higher level. Edgerton and Sabagh (1962) pointed out other positive features of the sheltered institutional setting for the high-level retarded child. They noted certain "aggrandizements" of the self that are available, such as the presence of inferior low-level children with whom they can compare themselves favorably, their far greater social success within the institution, and mutual support for face-saving rationales concerning their presence in the institution.

Not all of these positive effects of institutions appear beneficial, at least to outsiders. For example, in tasks that involved opportunities for non-retarded and retarded children to imitate models, the retarded children were more sensitive to models, displaying as a result a lack of creativity and spontaneity (Turnure & Zigler, 1964). It also seems reasonable to expect that in environments where a high degree of compliance has adaptive value, such as in total institutions, greater imitation would be found. In several studies (e.g., Lustman & Zigler 1982; Yando & Zigler, 1971), institutionalized retarded persons were found to be more imitative than those who lived at home.

In regard to the attachment-to-adults aspect of the outer-directedness formulation, there is some evidence that individuals who have not formed healthy attachments to adult caretakers will have an atypically low level of outer-directedness. Balla et al. (1980) found that institutionalized retarded individuals whose caretakers had negative attitudes concerning them were less outer-directed than those whose caretakers had positive attitudes. Thus, individuals who are responded to in a negative manner may learn to ignore cues provided by adults and thus become less imitative.

We see then that outer-directedness can have both positive and negative effects. There are undoubtedly many situations where a child is rewarded for careful attentiveness to adults. This attentiveness can also be interpreted to mean suggestibility, a trait frequently attributed to retarded persons.

And suggestibility could enable them to be easily misled. For example, slower students have been shown to conform more frequently to group decisions than brighter students, even when the group makes the wrong decision (Hottel, 1960; Lucito, 1959). Sanders et al. (1968) found that overreliance on external cues could prove detrimental in decision making. They employed a task where the child had to learn to discriminate between helpful and misleading cues in choosing the "correct" stimulus in a three-choice game. Even when the cue (a light over one of the choices) consistently indicated an incorrect choice, retarded children followed the signal. Outer-directedness can also result in distractibility, another trait frequently attributed to retarded persons. However, in an examination of retarded children's glancing behavior, Turnure (1970) found that it was motivated by information-seeking. He noted that the glancing behavior of retarded children was neither random and of a type attributable to a neurological problem, nor was it some automatic responsiveness to salient but irrelevant social stimuli.

Optimal problem solving requires a child to utilize both external and internal cues. The retarded individual's overreliance on external cues is understandable in view of his or her life history. The intermittent success accruing to retarded persons as a result of such a style, in combination with their generally lowered expectation of success in problem-solving situations, suggests the great utility that outer-directedness can have for those with attenuated intellectual abilities.

Self-concept

The self-concept construct has had a central role in general personality theory, but, surprisingly, has received relatively little attention in the mental retardation literature (Balla & Zigler, 1979). Traditionally, a person's self-concept has been viewed as heavily influenced by life experiences. Thus one might expect that both perceived intellectual inadequacy and pervasive stigmatization of retarded persons would result in their having lower self-concepts than nonretarded individuals of the same mental age. This supposition, however, has been only partially confirmed.

Another way to gauge the effect of experience of self-image is to compare retarded persons in different settings. For example, several investigators have compared institutionalized and noninstitutionalized retarded individuals on self-concept measures, but again, the results are mixed. For example, Gorlow, Butler, and Guthrie (1963) reported lower self-concepts in retarded persons living in institutions. The results of a similar study by Harrison and Budoff (1972) indicated that when the issue was one of self-involved competence, the institutionalized groups used their peers as a reference group and felt superior. In issues concerning social status and affect, however, this group used the world at large for their frame of reference, and felt inferior.

An alternate view to the self-concept as a function of life experience is the developmental approach proposed by Zigler and his colleagues (Achenbach & Zigler, 1963; Katz & Zigler, 1967). The central argument in this work is that the development of an individual must invariably be accompanied by a growing disparity between the assessment of the real self-image and the ideal self-image. This is due, for example, to the individual's growing capacity to experience guilt, a capacity that accompanies a growing understanding of social demands, morals, and values. The difference between the individual's perceived self and ideal self therefore becomes greater with higher levels of development.

A comprehensive understanding of the self-image construct appears to require a synthesis of both developmental and experiential positions. Several studies have given both positions empirical support. For example, Zigler, Balla, and Watson (1972) found that older nonretarded children had a more adverse self-concept than did younger nonretarded children, a finding consistent with the developmental approach. Consistent with the experiential position, however, was the finding that retarded children had lower ideal self-images than did their nonretarded peers matched on both CA and MA. This result has since been replicated (Leahy, Balla, & Zigler, 1982). These findings concerning the self-image of retarded persons seem to indicate that one consequence of being identified as retarded is a lowering of goals and aspirations, an interpretation certainly consistent with the expectancy-of-success literature cited earlier in this chapter.

Summary

Much of the research on motivational and emotional factors in the performance of retarded people is still more suggestive than definitive. It is clear, however, that such factors, in interaction with cognitive ability, play an extremely important role in determining the retarded person's behavior. Moreover, these factors seem much more open to environmental manipulation than do the cognitive processes. We would like to think that if ways were found to change certain personality problems in retarded persons they would be better able to use their cognitive capacities to a fuller extent.

What then is the burden of the total body of evidence concerning personality in retarded persons? First, proven differences in motivation between retarded and nonretarded persons must be kept in mind when interpreting all research comparing these groups. We must always ask what incentives the researchers offered, what opportunity there was to interact with the adult examiner, etc. Second, knowledge of what motivates retarded people can be helpful in our everyday encounters with the retarded at work, at school, and in clinical settings. For example, in administering an IQ test we cannot assume that the retarded child enjoys meeting the challenge of more difficult items, feels confident enough to venture a guess, or even cares to perform for us. We must treat each case separately, looking for appropriate motivational incentives on the basis of unique social and intellectual histories. As we hope we have shown in this chapter and in this book, we should let our knowledge of normal development serve as a guide.

Part IV

Intervention and treatment approaches

7 Principles of early intervention with organically retarded children

Probably no other area in mental retardation is as subject to as many different approaches and goals as is intervention. Developmental, behaviorist, and ecological intervention programs are among the choices available; and claims of interventionists range from modest improvement in the functioning of retarded individuals to the promise of near normality. In the following three chapters we will overview some of the theoretical and practical issues in intervening with different types of retarded children.

In this first chapter, we will discuss some of the domains of functioning open to intervention and several of the approaches being tried. Our focus will be on early intervention work with young, severely retarded children and their families. Next we will examine several well-known programs for familial retarded and at-risk children, and provide some thoughts on how to determine if a program is effective. The final chapter in this intervention section (Chapter 9) covers some procedures (patterning, vitamin therapy) that have become controversial, as well as some promising medical advances in the mental retardation field. Despite the wide range of topics covered, we realize that our treatment of the intervention issue is in no way comprehensive. Available programs are so numerous and diverse that only a small set of basic issues can be dealt with in these pages.

Behavior modification with severely retarded children

While we espouse the developmental approach to mental retardation, our position must be tempered when it comes to early intervention work with severely retarded children. There has been a long and distinguished history of teaching self-help skills to retarded children through operant procedures. Baker (1984) reviewed some of these efforts, and Table 7.1 presents several case studies that successfully employed operant procedures. In each study, "parents were taught to break the skill into components, model the steps,

139

Table 7.1. *Case studies of training with parents of developmentally disabled children*

Authors	Child (age in years); diagnosis	Target behavior	Program	Design	Results; follow-up (FU)
Adubato, Adams, & Budd (1981)	Jay (6), brain-damaged	Dressing	Clinic-trained mother who trained father	Multiple baseline	Increase in dressing, eating, and toy use
Arnold, Sturgis, & Forehand (1977)	Katie (15), retarded	Conversational skills	Mother prompt/reinforcement (6 sessions)	AB	Coded audiotapes showed significant improvement; 2-month FU
Barnard, Christophersen, & Wolf (1976)	Moe (4), retarded; Mark (3), severely mentally retarded with multiple handicaps	Self-injury: head banging Hand-biting	Overcorrection Overcorrection	AB AB	Reduction to almost zero for both 21- and 2-month FU
Brehony, Benson, Solomon, & Luscomb (1980)	Steven (7), severely mentally retarded	Throwing, sitting, compliance	Praise, punishment (6.5 hours training)	Multiple baseline	Considerable change and transfer to restaurant
Budd, Green, & Baer (1976)	Andrea (3), developmentally delayed	Noncompliance	Differential attention and time out (162 sessions)	Multiple baseline	Eventual success; 4-month FU
Casey (1978)	4 subjects (6–7), autistic	Communication, behavioral problems	Parents taught signing (20 sessions)	Multiple baseline	Significant changes; 2-month FU at school
Forehand, Cheney, & Yoder (1974)	John (7), deaf	Noncompliance	Reinforcement of skills and time out	AB	From 20% to 100% compliance at clinic; 3-month FU
Fox & Roseen (1977)	T (3.5), phenylkenonuria	Lofenalac refusal	Token economy	ABAB	Increased consumption maintained at 1 year
Frazier & Schneider (1975)	Boy (3), retarded	Acting-out behaviors	Time out	Multiple baseline	Very effective; 1-month FU

Study	Subject	Target behavior	Treatment	Design	Results
Gerrard & Saxon (1973)	Helen (2.8), deaf, autistic	Screaming, crying; sitting, attending	Team training in clinic		Screaming, crying reduced to zero; increased sitting and attending
Gross, Eudy, & Drabman (1982)	3 subjects (2.8–3.7), physically disabled	Arm extension	Model by physical therapist (40 minutes)	Multiple baseline	Coded videotapes showed good progress; 1-month FU
S. M. Johnson & Brown (1969)	Judy (2.8), developmentally delayed	Mother–child interaction, playing	Modeling (13 sessions)	AB	Change in mother–child behaviors during play
M. R. Johnson, Whitman, & Barloon-Noble (1978)	Girl (4), autistic behaviors	Noncompliance, nonfunctional speech	Positive attention, time out (5 sessions)		Change in both behaviors
Moore & Bailey (1973)	Girl (4) autisticlike behaviors	Response to requests	Social reinforcement, punishment (53 sessions)	Multiple baseline	Clear changes
White (1982)	Boy (13), moderately mentally retarded, deaf	Eating for weight gain	Contingency management	ABA	Weight gain; 2-year FU
Wildman & Simon (1978)	Paul (9), autistic	Social interactions	Family tutoring	ABA	Interaction increased during tutoring, not other times
Wiltz & Gordon (1974)	Boy (9), hyperactive, childhood schizophrenia	Noncompliance, destructive acts	Reinforcement, time out, 5 days in experimental apartment		Good decrease, carried over to home

Source: Baker (1984), with permission.

prompt and guide as necessary, reinforce successive approximations, fade prompts and reinforcers, and record progress" (Baker, 1984, p. 323). In addition to teaching self-help skills like dressing, eating, and toileting, several studies successfully employed operant techniques to eliminate destructive behaviors such as head banging or hand biting. This not only prevents harm but frees children to focus their energies on other, more constructive tasks.

Behavior modification techniques have proven particularly effective in teaching behavior to very low-functioning retarded children. As described by Werner (1948) and Zigler and Glick (in press, Chapter 2), low-functioning individuals often seem less able to generate internal mental concepts of their own; they are also more likely to become "caught" by external stimuli and by their own internal need states. Low-functioning retarded children may thus be well-suited to approaches that stress tangible rewards (food, prizes, etc.).

The teaching of self-help skills to severely retarded children is beneficial not only to the children but to the parents. First, parents come to have realistic expectations of their retarded child. When there is progress, however modest, parent-therapists gain some sense of control over a difficult child. Instead of guilty, they begin to feel efficacious, an important foundation for all future interactions with their child (see below).

Still, it should be noted that the proper role of behaviorist procedures is probably limited to the *processes* of intervention. Especially for the most severely retarded children, operant procedures are effective tools for teaching. However, the developmental sequence provides the most useful guide as to what it is that should be taught and in what order (with the possible exception of self-help skills). In future intervention efforts there may be a marriage of the two approaches, involving an operant approach to teaching (as well as other approaches to be discussed later), but with a content that is informed by developmental knowledge.

This merger of the two approaches is not without controversy, however. For example, Seibert and Oller (1981) argue that in language training the use of reinforcements is unnatural and a hindrance to the child's desire to communicate:

To reply [to the child's utterance] by saying "That's good talking," or by giving the child an M&M may provide reinforcement for vocalization, but these reinforcers miss the pragmatic target and waste a golden opportunity to expand the child's awareness of communicative possibilities. The [developmental] approach takes advantage of the child's desire for communication itself and tailors its reinforcers to include pragmatically appropriate responsive communications from the interventionist. (p. 83)

Despite this criticism, it seems that some joining of the two approaches remains possible. For example, when reinforcers are used they should be dispensed in as natural a manner as possible. The interventionist might also use operant techniques interspersed with other methods of intervention. We now turn to some developmental procedures currently being used in early intervention work.

The developmental approach to early intervention

As noted in Chapter 2, a major assumption in developmental theory is that the organism is active. The developmentalist sees the retarded child as an active learner, or "constructor" of the world, in spite of any mental or physical problems that the child may have. This viewpoint directly influences the methods of intervention chosen. The developmentally oriented therapist attempts to create an environment that stimulates the child's own internal process of discovery. The effort is to present more and more complicated problems for children to master by themselves. Although the behaviorist techniques of reinforcement and modeling are occasionally employed, the general method is to guide the child's own learning.

The goals of developmental interventions are also affected by the view that the child is an active learner. In contrast to more behaviorist programs, the aim is not an increasing number of behaviors, per se, but rather an increasing number and variety of mental operations. These operations can then be used to generate a variety of different behaviors in different situations. The developmentalist is therefore concerned with behavior only as it demonstrates the increasing range and flexibility of the child's internal mental abilities.

The example of teaching object permanence to a retarded child can illustrate this difference in emphasis. The behaviorist therapist tries to teach the child the behavior of uncovering an object hidden behind a cloth. The purpose is to teach the "uncovering behavior," an action that can then be used to uncover other objects, or objects hidden behind other types of coverings. The developmentalist also teaches uncovering, but for the purpose of helping the child to develop the concept of object permanence (the knowledge that objects continue to exist even when they are out of sight). Thus, the developmental therapist is further interested in whether the child will cry when the mother leaves the room, or will laugh when the mother playfully hides herself in a game of peekaboo (two situations that also bring out the concept of a permanent object). When the child realizes that objects continue to exist when hidden, this knowledge can be used to perform other types of behavior in different contexts.

Of course developmentally based interventions are rarely followed exactly as stated here. The therapist occasionally gives the child reinforcements or may even shape the child's behavior into closer and closer approximations of the desired action. These practices are more likely to be used in teaching behaviors that do not rely much on mental processes (e.g., toileting, grooming, and other self-help skills) or when dealing with the lowest-functioning retarded children. Still, the goal of the developmentalist will rarely be that the child merely acquire a behavior, and the method will generally allow at least some room for children to "discover" and practice by themselves.

Developmentalists also conceptualize the environment as active and in constant interaction (transaction) with the developing child. As discussed in Chapter 2, children develop their intellectual potential through their interactions over time with a wide range of environments. Only a history of an extremely poor environment will substantially lower IQ. The cognitive system seems to be buffered against minor or short-term environmental manipulations, at least for children in the normal range of intelligence.

For young, organically retarded children, however, there is much more of a need for an optimal or nearly optimal environment. The challenge to the interventionist is to provide conditions that as much as possible stimulate those concepts with which the retarded child is currently struggling. For the child who is gradually acquiring the concept of object permanence, the interventionist might hide a much desired object under a cloth or have the child's mother repeatedly leave the room in a loud and obvious way. Again and again, the attempt is to be one step ahead of the child, anticipating the particular skills the child will next develop from those he or she already possesses, and to help this development by presenting problem situations that are on the cutting edge of the child's capabilities. Indeed, it is the challenge to be always exactly in the right place for the child, presenting problems that are neither too easy nor too hard, that makes the interventionist's job so difficult.

This ability to modulate the intervention to the child's level of development implies a thorough knowledge of the developmental sequence in each domain of functioning. This similar sequence hypothesis, discussed in a research sense in Chapter 2, provides the "staged curriculum" (Kaye, 1982) for the early interventionist. Once one knows that skill A precedes skill B in normal development, and that retarded children follow the normal developmental progression, then the best way to help the child acquire skill B is first to introduce skill A. The assumption is that A is a prerequisite necessary to the development of B, so both skills should be presented in the same order as they appear in nonretarded children.

A good example of how a knowledge of developmental sequence informs intervention efforts is seen in language training. In many behaviorist-oriented programs (e.g., Sailor, Guess, & Baer, 1973), the child is taught functional language, or language presumed to be useful in getting one's needs met by others. Instruction proceeds from simple functional words (e.g., "yes," "no," nouns), to more complicated functional phrases and sentences ("I want X").

In contrast, developmental programs (e.g., MacDonald & Blott, 1974; McLean & Snyder-McLean, 1978; Miller & Yoder, 1974) begin with several of the meanings that are present in the early utterances of young (i.e., 18- to 24-month-old) nonretarded children. For example, the retarded child might first be exposed to the idea of recurrence, learning to say "more" while pointing to a desired object, later to say "more juice," and eventually to produce grammatical sentences to express the child's needs. The assumption is that retarded children will develop faster if they proceed along the universal sequence in which language is normally acquired, and that this language will eventually prove functional for the retarded child.

Finally, we should mention that the issue of similar reactions to outside experience is also an important consideration in early intervention work with retarded children (see Chapter 6). In particular, research with normally developing infants (e.g., Shultz & Zigler, 1970; Yarrow, Morgan, Jennings, Harmon, & Gaiter, 1982) has shown that children are interested in mastering their environments from the first months of life. Shultz and Zigler (1970), for example, found that infants spend the greatest amount of time gazing at stimuli that are sufficiently challenging (given their level of cognitive ability); stimuli that are too easy or too hard are not preferred. Similarly, Yarrow et al. found that the degree to which infants persist at a task is related both to their degree of success at that task and to their scores on the Bayley test of infant development. These authors noted,

Infants who work assiduously at perfecting their skills may become more competent; in turn, competent infants derive greater satisfaction from working on skills, and thus are more likely to practice them. It does not seem to be a circular process, but a sequential and hierarchical one in which mastery motivation facilitates consolidation of skills and leads to the emergence of new ones. (1982, p. 140)

Indeed, the idea of mastery and self-competence is as important in infancy as it is at other times in a person's life.

The motivation to master one's environment also plays a salient role in early intervention work. The therapist is continually engaged in fostering success and feelings of success in the child, through the child's solving progressively more difficult problems. By definition, however, the introduction of more difficult problems makes failure more likely for the retarded child, while it simultaneously makes success more rewarding. The therapist must attempt a delicate balance between helping the child to develop cognitively (by risking failure at more demanding tasks) and promoting the child's feelings of self-efficacy.

We now turn to the areas of cognition and language, two domains in which developmentally-based intervention curricula are currently being implemented. Although the specification of complete curricula is beyond the scope of this book, some examples of programs in these areas can serve to flesh out our concept of intervention from a developmental perspective.

Intervention to enhance sensorimotor cognitive functioning

Thanks to the careful observations of Jean Piaget, developmental psychologists probably know more about the sequence of cognitive development in the first few years of life than at any other age. Briefly stated, Piaget (1954, 1966) has described the universal sequence of development in six sensorimotor domains: object permanence, means-ends, spatial ability, causality, imitation, and appropriate uses of objects. These skills, typically acquired in the first two years, seem essential to human thought. Means-ends (the use of a person or object to reach a particular goal) and causality (the understanding that people can cause events to occur) lead to concepts that are crucial in meeting, and getting others to meet, one's personal needs. Imitation skills (gestural and vocal) have been implicated as a major mechanism in both human and animal learning (Kaye, 1982; Piaget, 1954). The capacity for the "appropriate uses of objects" (the knowledge that certain objects are used in certain ways), which ultimately leads to symbolism, is necessary for the mastery of language and other sign-symbol systems. Knowledge of the spatial world seems important for the everyday navigation of one's environment. Even object permanence seems to be an important accomplishment. Flavell (1977) has gone so far as to state, "If any concept could be regarded as indispensible to a coherent and rational mental life, this one [object permanence] certainly would be. Imagine what your life would be like if you did not believe that objects continued to exist when they left your visual field" (p. 42). In short, the six domains of sensorimotor cognitive development described by Piaget seem among the most important developments of the human species, important in themselves and as prerequisite skills for all later cognitive developments.

There are now several scales used to measure development in each of these six domains. The most well-known of these is Uzgiris and Hunt's (1975) Ordinal Scales of Infant Development. The scale measures sensorimotor development along a series of graded steps; the six subscales, one for each domain, have a different number of steps through which the child develops. These subscales have been shown to be ordinal, in that normally developing children pass steps in each subscale in a fixed sequence (i.e., step 1 comes before step 2, which comes before step 3, etc.).

Research has demonstrated the applicability of Piagetian sensorimotor scales to retarded children (e.g., Rodgers, 1977; Woodward, 1959). For example, Kahn (1977) studied 63 severely and profoundly retarded children, 30 of whom lived in residential facilities and 33 of whom were home-reared. Their etiologies varied widely, with 22 Down syndrome children, several who suffered from anoxia or encephalitis or who were microcephalic, and 19 children who suffered from "unknown brain damage." Each child was tested on the object permanence, means-ends, causality, spatial, schemes, and imitation subscales of the Uzgiris-Hunt scales. Kahn found that each of the six subscales formed a scale with ordinal sequence, such that a child who possessed skill C also demonstrated skills A & B in that domain. In fact, even in this sample of severely and profoundly retarded children of varying etiologies and living situations, few if any instances were found of a child possessing a higher-level skill in the absence of lower-level skills.

A more complicated picture emerges when sensorimotor development is examined longitudinally. Wohlhueter and Sindberg (1975) tested moderately, severely, and profoundly retarded institutionalized children at monthly intervals for a year. Instead of evidence of slow, steady development through Piagetian stages of object permanence (the only domain tested), three patterns were found: for one third of the children monthly scale levels varied widely; another third showed no change; and the remainder showed upward change similar to the development of nonretarded children. Children with EEG abnormalities (i.e., seizure disorders) were among those with a variable, up-and-down level of object permanence from one month to the next. In addition, Wohlhueter and Sindberg found a fair amount of skipping of steps, such that a child showing skill A one month might show skill C the next (without having shown skill B). Although this may be due to the one-month interval between testings, such findings were unexpected and demonstrate a need for more study of the course of sensorimotor development in young retarded children.

Piagetian sensorimotor skills may also be amenable to early intervention.

In a small-sample intervention study, Kahn (1977) first matched four pairs of severely and profoundly retarded children on age, etiology, and scores on the Uzgiris-Hunt scales. One child in each pair received individual training in object permanence for 45 minutes a day, three days a week for six months. At the end of the experimental period the four trained children had reached the highest-level item on the object permanence subscale of the Uzgiris-Hunt. They also advanced on all or most of the other Uzgiris-Hunt scales. One child in the control group also gained two steps on the object permanence subscale but showed decreases in another subscale. None of the other untrained children showed gains on any of the subscales. Kahn's results not only point to the possibility that intervention can improve sensorimotor skills in retarded children, but they also show that training in one area might generalize to other areas of functioning.

In recent years, various intervention programs have begun to employ Piagetian-based sensorimotor interventions with retarded children (see Dunst, 1980a; Haring & Brown, 1976). To date, few of these programs have been subjected to careful study; it is not yet clear that the Piagetian-based components of these programs form the key ingredients that promote early cognitive development. Still, the scalable nature of Piagetian sensorimotor skills, their importance in all human thought, and the significance of these skills to future developments all attest to their utility in early intervention work. Even behaviorists such as Switzky, Rotatori, Miller, and Freagon (1979) concede that "... in infancy and early childhood developmentally significant behaviors seem so basic to the child's interaction with the environment [that] they may serve as educational objectives" (p. 168). It seems likely that early intervention programs based on Piaget's sensorimotor domains will continue to increase in popularity, thereby making true developmentally based interventions the norm in the area of early cognitive functioning.

Linguistic and communication skills

The evolution of developmentally based curricula for language intervention has followed the changing understanding of language in the field of developmental psychology. To summarize briefly, 30 years of work in linguistics and psycholinguistics has taught us that language consists of a grammar (i.e., an ordering of words of appropriate form in a sentence), which provides meaning in terms of the sentence's actor, action, and object (semantics). In addition, each sentence has an underlying reason for being uttered (to demand, declare, question, or inform) and the entire package leads to the fulfillment of tangible or intangible needs. Thus, language consists of grammatical, semantic (meaning), pragmatic (purpose), and reward aspects.

The addition of each of these elements to the definition of language has had the effect of pushing back the time at which language (or more precisely, communication) is said to begin. At first, only children with grammar (i.e., sentences two or more words long) were thought to be linguistic. Later, children producing meanings through one-word sentences (sometimes accompanied by gestures) were considered to possess language. With pragmatics, even the 10-month-old child who could make demands by pointing or vocal "proto-imperatives" was considered to be communicative. It may even be that infants of every age are communicative; that there might not be such a thing as a nonlinguistic child.

This historical redefinition of language has begun to blur the distinction between early linguistic (or communicative) skills and sensorimotor cognitive skills. Consider the pointing behavior of a 10-month-old infant. This behavior demonstrates knowledge of the concept of means-ends, in that the point is intentionally used as a means by which the child gets the adult to retrieve an object (the end). However, a point can also be thought of as a pragmatic gesture, in that it communicates a demand to another person (Bates et al., 1975). Thus pointing is one among many behaviors that are both cognitive and linguistic, merging two domains once considered distinct. Stated another way, one can see how early linguistic behavior may be rooted in early cognitive skills.

This tie between the two domains of infant functioning seems more than coincidental. Bates and her colleagues (Bates, 1976; Bates et al., 1975) have shown that infants able to perform certain behaviors (especially means-ends and causality tasks on the Uzgiris-Hunt) are likely to engage in pragmatic behaviors (e.g., pointing, showing, consciously vocalizing their intentions to others); infants unable to perform these sensorimotor tasks also do not demonstrate intentional communicative behaviors. This relationship between cognition and early communication also seems true of several atypical groups. In a study of older severely disturbed children, Curcio (1978) found that abilities on three subscales of the Uzgiris-Hunt (means-ends, causality, and, to a lesser extent, imitation) seem necessary for the emergence of any communicative behaviors in this population. Disturbed children who possessed higher-level skills in these areas were also likely to possess some communicative skills (e.g., eye contact, some manual signs); those who showed only low-level skills in these areas demonstrated no ability to communicate. Mundy et al. (1984) found similar results in a study of retarded children: Those who possessed skills in means-ends and in schemes for relating to objects were likely to show some communicative abilities, whereas those without such skills invariably did not possess any early communicative behaviors (see also Kahn, 1975). Even in a sample of children who were at the one-word stage of language production, Snyder (1978) found that the language-delayed children were deficient in means-ends skills when compared to normally developing children who were also at the one-word stage.

It seems, then, that specific sensorimotor abilities may be the direct prerequisites of early communicative (and later linguistic) development, in both retarded and nonretarded children. In particular, abilities in the areas of means-ends and (possibly) causality seem indispensable for early intentional communication. Later language, which involves more symbolic and relational abilities (i.e., relating words to each other in sentences), may require a different set of sensorimotor skills (e.g., object permanence, spatial, appropriate uses) as their particular prerequisites (Leonard, 1979).

Functional language training and the problem of generalization

Before discussing the programs that have used these findings to enhance early language skills in retarded children, let us first examine those programs that emphasize training in functional language. These programs, briefly discussed earlier in this chapter, are generally behaviorist in orientation and, as a rule, focus on teaching linguistic behaviors that the designers consider to be functional for the retarded child. They generally employ the following four-step training process. First, they teach the child to attend to the teacher. Next, nonverbal imitation is taught, followed by training in the imitation of vocal sounds. Finally, functional speech is trained. Each of these behaviors is taught through the operant procedures of reinforcement, shaping, and fading (see Harris, 1975).

Although a large number of studies have reported success in teaching nonverbal children these four behaviors, "the major problem of language training programs based primarily on the operant paradigm has been the failure to attain spontaneous generalization of trained language" (Mahoney & Snow, 1983, p. 253). Thus, children in operant programs may learn the specific behaviors taught, but generally they have not been able to apply these behaviors to new contexts.

The reason for this lack of generalizability may be found in the basic approach of operant therapists toward the development of language. The following comment (describing the choice of curricula in teaching functional language) is typical: "Generally, the subject is first taught noun labels and then other forms of grammar. There are, however, no data to aid in de-

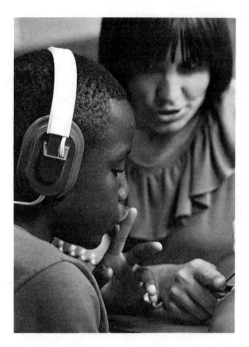

Photo 4. Speech therapy. (Photograph courtesy of Elwyn Institutes, Elwyn, Pennsylvania)

ciding the proper temporal sequence for introducing various grammatical forms. The only guidelines thus far are convenience and developmental norms" (Harris, 1975, p. 571). Data about the normal developmental sequence (developmental norms), and even about the prerequisites to linguistic functioning, are de-emphasized; the rationale for teaching skill B after skill A appears to be the therapist's own idea as to which task is easier for the retarded child to master.

There is some evidence of improved generalizability when the child's initial level of functioning is considered by the interventionist. Mahoney and Snow (1983) gave 14 Down syndrome children, all at the one-word stage of language, a developmentally-based language intervention over a six-month span. The administration of the intervention gradually passed from the therapist to the child's mother. Assessment data (collected before and after intervention) consisted of the Bayley Scales of Infant Development (Bayley, 1969), the Uzgiris-Hunt scales, and several measures of linguistic functioning. In addition, mothers reported the number of words that their children spontaneously produced three or more times in appropriate contexts.

Results revealed that all of the children progressed in their language skills, but that those who were highest in cognitive ability (on the Bayley and Uzgiris-Hunt scales) at the beginning of the study advanced more in their use of spontaneous language. Mahoney and Snow concluded that "the impact of intervention on spontaneous expressive language did appear to be related to children's level of cognitive functioning. Thus, cognitive status seems to be a critical factor for the generalized use of spontaneous communication" (1983, p. 253).

Admittedly, the Mahoney and Snow study was correlational; there was no control group that received no therapy or a competing therapy. Only in a study of this type could one unequivocally state that a certain level of cognitive development is necessary before generalization will occur. Still, considered in conjunction with studies comparing the linguistic development of children with and without certain sensorimotor abilities, this study indicates the need to pay closer attention to the developmental level (and sequences) in early intervention work with retarded children.

Developmental programs

In contrast to operant programs, the sequence of normal language development forms the core of the major developmental intervention programs – those of Bricker and Bricker (1974), MacDonald and Blott (1974), McLean and Snyder-McLean (1978), and Miller and Yoder (1974). Proposed at various times in the past 15 years, these programs incorporate, each to a different degree, the grammatical, semantic, and pragmatic aspects of normal language development. The first three programs, for example, attempt to foster the development of the 14 semantic categories found in children's earliest two-word utterances (Bloom, 1970; Schlesinger, 1971). Such concepts as existence ("that ball"), non-existence ("allgone baby"), recurrence ("more milk"), location ("book table," for "the book is on the table"), possession ("Mommy['s] sock"), and actor-action ("Daddy come") are all taught. The Bricker and Bricker program aims more at teaching those Piagetian sensorimotor skills which, as we learned earlier, seem to be prerequisites to later grammatical speech. The other programs (e.g., Miller and Yoder) specifically state that their curricula are applicable only to children who are already beginning to utter some words and do not attempt to teach sensorimotor skills. For a critical review of each of these programs, see McLean and Snyder-McLean (1978, pp. 212–232).

The methods used in these programs vary widely. The Bricker and Bricker program is probably the most behaviorist in its method of instruction, even though the content emphasizes sensorimotor skills. The other three programs emphasize to the child the use (pragmatics) of language, the understanding that putting words together in a certain order allows one to inform, request, or declare. (For an elaboration of the role of pragmatics in early language intervention, see Seibert & Oller, 1981.) These programs promote the development of language in an interactive context, with the child learning language in natural interactions with the mother and other salient adults. The goal is to help the child generalize the use of language to "real-world" situations by actually teaching it in a natural setting.

The differences in these major developmental language interventions suggest that the area is in flux at the present time. As interventionists assimilate changing theories of language and its development, as well as the new research on cognitive prerequisites to particular linguistic achievements, the intervention programs will change as a result. Still, the assumptions and goals of developmentally-based programs will remain constant. These are well summarized by McLean and Snyder-McLean:

We are suggesting that the child acquires language through interactions with his environment and that from these interactions he derives the cognitive [i.e., sensorimotor] and social [pragmatic] bases which underlie his mastering of the linguistic code of his culture. Further, we are suggesting that this specific linguistic code is acquired through the child's participation in a dynamic partnership with the mature language users in his environment. (1978, p. 111)

We will now explore the nature of this "dynamic partnership" between mother and child in early intervention programs.

The role of mother–child interaction in early intervention work

Just as the study of language has changed in recent years, so has the examination of the social environment of children. Prior to the 1970s, the results of the interactions between parents and their offspring were thought to be pretty much unidirectional: Parents affect children, socializing them into adult society. Although the area of socialization remains important (see Zigler, Lamb, & Child, 1982, for a review of the subject), recent years have added the recognition that parents (usually mothers) and children both influence one another (see Bell, 1968). Starting directly after birth, a highly predictable pattern of mother–child interaction occurs (Als, 1977). Mothers talk to, smile at, or stimulate an awake infant, but they are quiet and gentle with a fussy baby. Similarly, the positions in which the mother holds the baby vary depending on the infant's state.

At later ages, mothers and infants achieve "synchronous" interactions by the mother varying her behavior in response to the infant. For example, in play between mothers and their 3-month-olds, Brazelton, Koslowski, and Main (1974) describe how the mother first gets the infant's attention, then gradually accelerates the pace and strength of her behavior (e.g., louder speech, more abrupt movements). Infants become more and more excited as a result. However, when the baby begins to show signs of being overstimulated, the mother slows and softens her behaviors, allowing the infant to remain attentive at an optimal level of arousal. The entire process of interaction resembles two rising and falling curves of behavioral intensity. These curves are nearly in unison, as both partners respond to the behaviors of the other (see also Stern, 1974).

Field (1978) characterized the mother's role in these interactions as possessing the "three R's": responsivity, repertoire, and rhythm. A mother must be responsive to the behaviors and states of her infant, possess a repertoire of behaviors large enough to keep and hold the infant's interest, and deploy these behaviors in rhythm with the ebb and flow of infant attention. Goldberg (1977) adds the need for mothers to have an ability to "read" their infant's state and behaviors so they can respond accordingly. Although rarely achieved as ideally as stated here, the synchronous, perfectly calibrated interactions described by these workers form the prototypical pattern of mother–infant interaction.

The goal of these interactions is to induce a feeling of efficacy in both partners. The mother is happy that she can elicit behaviors from the infant, that the infant is actually responding to her. The baby is happy to be able to influence the mother, and begins to realize that he or she can have an effect on others. Thus there is a process of "mutual efficacy" (Goldberg, 1977) at work in all good mother–infant interactions; both partners feel that they have some control over the behaviors of the other.

This feeling of efficacy is sometimes lacking in interactions between mothers and their retarded children. Consider the finding that mothers commonly go through a kind of mourning process at the birth of a retarded or otherwise defective child (Solnit & Stark, 1961). First there is an initial period of shock ("this could not be happening to me"), then sadness or anger; gradually there is a reorganization of emotions as parents come to accept and commit themselves to their retarded child (see Blacher, 1984, for a review of research findings). However, the progression from shock to sadness to reorganization is not always this straightforward. In particular, Emde and Brown (1978) found that parents of Down syndrome infants often experience a new wave of sadness at about 4 months, when it becomes evident that their retarded baby is behind in development compared to other infants. These workers also found that mothers able to elicit smiling and cooing behaviors from their infants at this time are more likely to be emotionally attached to their babies later; a feeling of efficacy seems to help them to deal with the child's problems.

The retarded infant may likewise develop feelings of helplessness due to his or her inability to influence parental behaviors. Jones (1980) found that mothers of Down syndrome infants respond less to the interactive initiations of their infants than do mothers of normally developing infants who are at the same mental ages. In vocal interactions before (Berger & Cunningham, 1983) and after (Jones, 1980) 6 months, mothers and their Down syndrome infants also clash more often, as both attempt to speak at the same time. Although this difference in maternal behaviors may be partially due to particular characteristics of Down syndrome infants (they seem to be less clear and "readable" in their interactive behaviors; Cicchetti & Sroufe, 1976), the net result is a style of interaction in which the mother is highly directive. When the mother plays such a dominant role, both partners are denied the feeling of efficacy.

Still, it must be emphasized that mothers and their retarded children can and do engage in interactions that are mutually contingent and satisfying. In a study comparing developmentally retarded infants and their mothers to normal infant–mother pairs, Vietze, Abernathy, Ashe, and Faulstich (1978) found that the majority of interactions were contingent in both groups. The vocalizations of mother and child usually followed one another, in much the same pattern as found in prelinguistic "conversations" between mothers and normally developing infants. Mothers also spoke to their retarded children using the same level of language as mothers of nonretarded children of the same mental ages (Rondal, 1977; see Marfo, 1984, for a review of findings). Thus, although there are some aspects of mother–infant interaction that differ when the infant is retarded, most interactions are not atypical.

From the standpoint of early intervention, the interactions between mothers and their retarded infants are important because of the need to engage the mother as the child's primary therapist. With this goal in mind, a program by Bromwich (1976, 1980) attempts to enhance the functions of early interaction on several levels. At first the mother is helped to enjoy her baby, to experience the joys of motherhood often denied mothers of retarded infants. Next, the mother's role as a sensitive observer of her baby is stressed, as in Goldberg's (1977) conclusion that the mother must be able to "read" her baby. Interactions that are mutually satisfying to mother and infant (promoting feelings of efficacy) are then practiced and their developmental functions explained. The final stage of Bromwich's model emphasizes the mother's own ability to create developmentally appropriate activities and experiences for the infant.

A specific example of this interactional approach to early intervention is seen in Hodapp and Goldfield's (1983) attempt to teach the mother of a severely retarded child to play two common mother–infant games. In previous work with normal infant–mother pairs, Hodapp, Goldfield, and Boyatzis (1984) had observed that mothers employ various "scaffolding" (Bruner, 1978; Wood, Bruner, & Ross, 1976) techniques in game playing with their 8- to 16-month-old infants. In the two games of roll-the-ball and peekaboo, mothers first set the stage for interaction by clearing away distracting objects and positioning themselves facing their babies. Next, mothers attract the infant's attention by vocal, perceptual (e.g., bouncing the ball on floor), or physical (e.g., tickling) means. Once involved in the game, mothers provide the appropriate contextual supports to help their children to perform game-relevant behaviors. They hold out their upturned hands for the child to return the ball in the roll-the-ball game and lean forward and vocalize while hidden behind a cloth in peekaboo.

Each of these procedures, stage setting, attention getting, and providing appropriate contextual support, was the focus of an intervention procedure with a severely retarded 2-year-old boy. For both the roll-the-ball and peekaboo games the mother was coached in exactly how far to sit from the child, how to get the child's attention, and how to provide contextual support. The sensorimotor content of each game was also pointed out; it was explained why uncovering (object permanence) and returning the objects (means-ends and causality) were important skills for the child to develop. A greater number of successful interactions (i.e., child returning ball or uncovering mother) occurred after this coaching. Although attempted in only a preliminary way so far, these procedures may form the content and processes by which "interactive" intervention programs operate. Indeed, it is likely that all sensitive early interventionists already employ such techniques with retarded children. One of the goals of this line of work is to make these procedures explicit to mothers and therapists, allowing both to use these methods more efficiently in their intervention work.

We must stress that interventions based on interactions between mothers and their retarded infants are relatively new. At present, only Bromwich's (1976, 1980) program comes close to providing a complete curriculum of interaction, but no data have yet appeared as to its effectiveness. Still, the appeal of such an approach is undeniable. Mothers are included as full partners in the intervention program, and there are emphases on parenting skills, mutual efficacy in interactions, and the use of interactive behaviors that facilitate development in several domains. We can expect that these programs will become more formalized in future years, and perhaps that fathers will be included to a greater extent.

Families of mentally retarded children

The recent focus on mother–child interactions is rapidly expanding to an interest in how the larger interpersonal environment (e.g., father, siblings, family unit) affects the child's development. As in the case of language and social interaction, this concern within the larger field of developmental psychology has affected how interventions are conceptualized, delivered, and evaluated. More and more programs are beginning to feature a family component (Family Support Project, 1983); several workers have gone so far as to assert that the family, instead of the retarded child, is the proper focus of early intervention efforts (e.g., Bronfenbrenner, 1975, 1979). While it is still too early to assess the implications of such calls, we will briefly discuss how retarded children affect their families, and how families can be integrated into early intervention work.

Effects of the retarded child on the family

The birth of any infant brings about many changes in the structure of a family. If the child is first-born, parents are likely to take on traditional roles, as the mother takes care of the newborn and the father becomes, temporarily at least, the primary breadwinner (Lamb, 1978). If the infant is latter-born, the opposite trend in marital roles occurs: the father takes care of the older children while the mother is away at the hospital. When she returns, her role as the newborn's primary caretaker still leaves the father with expanded family duties. Older children are also affected by the birth of a sibling. For example, pregnant mothers may provide less maternal warmth and shorter contact with their older children (Baldwin, 1947), and begin to expect more from them. In effect, children are being readied for the role of older brother or sister that they will soon assume.

These changes in family structure are the natural consequences of having a new child come into the family. Handicapped infants, however, present even greater and unanticipated problems to their families. As described earlier, parents looking forward to a "healthy, happy baby" undergo a process of mourning as they attempt to cope with their ambivalent feelings. On one hand, they feel failure and frustration at having produced a defective child; on the other, they are trying to love and provide for their new baby.

Even years later, parents of handicapped children are affected, both as individuals and as couples. Cummings, Bayley, and Rie (1966) compared questionnaire responses from mothers of 4- to 13-year-old retarded, chronically ill, neurotic (i.e., behavior disordered), and nonhandicapped children. They found that mothers of retarded children were more depressed, were more preoccupied with their children, and had greater difficulty in handling their anger at their children than did mothers of normal children. Fathers of handicapped children also showed increases in depression and scored lower in dominance, self-esteem, and enjoyment of their (handicapped) children (Cummings, 1976). In short, both studies found parents of retarded children to be more emotionally impaired than parents of nonhandicapped children (also see Erikson, 1969, and Friedrich & Friedrich, 1981). These findings may help explain why handicapped children seem to be at greater than normal risk for child abuse (Embry, 1980).

It remains unclear what the specific effects of a handicapped infant are on the marital relationship. In some cases, the experience of jointly rearing a handicapped child can pull the couple together. But a weakening of the relationship may also occur, particularly if the mother becomes overattached to the affected child, causing the father to withdraw from the situation (Hagamen, 1980). Solnit (1976) notes that "trauma such as the birth of a defective baby tends to magnify the weaknesses in a marriage more than it enhances the strength of the relationship" (p. 178), a view corroborated by the increased divorce rates among parents of handicapped children (Embry, 1980; Tew, Payne, & Lawrence, 1974).

The rest of the family indirectly faces the crisis of a handicapped child as well. In typical families with newborns, older children are often helped to accept the arrival of the new sibling by gaining a special relationship with the father (Legg, Sherick, & Wadland, 1975). When the newborn is retarded or otherwise handicapped, the father may not be emotionally available to the older children. For daughters, the joint effects of being the older child and of being female (i.e., the traditional caretaker) in a stressful situation may account for the higher incidence of emotional problems in the oldest sisters of retarded children (Gath, 1977, 1978). Older male siblings, by contrast, may "escape almost scot-free" (Fox, 1975, p. 217). Although rarely examined, the side effects of having a handicapped member of the family may be great indeed for parents and others in the family.

Retarded children also influence the demographic characteristics of their families. Culver (1967; also Farber, 1970) found that families with handicapped children were more likely to remain at the same socioeconomic level they had when the child was born. The earlier in the marriage the birth of the retarded child occurred, the more economically immobile the family became. One reason may be that families with retarded and physically handicapped children spend more for health care and special services, and have frequent, costly visits with doctors, special educators and other professionals (Richards & McIntoch, 1973). Add to these the standard expenses such as food and clothing incurred for any child, and it is easy to see why a mentally retarded child can have an adverse effect on family finances.

Reviews of research on the families of handicapped children have attempted to assimilate these data within a framework emphasizing the retarded child as a stressor within the family unit (Gallagher, Beckman, & Cross, 1983). This approach treats the family as a unit that possesses strengths and weaknesses but that also functions in a larger ecological context (including neighborhood, school, church, etc.). Crnic, Friedrich, and Greenberg (1983) summarized this combined stress-ecological approach as follows: "Family functioning cannot be considered simply as a response to a retarded child; rather, it is more meaningful to consider familial adaptation as a response to the child mediated by the coping resources available and influenced by the family's ecological environments" (p. 136).

Although the joint perspective of a stressor within several levels of ecology is complicated, some general statements can be made concerning the relationship between families and their retarded children. First, it does appear that the retarded child is a source of stress (Cummings, 1976; Cummings et al., 1966; Erikson, 1969). This stress may become more pronounced as the child gets older (Suelzle & Keenan, 1981) and is (presumably) more difficult to manage. Stress created by the presence of a retarded family member falls on each parent, on the parents' relationship, on siblings, and perhaps on others in the extended family.

Second, the stress seems to be mediated by a host of factors. For example, families that are more economically advantaged are better able to handle the stress of a retarded child than those who are less well off (Farber, 1970). Two-parent families cope better than one-parent families (Beckman, 1983), and mothers in successful marriages seem to cope better with caring for the retarded child than those in less successful marriages (Friedrich, 1979). The nature of the child's handicap also comes into play, as Holroyd and McArthur (1976) have found that mothers of Down syndrome children report fewer problems for themselves and their families than do mothers of autistic children.

Third, external environments can affect the impact of a retarded child on the family. Suelze and Keenan (1981) found that a family's support networks (e.g., other parents of retarded children, extended family, friends) can help family members cope with the stress associated with having a retarded child. Having an extended family nearby seems particularly important, as parents of retarded children often feel that strangers will not understand their child's special needs and therefore rely on their relatives for help and baby-sitting (Watson & Midlarsky, 1979). Although each of these mediating factors is in some sense obvious, they are all indeed helpful in lessening the stress felt by families of retarded children.

Intervention with families of retarded children

Many intervention programs have included the family in an informal manner, but with the recent interest in ecological approaches to child development several programs have begun to intervene systematically with families of retarded children. To date, only preliminary data are available on the effects of these programs. Dunst (1982) reported that parents receiving "high support" in a family-based early intervention program (the Family, Infant, and Preschool Program in western North Carolina) rated themselves higher on health/mood scales and felt themselves less burdened by excessive time demands imposed by their retarded children. Bronfenbrenner (1975) argued that interventions aimed at the families of at-risk children promote the fastest development in the children themselves (i.e., the greatest positive IQ changes); this assertion remains untested in interventions with organically retarded children.

These programs, and the recent interest in the family, bring up the larger issue of the appropriate focus of intervention for retarded children. At first glance, the retarded child is most obviously in need of help; he or she is cognitively, linguistically, and motorically behind in development and often progresses at slower and slower rates over time (Hodapp & Zigler, in press; Kopp & McCall, 1982). But mothers, fathers, and siblings of retarded children also need emotional support, information, and instruction in how to deal with the retarded family member. The issue of specifying the appropriate target of intervention remains one of the most troublesome in the entire field of early intervention, both with organically retarded and at-risk children. We will return to this issue in the next chapter, when we discuss the appropriate ways to assess the effectiveness of early intervention programs.

We realize that in this chapter we have dissected the "whole child" into various domains of functioning. This technique was necessary to elaborate on developmentally-based interventions in the areas of cognition, communication, mother–child interaction, and family functioning. The use of this technique was dictated only by the fact that each domain is complex enough to require explanation. In the next chapter, we return to a more integrated focus as we explore the nature and evaluation of several comprehensive intervention programs serving young retarded children and their families.

8 Early intervention programs and their evaluation

The idea that one can intervene effectively with retarded children has a long history. From Itard's experiment with the wild boy of Aveyron (see Lane, 1976) to the Iowa studies of the 1930s, the hope has been that one could take a child at risk for mental retardation, provide an extremely stimulating environment, and thereby ameliorate the effects of an adverse environmental or genetic history.

In recent years, workers have vacillated in their views as to the merits of such interventions. Influenced by Hunt's (1961) pronouncements that IQ could be substantially altered, workers in the 1960s came to have over-optimistic views of the achievements of early intervention programs. By the late 1960s and early 1970s, such optimism had faded; in its place came numerous proclamations that "early intervention has failed" (see Zigler & Berman, 1983, for a review of this change in attitude). Even to this day both views can be heard. A more balanced picture is necessary, one that takes into account who is intervened with, how the intervention is performed, and how it is evaluated.

In the present chapter we will examine this issue by reviewing several of the well-known programs of early intervention. We will explore the nature of the programs themselves – the characteristics of the children and families served, the nature and extensiveness of the interventions provided – and critically examine the various effects of these programs. We will also discuss how early intervention programs should be evaluated, detailing the various controversies involved in such a seemingly straightforward issue.

In contrast to Chapter 7, our focus in this chapter will be mainly on programs that serve children who are at risk for mental retardation. It seems safe to say that the majority of published programs have focused on these children. As Zigler and Balla (1982a) have noted, "Reports of programs with children who have actually been identified as retarded are much less frequent" (p. 12).

At-risk children also seem to be the focus of most of the controversies

162

in the early intervention field. For example, it seems almost self-evident that severely and profoundly retarded children should be taught the earliest sensorimotor, linguistic, social, and self-help skills (as discussed in Chapter 7). These behaviors are essential for all further functioning, lead to the child's becoming more adapted to his or her surroundings, and are prerequisites to later functioning in virtually every area. Familial retarded and at-risk children have little trouble attaining such basic skills (see Scarr-Salapatek, 1975; Lenneberg, 1967), however, and the question of which area or areas should receive attention becomes more problematic when intervening with this group. The related issue of the appropriate evaluation of programs serving at-risk children is similarly the subject of widespread debate.

Major early intervention programs for at-risk children

In the following pages, we briefly discuss the Abecedarian, Milwaukee, and Perry Preschool projects of early intervention with at-risk children. These programs constitute the most well-known and influential programs in the United States. Evidence from the Milwaukee project, for example, led to much of the early enthusiasm for the efficacy of intervention programs boosting IQ scores of low-income, minority children (e.g., President's Committee on Mental Retardation, 1973); similarly, the Perry program has recently received national attention for its reported effectiveness in facilitating children's increased adaptation to school and society (Hechinger, 1984; Weikart, 1984). Although our discussion of even these three programs cannot be comprehensive, we hope to provide some sense of how each program operates and how each has been conceptualized and evaluated.

The Abecedarian Project

Established in the fall of 1972 at the Frank Porter Graham Child Development Center in North Carolina, the Abecedarian Project "was begun as an attempt to bring together a multidisciplinary team of researchers who would address themselves both to demonstrating that developmental retardation could be prevented and to examining how various psychological and biological processes were affected by such preventive attempts" (Ramey & Campbell, 1977, p. 158).

Target children were identified through the use of a High Risk Index (see Ramey & Smith, 1977) developed by center personnel. Risk factors included mother's and father's educational status, the family income, father's absence, father's work record, maternal or paternal IQ, data on siblings and the extended family, and other characteristics of the family. Each factor received a different weighting (based on the authors' best guess of relative importance) and only children with the highest levels of risk were included in the study.

To date, four cohort groups have participated in the program of research. In each cohort, matched pairs of subjects have been randomly assigned to experimental (i.e., intervention) or control groups. Both experimental and control subjects in every cohort have received free nutritional supplements and health care. Only the experimental subjects have received the intensive early intervention program at the day-care facility. This intervention, begun in the first three months of life, has lasted until the child is ready to enter school and involves the child's participation in a systematic, child-directed program for 6–8 hours per day, 50 weeks per year.

Intervention curricula focus on teaching a wide variety of skills to experimental group children. Up to 3 years of age, children receive curricula consisting of over 300 items in language, motor, social, and cognitive areas. After age 3, the areas of science, math, music, prereading, and reading are emphasized. The teaching of children who are below 3 years old often occurs in one-to-one interactions (the child to staff ratio is 3:1 at this age); at later ages, teaching of small groups predominates (child to staff ratios are 4:1 or 5:1).

Although currently conceptualized (e.g., Ramey, MacPhee, & Yeates, 1982) in terms of general systems theory (Bertalannfy, 1968), all intervention efforts have been directed toward the high-risk children, rather than toward their mothers, fathers, siblings, or families. As a consequence, most of the results of the program also pertain to the children themselves. The most consistent result is that experimental group children have been found to perform significantly higher on IQ tests than control children at every age after 18 months. At last report (Ramey, Campbell, & Finkelstein, 1984), three of the four cohort groups had reached age 5, with experimental-group children outperforming control children by 8 IQ points (e.g., 100.4 to 92.7 on the Wechsler Preschool and Primary Scales of Intelligence [WPPSI] at 60 months). Figure 8.1 shows these results for the 74 children described in the Ramey et al. (1984) report. As the authors note, "the relative intellectual superiority of the educationally treated group is apparently due to the declining then stabilizing performance of the control group rather than to rising scores in the HRE [High Risk Experimental] group" (pp. 424-425).

Ramey and his co-workers interpret these results in terms of the cu-

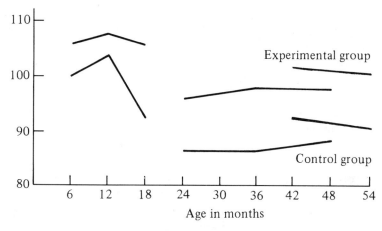

Figure 8.1. Comparison of experimental (treated) and control (untreated) groups of the Abecedarian Project. Curves starting at 6 months of age compare the two groups on the Bayley Infant tests (until 18 months) and on the Stanford-Binet (from 24 to 48 months). Lines beginning at 42 months compare the two groups on the McCarthy scales of children's abilities. (Original figure from Ramey, Campbell, & Finkelstein, 1984, used with permission; McCarthy scales data from text of Ramey, Campbell, & Finkelstein, 1984, and added by present authors)

mulative deficit hypothesis, the idea that because of poor environments high-risk children fall further and further behind in intelligence over time (see discussion of Jensen, 1974, in Chapter 4). "The pattern indicates a decline in intellectual performance [in the IQ scores of the control group] beginning at about 18 months and extending to about 36 months. The decline during that age period appears linear and therefore appears to support the cumulative deficit hypothesis" (Ramey et al., 1984, p. 427). These workers do, however, acknowledge that a straightforward cumulative deficit is not supported, in that the control children's IQs fall off only from 18 to 36 months and remain steady thereafter. It should also be noted that all comparisons of experimental and control IQs based on infant IQ scores are suspect; as mentioned in Chapter 4, infant IQ scores do not predict later IQs for any but the most retarded children.

A second finding in the domain of intelligence concerns the pattern of correlations between maternal and child IQ scores in the two groups of children. According to polygenic theory (and existing research data), mother–child correlations should approach .50 (see Chapter 4). However, the reasons for such mother–child correlations are unclear, as mothers and home-reared children share similar environments as well as half of their genes. In the few studies that have disentangled genetic and environmental influences – for example, the adoption studies of Scarr and Weinberg (1976, 1978, & 1979; see also Scarr & Carter-Saltzman, 1982) – the IQs of the adopted children rose considerably over those of their natural mothers (an effect of the environment), but the mother–child correlations still approached .50. Thus, it appears that while the IQ scores of the entire group of adopted children were elevated over the scores of their natural mothers (with whom they shared half their genes and none of their environment), their scores were still more closely related to those of their natural as opposed to their adopted mothers. This finding shows both genetic and environmental effects in the phenotypic intelligence levels of these children.

In contrast, the Abecedarian experimental children had IQ scores that were essentially uncorrelated with those of their mothers, while the control children showed the usual mother–child correlations. At 36 months, the mother–child correlation for experimental child–mother dyads was -.05; for control dyads the correlation was .43. Ramey and Haskins (1981) explain these findings as follows:

These data are consistent with the hypothesis that when mothers provide half the infant's genes and a substantial part of the infant's environment, one can predict a significant relation between the mother's and child's IQ, but when the mother provides half the child's genes and a relatively moderate part of the young child's environment, one cannot predict a relation between the mother's and child's IQ. (p. 17)

Other workers have offered alternative explanations for the lack of correlation between mothers and the experimental-group children of the Abecedarian Project. Jensen (1981b) suggests that the program itself may have taught specific items that were identical or similar to those found on the IQ tests (Bayley, Stanford-Binet, WPPSI) given to children in the program. If so, the Abecedarian children may not have changed in their intellectual abilities, but may have simply had prior exposure to test items. Ramey and Haskins (1981b) reply that the Abecedarian curricula were not similar to test items and that teachers were unfamiliar with the content of intelligence tests. With the exception of follow-up reports to see if these gains fade out over time (a common finding in the years after intervention programs have ended; Bronfenbrenner, 1975), there seems to be no definite way to judge the merits of the Jensen (1981b) or the Ramey and Haskins (1981b) arguments.

Other findings of the Abecedarian Project also deserve mention. In the area of children's social skills, experimental-group children have been found to be more socially confident (as measured by the Infant Behavior Record of the Bayley) than were control children at 6, 12, and 18 months of age (Ramey, Dorval, & Baker-Ward, in press). Farran and Haskins (1980) also found that the experience of participating in the intervention program helped to make experimental-group children more active and effective in their interactions with their mothers than were the children in the control group. For example, experimental-group children were much more likely to attempt to change the behaviors of their mothers (e.g., to ask their mothers to watch an activity) than were the control children. These increased social skills may not have helped the experimental-group children in their early grade school years, however, as kindergarten teachers rated the children in the experimental group as more hostile (and as more intelligent) compared to control children.

In addition, despite IQs in the normal range, nearly all of the children in the experimental group were assigned to the lowest academic group upon entrance into grade school, as were all of the control children. Although there have as yet been few graduates of the preschool program whose grade school progress has been evaluated, their achievement does not appear especially promising. Ramey and Haskins (1981c) speculate that, because graduates of the preschool program attend school with economically advantaged classmates, "the academic grouping of the public schools seems to pose a threat to any advantage enjoyed by children who attended the preschool program" (p. 108). Still, the results of this project show that IQ change, in and of itself, does not guarantee school (and life) success.

The mothers of children in the experimental group also seem to have been affected by the day-care program of their children. At 54 months, mothers of experimental-group children were found to have more education (11.9 years) than mothers of control children (10.3), even though education had been equivalent when children first entered the program. It is unclear exactly why this result occurred. It may have been that center personnel subtly conveyed their interest in education, or simply due to the fact that mothers of children in the experimental group were freed from child-care duties. Job attainment of experimental-group mothers also seems to have been positively affected by the child's placement in full-time day care (Ramey, Dorval, & Baker-Ward, in press).

It seems safe to conclude that the Abecedarian Project is "a thoughtful and well-done effort that represents an ideal case for testing the prospective value of the center-based, curriculum-heavy, preschool enrichment approach" (Zigler & Berman, 1983, p. 903). As these researchers noted, however, its small IQ gains may be possible with other, less intensive and less costly programs, programs that pay more attention to competence and family outcomes. (We discuss examples of such programs later in this chapter.) In addition, its effects on the lives of its children (e.g., school success) seem questionable, and only future follow-ups will demonstrate the ultimate achievements of this program.

The Milwaukee Project

As in the Abecedarian Project, the Milwaukee Project sought to identify children with the highest risk of mental retardation and to enroll them in an intensive program of early intervention. The main outcome measure for experimental children has been their scores on measures of IQ and various individual domains (e.g., language), both while participating in the program and now that they attend public schools. In addition, project personnel have also intervened with the mothers of experimental-group children, with the hope that these low-income mothers might become able to find employment and to parent their children more successfully.

The project began with a survey of mental retardation among the population of the city of Milwaukee. Certain low-income, inner-city neighborhoods were identified as the areas in which retardation among resident children was highest; approximately 22% of school-aged children had IQs below 75 in several inner-city neighborhoods. Even within these neighborhoods, the offspring of mothers who were themselves of low IQ (i.e., IQ of 75 or lower) were disproportionately likely to be among the school-aged retarded population (indeed, 45% of low-SES mothers accounted for nearly 80% of children with IQs below 80). Garber and Heber (1981) report that "If we could find a newborn child born into a seriously disadvantaged family where the maternal IQ was 75 or below, then according to our data the risk factor for retardation was 14 to 16 times as great as for the average child" (p. 73). This finding fits well with the polygenic model of intelligence discussed in Chapter 4.

The project itself involved 40 high-risk families, which were defined as low-SES, black families with a newborn child whose mother had an IQ of 75 or below. The 40 families were randomly assigned to experimental or control groups. The 20 control families were tested periodically over the next seven years, with no other services offered. The 20 experimental families were entered into a wide-ranging rehabilitation program with two emphases: an intensive educational program for the children, especially in the areas of language and problem solving; and a program of educational and vocational rehabilitation for the mothers.

The educational program for experimental-group children began shortly after the infants reached 3 months of age. Children were brought to a special neighborhood center daily, for eight hours a day, throughout the year. The center was staffed with teachers who were specifically trained to work with infants. Garber and Heber (1977) note that intervention was intensive, direct, and personalized to the specific needs of each child; no published curricula have been reported.

The maternal rehabilitation program focused on the training of job, reading, and home management skills to mothers of experimental-group children. Vocational training consisted of occupational training and of placement services, while reading instruction took place during adult education classes in the evening. Training in home management skills seems to have been less formal, with parents calling their individual parent worker during home- and work-related crises.

Results of the Milwaukee program are similar to those found in the Abecedarian Project, and may even be of greater magnitude. The IQ scores of experimental-group children have been approximately 20-30 points above those of control-group children at every testing after 18 months. Language gains by the experimental group seem particularly significant, as "differences [favoring experimental children] in language development are on the order of nearly 2 years" (p. 122) for the 3- to 6-year-old children of the Garber and Heber (1977) report.

The findings of different patterns of social interactions between mothers and experimental-group children are also similar to the Abecedarian results. Children in the experimental group supplied more verbal information to their mothers and initiated more verbal communication than did children in control dyads (Falender & Heber, 1975). In a sense, these higher-functioning children were themselves guiding their interactions with their mothers.

Follow-up reports of the Milwaukee Project have now examined children who have graduated from the program and attended grade school for several years. Children in both the experimental and control groups have declined somewhat in their IQ scores, but the 20-point differential remains (e.g., at 84 months, experimental children averaged 106 IQ, control children 85; Garber, 1975). In addition, one third of the experimental-group children are reported to have demonstrated some social or behavioral difficulties in the school setting. Thus, although Milwaukee Project children became more verbal and more assertive as a result of their preschool programs, these characteristics did not necessarily ensure their smooth transition to the elementary school environment.

The Milwaukee Project seems, then, to have increased the IQs of experimental-group children approximately 20 points over those of children from similar impoverished and high-risk backgrounds. Controversy continues to surround this project, however, as some have suggested that the two groups were not strictly equivalent at the start of the study (Page, 1972) and the project's results have only rarely been published (and almost never in peer-reviewed journals). The Milwaukee Project's effects on the life functioning of at-risk children and their families have also not been so clear-cut.

The Perry Preschool Project

Begun in 1962, the Perry Preschool Project is the oldest of the intervention programs discussed so far. It is the only program of the three that has provided information on the outcome of its subjects up to 19 years of age. It therefore allows an assessment of the long-term effects of a program of early intervention, including the results from various tests, from teacher and child ratings, and from the actual real-life outcomes of the children.

Also in contrast to the other two programs, the Perry Preschool Project began its intervention by selecting children who were already retarded, at least according to the AAMD definition in use at the time (i.e., IQ below 85; Heber, 1961). All 3-year-old children in certain low-income neighborhoods in Ypsilanti, Michigan, were located through door-to-door search and tested with the Stanford-Binet intelligence test. Children with IQ scores between 70 and 85, the so-called borderline mentally retarded, were then entered into the study (mean IQ = 79).

The IQs of eligible children were first rank-ordered, with one child admitted to the experimental group, the next to the control group. Slight modifications in this procedure were then made (to ensure equal numbers of boys and girls in each group, for example), but the two groups remained matched on IQ and other measures at the outset (see Schweinhart & Weikart, 1981, p. 23). Children in both groups came from families suffering from a variety of difficulties, including low-SES, crowded living conditions, one-parent families, high rates of parental unemployment and low levels of parental education.

The Perry Preschool provided a two-year intervention for five cohort groups of 3- and 4-year-old children. Experimental-group children were entered into the program over a span of four years (1962–65) when they were 3 years old, and spent the next two years in the program. Control children received only testing at specified intervals. The program consisted of high-quality, center-based day care for 2½ hours per day (12½ hours per week) and a 1½-hour weekly home visit; the school year lasted from mid-October until the end of May (30 weeks). The teacher-to-child ratio was 1:5 or 1:6, and a Piagetian-based curriculum was featured (Hohmann,

Banet, & Weikart, 1979). Thus, although the Perry Preschool Project provided an intensive preschool program, the length of the school day (2 ½ hours), length of school year (30 weeks), number of years spent in the program (two years), and the age at which children entered the program (3 years old) were all much different from either the Milwaukee or Abecedarian programs.

Results from the Perry Project are now available on a variety of measures for children up to 19 years of age. Concerning intelligence, the experimental-group children demonstrated a 10-15 point increase in IQ scores when they were 4 and 5 years of age, but they gradually lost their advantage over the control group in later years. By the age of 8, the experimental group advantage was minimal (2–3 points), and by 11 the two groups were identical. These findings are in accordance with the general finding of fade-out of IQ gains in the years after intervention programs have ended (Bronfenbrenner, 1975).

The program's effects on achievement test scores and on real-life outcome measures seem more promising. Experimental-group children outperformed control children on the California Achievement Tests at every age throughout the elementary and middle school years. "Differences favoring preschool [children] were between 5 and 7 percent of items passed from age 7 to age 10, but dropped to 2 percent at age 11. At age 14, there was a highly significant difference of 8 percent of items passed in favor of children who attended preschool" (Schweinhart & Weikart, 1981, p. 37).

In comparing the achievement test differences to the lack of differences on IQ tests, Schweinhart and Weikart (1981) point to the possibility that experimental-group children were more persistent in their test taking on this group-administered test. On a measure of task persistence, they note that experimental-group children attempted 89% of achievement test items, compared to 82% of items attempted by the control group (a significant difference). This effect of task persistence may not have occurred on intelligence tests due to the individualized nature of IQ test administration. This difference on achievement tests (but not on IQ) shows again the power of motivational factors in affecting children's everyday lives (Zigler, 1971).

Other measures of students' real-life progress and problems also differed between the two groups. By the end of high school, 39% of the control-group children had received special-education services for one or more years (the group averaged 2.1 years of special education), whereas only 19% of experimental-group children had received these services (the group averaged .92 years). Experimental-group children also reported that they had participated in a smaller number of delinquent behaviors than reported by control-group children, and teachers of experimental-group children rated them as having better relationships with other classmates and with their teachers than did control children.

These findings have recently been extended to 19-year-old children (Berrueta-Clement, Schweinhart, Barnett, Epstein, & Weikart, 1984). At this age, children who experienced the Perry Program when they were 3 and 4 years old were more likely than control children to have graduated from high school (67% of experimental group versus 49% of control group) and to have gone on to further academic or vocational study upon graduation from high school (38% to 21%). In addition, girls from the preschool group were about half as likely as control girls to become pregnant as teenagers, and experimental-group children were involved in 20% fewer arrests and detentions. At least on these measures of real-life success, then, the Perry Preschool Program seems to have begun a process that has positively affected experimental-group children long after the intervention itself had been completed.

Summary of findings from these three programs

We can make several, albeit tentative, statements concerning the effects of early intervention from descriptions of the programs discussed so far. We acknowledge that there may be other effects of early intervention programs on the functioning of at-risk children.

Risk factors. There seem to be certain specific indicators of a child's increased risk of retardation. Even when the socioeconomic status of children is equated, as in the Abecedarian and Milwaukee projects (where all children came from low-SES families), low maternal intelligence was most predictive of low IQ scores in the children. Both the Milwaukee Project (e.g., Garber & Heber, 1981) and the High Risk Index of the Abecedarian Project (Ramey & Smith, 1977) rate maternal IQ scores, or its proxy, highest level of formal schooling, as the best predictor of the child's later IQ. In addition, the High Risk Index employed in the Abecedarian Project rates paternal schooling (and IQ scores) high on its list of risk factors. This shows again the role of polygenic factors in intelligence.

IQ gains. Some gains in IQ scores seem to occur as a result of intensive programs of early intervention. These gains, in the neighborhood of 10–20 points, may (as in the Perry Project) or may not (as in the Milwaukee Project) fade out several years after the program has ended, but some permanent gains in IQ seem probable. IQ gains produced by the programs are most likely within the ± 12 points thought by many to be the reaction range of intelligence (see Cronbach, 1975; Gottesman, 1968; Zigler, 1970b; see also Chapter 4).

Style of interaction. Children who have received intensive day-care experiences over a period of several years become more assertive and more verbal in their interactions with others. This characteristic seems to help at-risk children to achieve more efficacious interactions with their mothers (Falender & Heber, 1975; Farran & Haskins, 1980), but may not necessarily help them in their adjustment to elementary school (Ramey & Haskins, 1981c).

Life success. Intervention programs can, but do not necessarily, improve the actual life success of at-risk children. This effect on degree of life success, seen most dramatically in the Perry Project (Schweinhart & Weikart, 1980, 1981), has also been demonstrated in Head Start and in other preschool programs for low-SES children (see Consortium for Longitudinal Studies, 1983; Lazar, Darlington, Murray, Royce, & Snipper, 1982; Seitz, Apfel, & Rosenbaum, 1981). As we will discuss later, however, positive changes in life success may not be the necessary outcome of early intervention programs, especially those (such as the Abecedarian and Milwaukee Projects) that are heavily cognitive in orientation, with the child as the sole focus of the intervention.

Diffusion effects. Early intervention programs, even those directed at the children themselves, may positively affect the education and work status of the mothers of at-risk children (Ramey, Dorval, & Baker-Ward, in press). Other investigators (e.g., Gray, 1977) have noted that the siblings of experimental group children, even though they themselves do not receive day care, may also indirectly benefit from the program.

Assessing the effectiveness of early intervention programs

In reviewing the Abecedarian, Milwaukee, and Perry Projects, it becomes clear that the evaluation of any program is not such a straightforward matter and that different programs have assessed their effects in different ways. For example, the Perry Preschool Project has examined a variety of achievement scores, teacher and child ratings, and educational outcomes, in addition to the IQ scores of its subjects. The Abecedarian Project has examined IQ, social interaction, and, more recently, school placement and success. The Milwaukee Project has focused mainly on IQ test results, although there have also been some evaluations of the children's school outcome and of the maternal intervention component of the program.

We provide below a listing of the various outcomes that we feel should be evaluated in any early intervention program with retarded children. To date, few if any programs have systematically evaluated on such a broad scale. However, it is our view that such assessments are necessary to ascertain if an early intervention program does indeed work for at-risk and retarded children. In our discussions below, we will discuss three levels of assessment separately: the child, the family, and cost-benefit analyses. We conclude this chapter with an example of one program that included many of the components that we feel are important to any successful early intervention program.

The child

IQ. IQ scores from standardized tests (e.g., WISC-R, Stanford-Binet, WPPSI) are among the most widely employed outcome measures in program evaluations (Zigler & Trickett, 1978). They are readily available, are standardized with known psychometric properties, and have an impressive track record of showing short-term 10–20-point gains due to early intervention efforts. In addition, no other measure has been found to be related to so many theoretically and practically significant behaviors (Kohlberg & Zigler, 1967; Mischel, 1968). Finally, the history of the nature–nurture argument as it concerns intelligence must be considered. As Zigler and Seitz (1982) have noted, "with such leading figures as Hunt (1971) reporting IQ improvements of 50 to 70 points as a result of early intervention, it became increasingly seductive to bet on improvement in the IQ as the bedrock outcome measure" (p. 598).

At the same time, IQ tests have also received a large amount of criticism. McClelland (1973) has estimated the correlation between IQ scores and everyday performance in life in the postschool period at only around .20. Zigler and Trickett (1978) have noted that, even in the school years, IQ scores and school success correlate .70, leaving half of the variance unexplained. As mentioned in Chapter 1, Mercer (1973a, 1973b) decries the use of IQ tests for minority children, and Kamin (1974) sees their widespread use as a tool of social injustice and political oppression. Finally, at least for mildly retarded persons, IQ has not been as powerful a predictor of ultimate adaptation and social adequacy as a variety of personality factors (McCarver & Craig, 1974; Windle, 1962).

Given such contradictory information, how should one assess the use of the IQ test as an outcome measure of early intervention programs? Used solely as an indicator of the individual's level of formal cognitive ability, the IQ test appears to be most free of criticism (as compared to its other uses). But overall, "We do not feel the IQ score is as good as the IQ champions would seem to believe, nor do we feel it is as bad as some of its critics have stated" (Zigler & Trickett, 1978, p. 790). It should be one, but not the main, outcome measure used to assess the effectiveness of an early intervention program.

Social competence. The real goal of any early intervention program is to promote social competence in its subjects. Broadly defined, social competence involves the child's degree of success in meeting societal expectations (which differ at different ages) and the child's self-actualization or personal development (Zigler & Balla, 1982e). The construct has proven difficult to apply in practical terms, however, with some workers (e.g., Zigler & Trickett, 1978) disagreeing with present measures of social competence, and others (Anderson & Messick, 1974) viewing the construct as impossibly vague.

Despite such caveats, we propose at least the following four areas of social competence: the child's health and well-being, the child's formal cognition, the child's academic achievement, and the motivation and personality development of the child. Each area is an important outcome of any intervention program, and each is easily measurable.

To date many early intervention programs have concerned themselves with one or more of these four areas of social competence, few with all four. For example, the Abecedarian Project specifically provided both the control and experimental families with free nutritional supplements and health care. Although the rationale for this practice was to lessen the effects of one group receiving more attention than the other, there does seem to have been an acknowledgment that a child's health status is important. Similarly, Head Start has historically featured a strong commitment to the health of its children, as its founders considered children's health needs an important factor in their development (see Zigler & Valentine, 1979). In the theoretical literature as well, health has received attention as an important influence on children's functioning. Jensen (1980) has argued that intrauterine and nutritional and health factors are more influential on intellectual development than many of the social and cognitive factors that one usually associates with the term *environment*. In short, there is an important, if often overlooked, health component to the optimal functioning of any child, retarded or normally intelligent. (See North, 1979, for a discussion of the physical health measures that have been used in assessments of early intervention programs.)

Similarly, the academic achievement of children who participated in early intervention programs has been examined in several programs. The Perry

Project is probably the clearest example in this regard, with the later academic achievement of its experimental-group children among its most powerful effects. Even years later, children who experienced the two-year day-care intervention of the Perry Preschool performed better on achievement tests and received special-education services less often and for shorter periods of time than did control children.

Finally, motivation and personality measures similar to those discussed in Chapter 6 could be included in the assessments of early intervention programs. We are aware of the measurement problems involved in assessing motivational and personality attributes, but we do not view these problems as insurmountable. In the light of our own evaluation efforts, we suggest that emotional and motivational measures be selected from the following collection.

1 Measures of effectance motivation, including indicators of preference for challenging tasks, curiosity, variation seeking, and mastery motivation.
2 Outer-directedness and degree of imitation in problem solving.
3 Positive responsiveness to social reinforcement.
4 Locus of control.
5 Expectancy of success.
6 Verbal attention-seeking behavior.
7 Aspects of self-image, including real and ideal self-image.
8 Measures of learned helplessness.
9 Attitude toward school.
10 Creativity.

Details of each of these measures can be found in the studies reviewed in Chapter 6 and by Zigler and Trickett (1978).

In addition to these direct measures of motivation and personality attributes, there are a variety of indirect measures of program effects that relate to the child's personality. These include the incidence of juvenile delinquency, incidence of teenage pregnancy, incidence of child abuse, being in school rather than out, being in the appropriate grade for age, and being self-supporting rather than being on welfare. These factors have been found to be affected by early intervention efforts, both in programs reviewed earlier (e.g., Schweinhart & Weikart, 1980, 1981) and in those studied by members of the Yale group (to be discussed later in this chapter).

The family

As mentioned in the previous chapter, the family of the retarded and at-risk child plays a large role in the child's development. Several early intervention programs (see Family Support Project, 1982) are now including the family as an integral part of their early intervention efforts. Regardless of the focus of the intervention, however, a program's effects on the family should be evaluated.

In the programs discussed so far, we see that there are often important effects on the mothers of at-risk children due to their child's participation in an early intervention program. The Abecedarian Project found that mothers of experimental children had more education when the children were 54 months old than did mothers of control-group children. In addition, in both the Abecedarian and Milwaukee projects, experimental-group mothers more often spoke with their children and interacted with them for longer periods of time.

On the broader family level, as well, interventions may be helpful and should be evaluated. At present, few if any intervention programs systematically evaluate changes in the functioning of the fathers of at-risk children in the programs. Similarly, program effects on the relationship between mother and father, and on the role of the extended family, have yet to be assessed in most early intervention programs. Sibling work is limited to Gray's (1977) finding that the nontreated siblings of experimental-group children increase in their IQ scores; few measures of achievement, motivation-personality, or life success are available for the siblings of at-risk children who have participated in early intervention programs.

It seems reasonable to conclude that evaluations have barely begun of the families of at-risk children who have been involved in early intervention programs. Programs founded in the late 1970s and 1980s can be expected to systematically evaluate the families in their programs, as can the later reports of the Abecedarian, Perry, and Milwaukee programs.

Cost–benefit analyses

Although many debates center around the benefits to society of early intervention programs versus the costs of such programs, few programs have been subjected to systematically performed cost–benefit analyses. Of the programs discussed so far, the Perry Project is the only one to have included cost–benefit analyses, and the results are encouraging. Schweinhart and Weikart (1981) report that in the Perry Project the "benefits of two years of preschool education in 1979 dollars were $14,819 per child against a two-year program cost of $5,984 per child ($2,992 per year) – a 248 percent return on the original investment" (p. 69). Such benefits include a reduced cost of public education for the children who attended the program (fewer of these children required expensive special services), larger projected lifetime earnings, and the value of mothers' released time while the child attended the program.

The Yale Project

Most of the projects discussed thus far can be considered child-focused in their emphasis. In addition, all have been primarily concerned with intellectual development, few with more real-life measures. Thus, for example, the Milwaukee Project has mainly focused on the child's IQ and language abilities, the Abecedarian on the child's IQ. Although some of these programs have recently discovered other outcomes (e.g., changes in maternal education levels; Ramey et al., in press), most of their interventions and evaluations have not been devoted to such effects.

An exemplary program that featured an entirely different focus was the Yale Project. From 1967 to 1972, Sally Provence and her colleagues mounted the Yale Project, a family support program involving social-work services, pediatric care, voluntary day care, and psychological services to approximately 20 low-income families. The program began prenatally and continued until the child was 30 months (see Provence & Naylor, 1983, for a description of this program). The emphasis of the program was on helping mothers to work with their children themselves, as opposed to the center-based Abecedarian, Milwaukee, and Perry projects. In addition, even during the intervention program, most emphasis was placed on the child's adaptation, not on IQ or cognitive stimulation per se.

In terms of child outcomes, the Yale Project (which also features the strength of not being evaluated by the same investigators who mounted the program) has shown that the major effect of early intervention can be the children's increased school and life success. Although intervention-group children had greater IQs than did control-group children at 30 months (Rescorla, Provence, & Naylor, 1982), and at 5 years (Trickett, Apfel, Rosenbaum, & Zigler, 1982), there were no differences in WISC-R IQ performance at the 10-year follow-up (91.7 for intervention group, 93.3 for controls; Seitz, Rosenbaum, & Apfel, 1985). Most importantly, however, the 10-year follow-up showed that the intervention group – particularly the boys — had outperformed the control group on a variety of school and adaptive measures. Experimental-group boys received fewer special services from their schools, attended school more regularly, and were considered better adjusted by their teachers. Control-group boys, in contrast, were much more likely to have demonstrated serious absenteeism and were less often considered well-adjusted by their schools (Seitz et al., 1985). This program, geared from the beginning toward adjustment of the children, seems to have had a lasting impact in this area.

The Yale Project's family results are equally striking. As shown in Table 8.1, the mothers of experimental and control-group children differed in

Table 8.1. *Comparison of experimental and control family characteristics 10 years after the completion of the Yale Project*

	Groups	
	Experimental	Control
Years of maternal education	13.0	11.7
Number of children per family	1.67	2.2
Proportion of families that are self-supporting	13/15	8/15
Amount of community services resources expended per family, per year[a]	$700	$2,705

[a]Estimated in 1982 dollars.
Note: All comparisons significantly different between the two groups.
Source: Information from Seitz, Rosenbaum, & Apfel (1985).

several respects 10 years after the program had ended. Levels of maternal education averaged 13.0 years in the experimental-group mothers, 11.7 years in control mothers. The fertility rate of mothers who participated in the program continued to remain low years after the end of the program, and their rates of self-support (defined as total monetary self-sufficiency) were higher for experimental-group mothers than for control mothers (Seitz et al., 1985). Taken together, the Yale Project's interventions produced more educated and more employable mothers who were receiving a lesser amount of social services, every year, for themselves and their (smaller) families.

In monetary terms, the benefits of the Yale program vastly outweigh the costs necessary to mount it. Seitz et al. (1985) estimate that the Yale Project cost $20,000 (in 1982 dollars) over its 30 months of operation. However, considering the smaller family size in experimental-group families, the increased employability of experimental-group mothers, and the decreased use of special educational services by experimental-group children, these workers estimate that the total differential between control and experimental groups equaled $40,000 per year (i.e., summed over all 20 subjects). "In comparison with costs, the project currently appears to be paying itself off at the rate of at least two families per year" (Seitz et al., 1985, p. 389). The long-term payoff of the Yale Project can be expected to continue, and possibly even increase, as the children from the program grow older and assume adult responsibilities.

On a variety of measures, then, the Yale Project must be considered successful. Children who participated in the program have shown better social adjustment years after the end of the intervention and the children's families are better off. The costs of the project seem to be reasonable, especially in light of benefits that accumulate with each passing year. This sort of family-based approach seems, in light of all of the available evidence, a better approach to early intervention for at-risk children than those programs that are more center-based, cognitively oriented, and child-centered. As Zigler and Berman (1983) noted in comparing the Yale Project to the Abecedarian Project:

> if equal benefits can be derived from the far less expensive family support approach, and if these benefits extend to the family on a long-term basis, then this alternative appears to hold the advantage. Additionally, because a family support program does not separate a child from the family except at times and by choice, such a program minimizes the discontinuity between children's environments at home and school and is more in keeping with current values in our society. (pp. 903-904)

Summary

In this chapter we have presented an overview of three of the most widely known programs of early intervention, the Abecedarian, Milwaukee, and Perry projects. Each program provided an intensive and long-term intervention to children who were either suspected of being at risk for retardation (Abecedarian, Milwaukee) or who were already identified as retarded in their early years (Perry).

Results demonstrate that children involved in these programs achieved higher IQ scores (although the magnitude and duration of such changes remain unclear), better interactions with their mothers, and, in some programs, better school adjustment and life success. It seems clear from the Abecedarian and Milwaukee results, however, that higher IQ scores do not necessarily ensure better school adjustment for children who have graduated from an early intervention program.

We have concluded this chapter with our own recommendations as to how one should evaluate early intervention programs. Three levels of evaluation, the child, family, and society, were discussed. As concerns the child, we propose that the goal of any early intervention program should be to increase the child's social competence, which is defined as the child's success in meeting societal expectations and the child's self-actualization or personal development. Four aspects of the self-competence construct were discussed: health, formal cognition, academic achievement, and motivation and personality development. We also discussed the various program effects on families and advocate the adoption of family-support programs such as the Yale Project in future early intervention efforts.

9 The search for miracle cures

The previous two chapters reveal a surprising number of areas in which workers can aid retarded people. A person's thinking, language, social skills, and motivation are open to developmental interventions. Behavior modification techniques promote self-help skills and adaptive behavior in even the most severely retarded individuals. The family systems approach helps to anticipate and alleviate problems in the families of at-risk and retarded children. Overall, improvements can be made in a wide array of domains through psychological interventions.

Still, there is the gnawing feeling that all of our best efforts produce only the slowest of progress in any area. We have not "cured" mental retardation with any of these procedures, and no cure seems imminent. At best we have succeeded in improving the lives of retarded individuals to a modest degree.

In recent years, proponents of several widely publicized treatments have proposed to change this situation. These therapies purport to bring about quick, dramatic, and lasting improvements in retarded persons. Some of the therapies have been said to be effective even with the most severely retarded individuals, those for whom traditional interventions are least useful. Two therapies in particular, the Doman-Delacato technique and vitamin therapy, have reportedly produced significant changes in IQ and in adaptive behavior with retarded and brain-damaged individuals. Glenn Doman declared that with his therapy "the rate of neurological growth changes from an average of 35% of normal to an average of 210% of normal" (quoted in Warshaw, 1982, p. 124). Similarly, Harrell, Capp, Davis, Peerless, and Ravitz (1981) described the progress of a 7-year-old boy with an IQ of 25-30 who received vitamin treatments for a prolonged period; he "read and wrote on the elementary school level, was moderately advanced in arithmetic, and, according to his teacher, was mischievous and active. He rode a bicycle and a skate board, played ball, played a flute, and had an IQ of about 90" (p. 574). Clearly, if such claims are valid,

181

these therapies should be prescribed to all retarded children, since their benefits are well beyond those possible with more traditional methods.

In this chapter we will try to evaluate both the Doman-Delacato and vitamin therapies as fairly as possible. Since our conclusion is that neither substantially improves functioning in retarded individuals, we debated giving these approaches any additional attention. However, it is our view that such therapies must be evaluated, especially given the media coverage each has received, the magnitude of the purported effects, and the hopes and vulnerabilities of families of retarded persons to any treatment that essentially promises to cure retardation. We end this chapter with a short discussion of phenylketonuria, an example of a true advance in the field of mental retardation.

The Doman-Delacato procedures

Begun in the late 1950s by physical therapist Glenn Doman and educational psychologist Carl Delacato, the Doman-Delacato "patterning" technique is now widely used to treat mentally retarded and brain-damaged children. Proponents of the patterning treatment assert that the neurological development of brain-damaged and retarded children has been attenuated or arrested at relatively immature stages of development. They argue that if lower-level functions are not adequately mastered, then higher-level abilities cannot be organized properly. Thus a child with perceptual or language difficulties must go back to the very early developmental tasks and begin with relearning to creep or crawl, even if that child can already walk.

The patterning treatment involves first finding the supposed developmental stage at which impairment of neurological growth took place. The child is then retrained from that point through the higher stages until correct neurological organization is achieved. This retraining consists of leading the child through a series of exercises. Three to five volunteers at a time manipulate the child's limbs and head in patterns that allegedly simulate the prenatal and postnatal movements of nonretarded children. According to the theory, if a child makes certain motions frequently enough, previously unused brain cells will become programmed to take over the functions of the damaged cells.

In addition to several books and journal reports, articles about the Doman-Delacato procedures have appeared in popular periodicals like *Look, Good Housekeeping, Reader's Digest,* and the *New York Times.* Under titles such as "Miracle in Pennsylvania" and "The Miracle Boy," many of these articles featured one or two children who made "miraculous recoveries" following these procedures. Most of these reports ignored the scientific controversy over the techniques, although more recently several popular articles have questioned their power to make retarded children "normal" (e.g., Warshaw, 1982), or to turn normal infants into "geniuses" (Blais, 1982; Brinley, 1983).

Given all this fanfare, it is important to scrutinize carefully studies of the Doman-Delacato approach. But first we will discuss the neurological principles underlying the therapy and more fully describe the procedures themselves.

The neurological theory of patterning

The Doman-Delacato technique is based on the idea that children progress along a certain sequence of developments in the motor domain, and that these advances reflect brain organization. Doman and Delacato feel that these developments do indeed form an invariant sequence of stages, the violation of which adversely affects later developments in numerous domains. These stages are also thought to follow a broad evolutionary progression, leading to adult human functioning. Thus, the human infant successively learns to perform the movements of swimming (fish), homolateral crawling (amphibians), cross-pattern crawling (reptiles), gross walking (primates) and, finally, cross-pattern walking (mature human cerebral functioning and hemispheric dominance).

Pathologies of various types are thought to reflect a failure to master earlier motor levels. Thus, if the child is unable to practice and master crawling or creeping, walking will later be affected, as will linguistic and cognitive abilities. Intervention, in the form of the patterning treatment, consists of the following:

(a) permitting the child normal development opportunities in areas in which the responsible brain level was undamaged; (b) externally imposing the bodily patterns of activity which were the responsibility of damaged brain levels; and (c) utilizing additional factors to enhance neurological organization. (Doman, Spitz, Zucman, Delacato, & Doman, 1960, p. 257)

On the surface, this theoretical justification has some appeal. It seems reasonable that failures or inadequate developments at lower levels might affect later progress. Similarly, it is not illogical to assert an invariant stage sequence to motor development. Even the idea that ontogeny recapitulates phylogeny (i.e., that the development of the infant is parallel to the history of human evolution) is not too farfetched, and was advanced by Haeckel in the late 19th century (see Dobzhansky, 1962). The use of recapitulationist theory in explaining development and in intervening with retarded children might also make some sense.

However, several major flaws of the Doman-Delacato perspective become apparent on closer inspection. Throughout the natural sciences, Haeckel's recapitulationist theory has now been discarded. Indeed, "the history of biology is replete with considerations of the weaknesses of recapitulationist theory and no substantial support for the general viewpoint can be drawn from current consideration of the nervous system and its development" (Cohen, Birch, & Taft, 1970, p. 304). The problem, as Dobzhansky (1962) explains, is that "embryos of one animal do not resemble adult forms of other animals, only their embryos" (p. 162). Thus, while vestiges of other animals can be observed in the prenatal stages of higher animals (e.g., the tail of the human embryo), their use as a description of human development (ontogeny) is suspect.

Second, the stagelike character of motor development has not been strongly supported, nor do prior motor achievements appear necessary for later motor developments. Many children show reversals in the usual sequence from crawling to creeping to walking, yet they show no disabilities in later motor, cognitive, or linguistic developments (Cohen et al., 1970). In a study of Hopi Indian infants, Dennis and Dennis (1940) found that babies strapped to cradle boards in the first year of life (a time when most babies crawl and creep) showed no delays in walking compared to a control group of uninhibited Hopi babies. Further, many cerebral palsied and otherwise motorically handicapped children possess cognitive and linguistic skills in the normal and even in the superior range, demonstrating that motor skills are not necessarily related to intellectual development.

Third, there is the issue of the patterning of behavior. According to Delacato (1965), "We have been able to take children who deviated from normal development (severely brain injured) and through the extrinsic imposition of normal patterns of movement and behavior, have been able to neurologically organize them sufficiently so that they could be placed within the human development pattern of crawling, creeping, and walking" (pp. 77-78). However, there is no evidence that such "impositions" affect neurological organization. It is probably very different for a child to crawl voluntarily and to be passively forced to engage in crawling movements. Indeed, such a passive view of the child is rejected by most theorists of child development (see Chapters 2 & 7).

Finally, there is the issue of possible harm done to children who undergo patterning. In this vein, Freeman (1967) notes that "Some brain-damaged children who begin to sit or walk before the Institutes [i.e., the Institutes for the Advancement of Human Potential, run by Doman] decide they have properly mastered the preceding stages of mobility are prevented from doing so by a variety of ingenious devices" (p.84). It is not as yet clear whether children forcibly forbidden to perform higher-level behavior incur further developmental harm. On the other hand, although the theoretical base of the Doman-Delacato program may be weak, it is possible that the procedures may nevertheless prove effective in promoting development in retarded children, an issue to which we now turn.

Research on the Doman-Delacato procedures

The original report of the patterning techniques was presented in 1960 by Doman, Spitz, Zucman, Delacato, and Doman in the *Journal of the American Medical Association*. This study is the main scientific publication to date of the Doman group at the Institutes for the Advancement of Human Potential (IAHP), although several books have also appeared. The study involved 76 brain-damaged children, ranging in age from 1 to 9 years. Children had various impairments, and the severity of brain damage ranged from mild to severe. The length of treatment for these children ranged from 6 to 20 months, with a mean duration of 11 months. All children were categorized as to their level of mobility on a 13-point scale created by the investigators. The scale ranged from no mobility (the 0 level) to cross-pattern walking (Level 13). No control or comparison group was employed.

Treatment in this and other patterning studies consisted of the following:

1 *Patterning* – manipulation of limbs and head in a rhythmic fashion. Each child's level of crawling determines whether the patterning is (a) homolateral (left leg and left arm flexed simultaneously and in the same direction in which head is turned) or (b) cross-pattern (left leg and right arm flexed simultaneously with the head turned to the right).
2 *Crawling and creeping* – Crawling is defined as forward bodily movement with the abdomen in contact with the supporting surface. Creeping is locomotion with the abdomen raised from the surface.
3 *Receptive stimulation* – one or more types of each of the following: visual stimulation (flashing lights, tracking, convergence); tactile stimulation (feeling various textures, shapes, etc.); and auditory stimulation (listening to various noises, sounds, and words).
4 *Expressive activities* – a variety of manual activities (e.g., picking up objects), the goal of which is to develop manual and tactile competency. Creeping and crawling are also considered expressive activities.
5 *Masking* – breathing into an oxygen mask to increase the amount of carbon dioxide inhaled, which is believed to increase cerebral blood flow.
6 *Brachiation* – swinging from a bar or vertical ladder.

7   *Gravity–antigravity activities* – rolling, somersaulting, and hanging upside down.

Each of these activities is presented to all children, depending on their motor level, several times each day, for several minutes at a time.

Results showed that the mean improvement in mobility was 4.2 levels on the 13-level mobility scale. While none of the children could walk at the start of therapy, 11 began to walk independently over the course of the study. The amount of overall improvement did not appear related to the age children began receiving patterning, although 9 of the 11 children who began to walk were below 2 years of age when the study began. Doman et al. (1960) conclude that "We found significant improvement when we compared the results of the classic procedures we had previously followed with the results of procedures described above. It is our opinion that the significance of the difference tends to corroborate the validity of the hypothesis set up as the theoretical basis for the program" (p. 261).

Closer examination of the results reveals a multitude of methodological errors and overstatements of findings. The major flaw is that, despite the comparison to the results of "classic procedures" employed earlier, the study had no control group, or group of children who did not receive patterning over the 11-month span. Thus, progress in the experimental group cannot be compared to gains that would have occurred with no intervention. While the prognosis for brain-damaged and retarded children is not always hopeful, most show some developmental progress over the course of a year, even if no treatment of any type is provided. Comparing the children of the Doman et al. study to a group of similar children who were not treated, Cohen et al. (1970) found no differences in the two groups over 11 months. Of the 16 children in the Doman et al. study under the age of 18 months when therapy began, 9 (56%) were walking at the end of the therapy period. Of 119 retarded and brain-damaged children seen by Cohen et al. at the Einstein Clinic in New York City, 70 (59%) achieved independent walking. As summarized by Cohen et al.,

On the basis of these clinical experiences with essentially untreated children exhibiting delays in motor development, the results reported by the advocates of patterning appear singularly unimpressive and lead to the possible inference that the reported changes were at least as much a function of maturation over time as they were improvement induced by treatment. (1970, p. 306)

Similar evaluations by these authors of gains made in language by patterned children (reported in Delacato, 1963) lead to the identical conclusion: patterned and untreated children make almost identical gains in language over a one-year period.

In actuality, it is difficult to determine just how much the Doman et al.

children really did advance while undergoing patterning. The investigators rated mobility on a scale of 13 levels ranging from no mobility to walking. This would correspond to ages from birth to about 15 months in average children. Doman et al. reported their children increased about 4.4 levels over the 11-month treatment period. By assigning average ages at which different levels develop in normal children, then by examining how far each patterned child progressed (from Table 4 of the Doman et al. report), we calculate the gains of children in the Doman et al. study to be approximately 4.59 months over the 11 months of the program. The rate of progress attained, approximately .42 months per month of therapy (i.e., 4.59 months progressed divided by the 11 months of therapy), is perfectly expectable in a group of retarded children. We therefore must agree with Cohen et al. (1970): The gains of the patterned group are probably not different from those expected by maturation alone.

While the Doman et al. study was too flawed to allow any valid conclusions about the efficacy of patterning, a flurry of studies on its effectiveness appeared in the late 1960s and throughout the 1970s. Many dealt with the treatment's effects on reading and will not be reviewed here (see Robbins & Glass, 1969). Others were poorly designed, involving at least one of two obvious flaws. The first mistake, called "regression to the mean," occurs when the experimenter does not randomly assign subjects to experimental and control groups, but gives the therapy only to the lowest-functioning children. The experimental group will "improve" more than the higher-functioning controls solely because extreme scores always become less extreme on the second testing. No effect of therapy is necessarily involved; the regression of extreme scores toward the mean is but a statistical artifact. The second common mistake in many of these studies lies in "teaching to the test," that is, testing exactly what has just been taught (as in the Doman et al. study). In this way, no conclusions about the child's "underlying brain organization" can be drawn; the child has simply had more practice on the specific test items by the second testing, since this is what the therapy involved.

Two of the better-designed studies on the effects of patterning do deserve mention, however. Sparrow and Zigler (1978) placed 45 severely retarded children into three groups of 15 each, all matched on CA, MA, IQ, and other characteristics. The first group received the patterning treatment for two hours per day, five days per week over a one-year period. The second group received a so-called motivational treatment for an equivalent amount of time. This treatment was "geared toward improving motivation by simply creating a warm relationship with an adult who provided continual positive reinforcement" (Sparrow & Zigler, 1978, p. 143). A third group received no treatment other than the standard care provided for residents at the institution.

Development was assessed with a plethora of measures, including the Institutes' Developmental Profile and tests of general intelligence, motor development, language, affective and social behavior, and maladaptive behavior. All together, there were 22 separate scores covering virtually all areas of functioning in these severely retarded children. By the end of the year, however, no overall differences were found among the three groups. On only one of the 22 dependent measures, time not attending to the relevant aspects of the environment, did the two treatment groups (patterning and motivational treatments) differ from the control group. Even this finding could have been due to chance, as there were 22 measures and 1 in 20 analyses could be expected to show differences by chance alone. Sparrow and Zigler (1978) concluded, "No evidence was found that [patterning] treatment resulted in any improvement in the children's performance over what would be expected on the basis of attention (as assessed by the performance of the motivational group) and maturation" (p. 148).

In a second study, Neman, Roos, McCann, Menolascino, and Heal (1974) examined the effects of patterning on moderately retarded institutionalized children. The children were carefully selected for age (M = 15 years), IQ (above 30), diagnoses (no Down syndrome, blind, or deaf children), and "neurological level" (from the Institutes' Profile of Development). They were then randomly assigned to one of three conditions of 22 children each: Experimental 1, a patterning group; Experimental 2, a group that received a "less structured" curriculum of physical activities and caretaker attention; and Control, a group that received no therapy of any type. The study lasted for seven months, with therapy given two hours each weekday for the first two and a half months, and seven days a week thereafter.

Dependent measures included tests of intelligence, language, visual perception, and motor abilities. Overall, 46 scores were obtained for each child at each testing. Testing occurred four times: before the therapy period began, three months later, immediately following the end of therapy, and three months after the therapy was completed.

While the results of this study were complicated, several relatively clear-cut findings did emerge. First, there were no dramatic cases of individual improvement, nor were there changes in global intelligence. In addition, "with two exceptions, no significant changes in motor performance were observed." However, "significant improvement associated with the sensorimotor group [Experimental 1] was seen most strongly with the Profile of Development," and "some significant improvements associated with the Experimental 1 program were observed in language development and spatial perception" (Neman et al., 1974, p. 381). The researchers concluded, "The question raised in the present study – does sensorimotor patterning have a measurable effect in any behavioral domain — has been answered affirmatively" (p. 382).

Although the Neman et al. study is an improvement over many others on the effectiveness of the patterning therapy, Zigler and Seitz (1975) cite numerous areas in which the Neman et al. study remains open to serious methodological criticism. First, it is unclear whether the Experimental 2 group received equal amounts of time and caretaking energies as did the Experimental 1 group. (This question is raised because we were told the patterning group's program was "individualized" while that of the Experimental 2 group was not.) Second, the major finding of "significant improvement" in the patterning group was on the Profile of Development. However, the tasks on this measure are virtually identical to the therapy these children received (the therapists "taught to the test"), which weakens the results substantially. Third, the use of the Developmental Profile as a sensitive measure of neurological level must itself be questioned, since the instrument shows gains of 4–6 months in "neurological level" when the child passes only one or two more items. Given that testers may not have been "blind" to the treatment condition of each child, a tester suspecting that a child received patterning would need only give credit for one or two close items in order for the child to show a gain of from 4 to 8 months in neurological age. Finally and perhaps most importantly, Zigler and Seitz (1975) questioned the statistical analyses used by Neman et al., analyses that increased the possibility of finding differences in the three conditions due only to chance (the gains in language and spatial perception seem most likely to have been due to chance). Weighing all of these methodological flaws, Zigler and Seitz (1975) concluded that "the positive findings of the sensorimotor training program should be discounted" (p. 491). The interested reader is referred to the original study by Neman et al. (1974), the criticism of that study by Zigler and Seitz (1975), and the Neman (1975) reply to that criticism for firsthand discussions.

Possible harmful effects of the patterning treatment

Any human treatment should first be assessed against the principle of *Primum non noscere* (first not to injure). To date there is no evidence that patterning causes any harm, although Freeman (1967) questioned the effects of not allowing children to perform behaviors they appear ready to perform, simply because the therapist wants sufficient "neurological organization" to take place first.

However, the retarded child is not the only one affected by therapy. Parents and other family members are the ones who implement therapies, pay for them, and have expectations as to the outcomes. In this broader sense the Doman-Delacato therapy may indeed cause injury to its participants.

Let us look closer at the patterning procedures. Patterning can be described as a time-consuming, rigidly applied, rigorous, and expensive therapy. It must be administered to a child on an individual basis exactly as mandated, for hours every day, 365 days a year. Dozens of trainers are required, as the techniques require three to five persons to manipulate the child's arm and legs in rhythmic patterns. Even if these trainers are unpaid volunteers, the treatment itself is expensive since courses and materials from the Institutes must be bought.

In view of such difficulties, it is doubtful whether the patterning treatment can be executed perfectly. When the program does not deliver its promised effects, parents may feel that it is their fault, since they might have done a pattern wrong one day or missed a session (which is highly probable since so many are required). Warshaw (1982) describes the feelings of one parent who received little consolation from the Institutes' personnel:

Their attitude was, "You have failed; we have not," says Polly Spare of Doylestown (PA), who worked devotedly for almost three years patterning her brain-injured son, Chris. Chris was later institutionalized. When his patterning failed, Chris' mother says, Institutes' personnel "were not available to discuss what else they could do." (p. 187)

Such stories of parents made to feel guilty when their children did not respond to patterning are commonplace in recent articles about the Doman-Delacato procedures (e.g, Blais, 1982; Brinley, 1983; Warshaw, 1982).

The effects of the patterning regimen on other family members may also be detrimental. In Chapter 7, we learned that siblings of retarded children have a greater-than-average risk of suffering emotional problems (Gath, 1977, 1978). One explanation may be that parents give inordinate amounts of time and care to their retarded child, while the other children receive less parental attention and emotional support. We suspect that the patterning treatment may exacerbate this problem. In patterning, most if not all of the parents' efforts and resources (financial and emotional) are focused on the child. Parents, volunteers, and perhaps the siblings themselves all work unceasingly to help the child. There is little time or energy to give to the needs of other family members, which naturally take a lower priority. These families may suffer irreversible consequences to their personal relationships and family functioning as a result of the Doman-Delacato program.

Finally there is the issue of guilt and dashed hopes in families that have attempted patterning:

Perhaps the worst result of all is that a decision to end treatment, despite its legitimate basis, may leave parents laden with guilt. Any family with an exceptional child often feels that it is somehow their fault that their child is not normal. To add to that guilt by offering them, as their only hope, a program which may be impossible to carry out over an extended period of time is simply cruel . . . The old saw about the cure being worse than the disease may prove sadly true for families who try patterning. (Zigler, 1981, p. 390)

Our conclusion is that the patterning treatment has not been shown to produce impressive gains for retarded or brain-damaged children. None of the few studies that have carefully examined the program has shown large gains in any area, with any type of child, and even the few controversial gains reported are in selected areas of functioning (e.g., the "neurological age" of the IAHP's Developmental Profile). The impression that patterning may be worthless or even harmful is shared by the American Academy of Pediatrics, the American Association on Mental Deficiency, the National Association for Retarded Citizens, and other professional groups. Many professionals in child development and in mental retardation have also expressed grave reservations about the efficacy of the Doman-Delacato procedures. In view of these opinions and the time and cost of the Doman-Delacato program, there does not appear to be any justification for its continued use.

Vitamin therapy

Another therapy to receive widespread interest in the mental retardation field is the vitamin therapy work of Ruth Harrell and her colleagues. While the practice of treating retarded children with vitamins has been discussed for a long time (see Williams, 1956), vitamin therapy received renewed attention after a study by Harrell et al. in 1981. This study purported to show substantial IQ gains in retarded children who received large daily doses of vitamins. After reviewing the theoretical background for the treatment (i.e., the concept of genetotrophic disease), we will discuss the Harrell et al. study and the many attempts to replicate these findings.

The concept of genetotrophic disease

The starting point for nutritional therapies is the idea that each person has individual nutritional requirements, that "each individual's nutritional needs have been genetically predetermined and that the logical direction for the clinician to follow is to identify those needs and those individuals who may be at risk of not meeting those needs" (Raitan & Massaro, in press). It follows that there are certain diseases, called genetotrophic diseases, brought about or affected by an increased or decreased supply of certain nutrients. Examples of conditions of this type include anemia (i.e., iron deficiency), diabetes (insufficient insulin production), lactose (milk) intolerance, and, to a certain extent, high blood pressure. Each is cured, controlled, or lessened in its effects by dietary changes.

As applied to mental retardation, the concept of genetotrophic disease implies that dietary changes can alleviate the effects of certain types of retardation or prevent them from occurring at all. The best example is phenylketonuria (PKU), a genetically caused defect in enzyme production that can be treated by a phenylalanine-free diet (to be discussed later). The success of dietary treatment for PKU, and the finding that Down syndrome children have different blood levels of certain nutrients compared to nonretarded children (Matin, Sylvester, Edwards, & Dickerson, 1981), both lend some credence to the genetotrophic concept as it applies to mental retardation.

The Harrell et al. study

The study by Ruth Harrell and her co-workers was an attempt to increase functioning in retarded children by giving them high doses of certain nutrients. The impetus for the study was a reported case in which the IQ of a 7-year-old boy changed from 25 to 90 (with concomitant changes in social skills) after he received vitamin supplements. Harrell and her colleagues first selected 22 retarded children (mean CA = 9.2 years) and asked an outside consultant to form two groups "matched primarily on IQ." The consultant placed 10 children in Group 1, 12 in Group 2. Several children dropped out during the course of the experiment, leaving only 5 in Group 1 and 11 in Group 2.

The study consisted of two experimental periods, each lasting four months. During the first phase, the children in Group 1 received vitamin supplements while those in Group 2 received placebos. During the second phase both groups received supplements. Intelligence tests were administered at the beginning of the study and at the end of each phase.

The results showed that after four months, the five children of Group 1 increased in IQ while the 11 children in Group 2 did not. After the second phase, when all children had received vitamins, both groups increased in IQ over prestudy levels. For Group 1, the average IQ changed from 46.3 to 59.8 over the eight months that these children received vitamins; over the four months that Group 2 children received supplements, the average IQ changed from 44.7 to 58.7. Harrell et al. (1981) concluded that "our exploratory double-blind study supports the hypothesis that mental retardations in part have genetotrophic origins and that suitable nutritional intervention can improve the IQ and functioning of severely retarded children" (p. 577).

Although these results are suggestive, at least two problems with the Harrell et al. study must be mentioned. One is the small number of children who remained in Group 1; any results obtained with only five subjects are suspect. A larger problem is posed by the skewed attrition rates in the two groups. Half of the children who began vitamin therapy at the start of the study dropped out, but only one child in the larger group who initially received placebos was lost. The children remaining in Group 1 may have been those showing the most improvement, or those most motivated to try the therapy, or even those suffering the least side effects.

Another significant problem is that Harrell herself was one of the two examiners who administered the intelligence tests. While she may or may not have known which children received vitamins during the first phase, after the second phase she knew that every child had received supplements. This was therefore not a double-blind study, or a study in which each child's experimental condition is unknown to him- or herself and to the examiner. The scores on tests given by Harrell were, in fact, generally higher than those obtained by outside examiners who did not know which children received which treatment. The effect of this procedural error is that any difference due to the vitamin therapy may have been magnified, although it is difficult to determine to what extent. Still, the Harrell et al. findings are intriguing and have led several researchers to attempt to replicate the work.

Replications of the Harrell et al. study

The excitement over the Harrell et al. results has now led to at least six attempts to replicate their findings. In each of these studies, a vitamin supplement identical to that used by Harrell was given to half of the retarded sample, placebos to the other half. The replication studies also attempted to improve on the Harrell design by ensuring a double-blind procedure – no examiners, children, parents, or teachers knew whether any particular child was receiving vitamins or placebos. In addition, several of these studies employed multiple dependent measures to determine exactly which areas of intelligence (if any) were affected by the vitamin supplements.

Table 9.1 describes the six studies. They varied widely in the etiologies of the children employed, their ages, IQs, and MAs, and in their living settings (institutions versus homes). Several studies also examined the prestudy and poststudy nutritional status of the children. As can be seen in the table, all of the studies led to the same finding. There were no IQ differences between those children who received vitamins and those who did not. In fact, in four studies the vitamin groups showed slight decreases in IQ from pretreatment to posttreatment testings. The vitamin groups in the remaining two studies showed only marginal (nonsignificant) IQ gains.

Even though the vitamin groups generally remained the same, it is nevertheless conceivable that individual children with certain disorders might have benefited from vitamin supplements. This notion was suggested by the original Harrell study, in which Down syndrome children increased in IQ more than the group as a whole. However, as Table 9.1 indicates, none of the replication studies supports even this more limited benefit of vitamin supplements. Of the studies that reported individual changes as well as overall group means, none reported a gain of over 10 IQ points for any child receiving vitamins (although one child in the placebo group increased 19 points in the Weathers study). Thus, even the possibility that vitamins affect particular types of retardation is not supported by these studies.

The conclusion must be that vitamin supplements do not improve intellectual functioning. Although suggestive, the original Harrell et al. study was too flawed to prove the efficacy of vitamins in boosting IQ, and later, more carefully done studies have been unable to replicate her findings. These studies also found no substantial increases in IQ for individual children. Undoubtedly, more studies will soon be published in this area, but the hope that vitamins will greatly increase intellectual functioning in retarded persons seems unfounded.

Other nutritional therapies

The vitamin therapy tested by Harrell and her co-workers is but the latest in a long line of attempts to cure mental retardation through nutritional supplements. From the 1940s to the present, glutamic acid, tranquilizers, stimulants, and other compounds have been given to retarded persons. For a short period, each has been heralded as the poten-

Table 9.1. *Attempted replications of the Harrell et al. vitamin study*

Study	Subject characteristics	Treatment length	IQs	Extreme changes	Comments
Bennett, McClelland, Kriegsman, Anarus, & Sellas (1983)	$N = 20$ (10–V; 10–Pl) CA = 10 years Down syndrome	8 months	Vitamin subjects pre = 53.1, post = 52.5 Placebo subjects pre = 45.2, post = 46.0	None over 10 pts.	No significant differences between groups on Stanford-Binet, PPVT, ITPA, physical, hearing, or nutritional measures. Matched pairs design, on CA, sex, SES. Double-blind. Placebo subjects slightly younger and of lower IQ (might lead to better performance). Home-reared children.
Ellis & Temporowski (1983)	$N = 40$ (19–V; 21–Pl) CA = 29 Some Down syndrome, others "problematic"	7 months	Vitamin subjects pre = 26.5, post = 25.1 Placebo subjects pre = 26.2, post = 25.1	None over 9 pts.	No group differences. Significant decrease in IQ over time (both groups). ABS subscale shows no group differences. Matching techniques unreported (by CA & IQ, by group?). Testers blind to subjects' groups. Institutionalized adults.
Smith, Spiker, Peterson, Cicchetti, & Justice (1984)	$N = 56$ (28–V; 28–Pl) CA = 11 Down syndrome	8 months	Vitamin subjects pre = 45.0, post = 43.9 Placebo subjects pre = 46.2, post = 45.0	None over 9 pts.	Pairs matched on IQ, age, sex, & type of education program. Testers blind to subjects' groups; no tester retested same child. Decreasing IQ over time. No group differences on WISC-R, WISC-R subtests, motor, or visual tests. Home-reared children.

Study	Sample	Duration	Scores	Gains	Comments
Weathers (1983)	$N = 47$ (24–V; 23–Pl) CA = 6–17 Down syndrome	4 months	Vitamin subjects pre = 45.6, post = 46.4 Placebo subjects pre = 45.4, post = 48.9	One control subject gained 19 pts. (no info on others).	Matching on IQ, CA, early stimulation experiences, and prior nutritional supplementation. Testers blind to subjects' groups. No group difference on Stanford-Binet, Visual-Motor Integration, or weekly parent behavior records. Home-reared children.
Ellman, Silverstein, Zingarelli, Schafer, & Silverstein (1984)	$N = 20$ (10–V; 10–PL) CA = 21 Varied	6 months	Vitamin subjects pre = 39.3, post = 40.5 Placebo subjects pre = 38.8, post = 39.5	None over 9 pts.	No group differences on Leiter or Likert ratings of behavior. Subjects assigned to one of two matched groups on basis of CA, sex, diagnosis. Double-blind.
Coburn, Schaltenbrand, Mahuren, Clausman, & Townsend (1983)	$N = 58$ (18–Pl; 20–V1; 10–V2)	20 weeks	Vitamin subjects pre = 27.9, post = 27.0 Placebo subjects pre = 30.4, post = 30.5		Four groups: 1 Harrell's therapy, 1 RDA vitamins, & 1 B vitamins, 1 placebo. Averages estimated by authors. No group differences on Stanford-Binet. Matching procedures not reported. Averages for placebo versus Harrell vitamin groups.

tial "magic bullet" (Yannett, 1953) that would supposedly cure retardation.

Usually, early clinical and case reports supported the use of the particular supplement. For example, in the case of glutamic acid, Louttit (1965) reported that "during the decade from 1946 to 1956 over four dozen studies appeared in the literature, approximately two out of three supporting the hypothesis that glutamic acid therapy has a beneficial effect on intellectual performance among the retarded" (p. 495). With time, however, each of these supplements has been proven ineffective. Again concerning glutamic acid, Astin and Ross (1960) noted that "positive effects tend to be reported in studies not employing a control group"; in contrast, "the more carefully designed studies tend to be negative almost without exception" (p. 433). (Although see Vogel, Broverman, Draguns, & Klaiger, 1966, for a call to reopen the question of the effects of glutamic acid on intelligence.) A similar pattern of early hope based on uncontrolled studies, followed by a dashing of that hope once more exacting studies were performed, seems to characterize the history of a variety of dietary supplements given to retarded people.

One reason why nutritional therapies appear doomed to failure is that they are based on the notion that nutrition is a critical factor in determining intelligence. This seems not to be the case. In fact, studies performed in third-world countries have demonstrated that only severe and prolonged malnutrition causes a lowering of IQ (and even this finding is currently being debated; see Bejar, 1981). As discussed in Chapter 4 with respect to the nature–nurture issue, nutrition, like most aspects of the environment, does not seem to be linear in its effects. Thus, children from very impoverished backgrounds (in this case, where high levels of malnutrition exist) probably do suffer some impairment in cognitive functioning. From the levels of "barely adequate nutrition" to "well fed," however, no effects on intelligence are discernible. In statistical terms, nutrition does not appear to account for much of the variance in differences in level of intelligence. It is but one aspect of the environment, and the environment accounts for only a portion of the variability in intelligence.

The case of phenylketonuria

While it is unlikely that one vitamin or nutrient will help in all types of retardation, a single agent is responsible in certain circumscribed disorders. Such is the case in phenylketonuria (PKU). The PKU story describes one of the major advances in the field of mental retardation; it is also a tale of providential accident. Asbjorn Følling (1934), a Norwegian physician, noted that several retarded children brought to him had a musty odor. During routine tests he discovered that when he added ferric chloride to their urine, it turned green instead of the usual red (see MacMillan, 1982). Dr. Følling guessed (and was subsequently proven correct) that these children suffered from an inability to convert the amino acid phenylalanine to tyrosine, because of a deficiency in a specific enzyme produced in the liver.

In essence, Følling had discovered a true genetotrophic disease, one we now call an "inborn error of metabolism," caused by an overabundance of a substance that is toxic in large doses. In PKU, a genetically caused inability to metabolize phenylalanine causes a buildup of the substance in the blood to 20–30 times normal levels (Woolf, 1970). A poisoning of the brain then takes place, resulting in a rapid decline in intelligence from near normal levels to severe and profound retardation over the first several years of life.

With this discovery, it was not long until a dietary treatment was devised. First suggested by Woolf and Vulliamy (1951), a diet containing only small amounts of phenylalanine proved effective in treating PKU. (Since this amino acid is necessary for growth and development, even children with PKU require small amounts.) The diet must be strictly adhered to and closely monitored throughout the early years. The success of treatment is related to how soon the diet is begun. Baumeister (1967) reviewed 167 reported cases of PKU and concluded that "favorable results occur most consistently in the group in which treatment was begun under 15 weeks of age" (p. 843). Indeed, the damage done by PKU toxicity appears to be completed by 3 years of age; when treatment was begun after 160 weeks, "the distribution of IQs is essentially identical to that of untreated phenylketonurics" (Baumeister, 1967, p. 844).

Since the sooner treatment is begun the better, early diagnosis of PKU is imperative. Today all newborns are screened about three days after birth, by a blood test called the Guthrie Test. At this time boys with PKU already show elevated levels of phenylalanine. However, newborn girls oftentimes do not yet show elevated blood levels. For this reason a second screening, performed two weeks after birth, is necessary for girls but is also given to boys. Another idiosyncrasy of the Guthrie Test is that it overidentifies premature infants, who often show elevated phenylalanine levels for short periods of time. Indeed, Holtzman, Meek, and Mellits (1974) found that for every infant found to have classical PKU, there were 18 false positives. In virtually every case, the babies falsely identified as having PKU actually had only transient elevations of the amino acid in their blood.

Although the diagnosis and treatment of PKU has all but eradicated its dire consequences, the treatment is far from perfect. Untreated PKU children have IQs averaging about 25 (Jervis, 1963). If treatment begins in the first few weeks of life, phenylketonurics have IQs in the 90s, a level slightly lower than their unaffected siblings (Berman, Waisman, & Graham, 1966; Dobson, Kushida, & Friedman, 1976). Of course, the diet does not correct the metabolic defect, but it prevents its most destructive effects. The diet can be difficult to adhere to, however, as many common foods contain phenylalanine. As children grow older and begin to enjoy the social pleasures of food, they do not want to appear different from their peers, and the temptation to stray from the diet increases.

Even with these problems in the identification and treatment of PKU, the discovery of its cause and management remains one of the greatest success stories in the history of mental retardation. The management of the effects of PKU also began a new field of research into other inborn errors of metabolism. Discoveries so far include maple syrup urine disease (so named because the urine smells like maple syrup), galactosemia, cystathioninuria, and lysinuria, all caused by metabolic disorders that prohibit the digestion of one or another specific substance (see Clarke & Clarke, 1974b). Although each of these diseases is rare, much success has been achieved in identifying afflicted children and in preventing the tragedy of mental retardation through dietary means.

Conclusion

The long search for miracle cures has taught one clear lesson: There is not, nor is there ever likely to be, one single cure for mental retardation. Where dietary treatments are involved, success has only occurred in specific disorders caused by errors in metabolism. Having identified a toxic substance in the blood or urine, investigators have been able to stop or slow brain cell damage through a diet specifically tailored toward lowering the toxicity. In contrast, the vitamin therapies that have been tried are neither specific to a single etiology of retardation nor individualized to the needs of each child. As such, they violate the very concept of genetotrophic disease (Reitan & Massaro, in press). These therapies attempt to cure many different types of retardation with a single elixir.

Still, it is seductive to search for and believe in a magic cure for mental retardation. Both vitamin therapy and the Doman-Delacato procedures, as two examples of attempts to find such cures, have excited many parents of retarded children and workers in the field. The widespread disappointment of parents who have tried patterning and vitamin therapies may help other parents to avoid the anguish and expense caused by such therapies.

As the father of one 7-year-old Down syndrome child said in relation to vitamin therapy (but equally true of patterning), "We had to give this a try, but now it is back more than ever to the hard, day-to-day work of helping our son function to the best of his abilities" (Bennett et al., 1983, p. 713).

Part V

Caring for retarded people

10 Institutionalization

A continuing problem in the field of mental retardation is where and how retarded people shall live. Almost daily, the media report that a parent group is suing to close a local mental retardation facility, that there is a scandal at a state institution, or that area residents are opposed to the opening of a group home in their neighborhood. In many of these cases, good arguments can be made for or against a particular practice. Indeed, as with many of the social issues raised by mental retardation, the questions regarding the residential placements of retarded persons are both complicated and of long-standing duration.

In approaching this issue, it is helpful to begin by discussing the historical background of institutions for retarded people. We then review studies of the effects of different types of institutions on their retarded residents. (The effects of institutions in general were covered in Chapter 6.) We end this chapter with a short discussion of deinstitutionalization, the practice of moving retarded persons from large institutions to smaller group-home or community settings.

The history of American institutions for the retarded

Settings specifically designed to care for retarded people originated more than a century ago. The first institutions appeared in the state of Massachusetts, where Samuel Gridley Howe established the first public facility in 1850 in Boston (this facility later became the Fernald State School in Waltham) and Harvey Wilbur founded the first private facility in 1848 in Barre (the Elm Hill School). By 1890, there were approximately 20 residential schools in 15 states (Haskell, 1944).

The opening of these institutions was harmonious with the optimistic spirit of the times – a general belief in the inevitable advancement of the social, political, scientific, and moral qualities of humankind. This spirit favored the development of the many social institutions and services that

203

arose in the middle and late 1800s. At this time, schools were founded for blind, deaf, and mentally ill persons, and the professions of social work, education, medicine, and nursing were all established. As Best (1965) notes, "Probably the world has never known, before or since, such a pouring out of sympathy for the afflicted of society, a more zealous resolve to speed their relief, nor a more ardent faith in the possibilities of education" (p. 185).

The founders of American "training schools" (institutions for retarded people) were also influenced by the 19th century belief in progress. In particular, they were excited by news of the "physiological education" developed by Édouard Seguin in France. Seguin's training program was based upon stimulation of the muscles and senses, and was considered capable of greatly boosting retarded functioning. Thus society's concern for retarded persons was joined with the new, widely acclaimed methods for treating retardation, and schools for retarded children were born.

In a larger sense, however, Seguin's most influential contribution to the training of retarded persons in the United States was not his sensory method, but his view of "moral education" (Kraft, 1961). This view, prevalent in the treatment of many types of "defective" individuals (e.g., the blind and the emotionally impaired) and consistent with 19th century thought, included "the effort to reestablish the equilibrium of the desires or drives of the disturbed individual, to change the conditions of the environment, and in a careful manner to replace the sick personality of the patient with the total consciousness of the therapist by a strong act of will" (Kraft, 1961, p. 402). Featuring the disavowal of inhumane therapies and of harsh discipline, moral education aimed for a loving relationship between the teacher and pupil and the gentle bending of the will of the retarded student to that of the teacher. Proponents of moral education assumed that teaching retarded children involved "reawakening" them into a normal human existence.

Moral education was obviously characterized by an overoptimism concerning how much the environment could improve retarded functioning. Early pioneers such as Seguin and founders of the first training schools such as Howe, Wilbur, and Isaac Kerlin generally believed that their programs could cure retardation, or at least greatly alleviate its effects. Although some of these men (e.g., Howe) occasionally expressed reservations as to the limits of treatment, the following quotation from *Harper's Magazine* is typical of 19th century views:

all except the lowest grade (are) improvable up to the level of the average mass of mankind; . . . (they are) susceptible of great improvement . . . to care for their

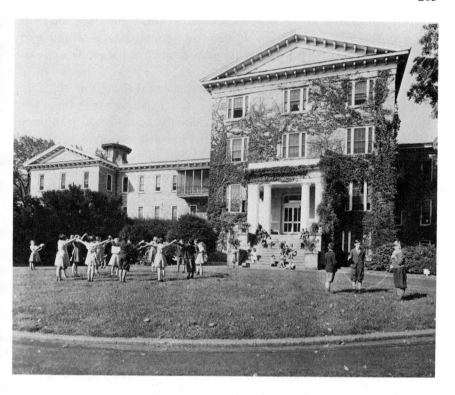

Photo 5. Recreational programs, 1930. (Photograph courtesy of Elwyn Institutes, Elwyn, Pennsylvania)

own safety . . . to distinguish between right and wrong . . . to acquire some forms of knowledge . . . and to reach a conception of their Maker and Redeemer. (from Best, 1965, p. 187)

At the same time, however, the very idea of teaching retarded people was new, and was therefore not readily accepted. In response to Samuel Gridley Howe's report calling for an educational facility for retarded children, his daughter recalls "There were people who laughed and said to one another: 'What do you think Howe is going to do next? *He is going to teach idiots!*' " (Richards, 1935, p. 172). State legislators were particularly wary of spending large sums on such uncertain ventures, and even after the establishment of a facility, its status remained tenuous. (The Kentucky legislature actually closed down a new facility for one year.) Administrators felt a need to "show results"; hence the practice of admitting only the "highest-grade defectives" to most institutions, the many public exhibitions of the skills learned by the residents, and the encouragement of visitors to the first residences, to come and "see for themselves." The glowing reports written by administrators of the early institutions were probably in part attempts to impress the public and state legislators.

Gradually, however, the early optimism concerning the effects of training on the functioning of retarded people began to fade. Although there were signs of improvement in many residents, administrators of early institutions concurred that only 10-25% eventually became self-sufficient members of the community (Wolfensberger, 1969). This rate of success was not as great as first predicted and therefore was seen as a failure. The emphasis began shifting from the residential school designed to teach retarded children during the school years to the long-term custodial facility.

It must be noted that the change from an instructional to a custodial focus was not spurred by malevolent motives. Institutional administrators were simply facing the fact that not all retarded children could be returned to the community as self-sufficient adults, and that there was a need for institutional care over the life span. Thus, in the 1880s Governor Benjamin F. Butler of Massachusetts spoke of the need to give retarded individuals "good and kind treatment; but not a school," and Wilmarth (1902) noted that "Institutions have changed their character, largely to furnish a permanent residence with congenial surroundings for those unfortunates" (from Wolfensberger, 1969, p. 96). Still, the loss of the original instructional focus was to prove harmful to retarded people in later years.

On the larger societal level as well, changes in attitudes toward retarded persons were occurring in the late 19th and early 20th centuries. Galton's studies of genius throughout generations of prominent British families and the rediscovery of Mendel's work led to an acceptance of genetic explanations of intelligence. Mendel's work in particular fostered the many studies of multigenerational subnormality during this period, such as Dugdale's (1877; 1910) study of the Juke family and Goddard's (1912) study of the Kallikaks. People began to believe that mental retardation was the inevitable and irreversible consequence of genetic inheritance. Other studies demonstrated that retarded people were overrepresented in prisons and retarded women were bearing disproportionate numbers of illegitimate children (see Davies & Ecob, 1959). Retardation came to be seen as a genetically caused phenomenon, peculiar to the lower classes of society, and closely associated with poverty, illegitimacy, and criminality (see also Doll, 1962; Baumeister, 1970; Scheerenberger, 1983a).

A second major influence on societal attitudes was the intelligence test movement. The first intelligence tests were created by the French psychologist, Alfred Binet, in 1905. The tests were introduced in the United States by Henry Goddard after he took over the Training School in Vineland, New Jersey, in 1906. The use of the Binet-Simon tests (and later of the Stanford revision, with its IQ measure) spread rapidly, and workers began to realize the extent of retardation in society. In addition, Goddard's yearly testing at the Training School demonstrated that "the vast majority of feeble-minded children are not changing and are not improving in their intelligence levels" (1913, p. 123), a finding that Walter Fernald called "the most significant . . . and the most discouraging that we have ever known" (1913, p. 127).

Genetic explanations for mental retardation, the linking of retardation to other social ills, and the knowledge of how prevalent and intractable retardation actually was led to what Fernald (1924; also, Sloan, 1963) called "the legend of the feebleminded." Fernald's own harsh but not atypical statement of 1912 reflects this view:

The feebleminded are a parasitic, predatory class, never capable of self-support or of managing their own affairs. The great majority ultimately become public charges in some form. . . . Feebleminded women are almost invariably immoral and if at large usually become carriers of venereal disease or give birth to children who are as defective as themselves. . . . Every feebleminded person, especially the high-grade imbecile, is a potential criminal, needing only the proper environment and opportunity for the development and expression of his criminal tendencies. (From Davies & Ecob, 1959, pp. 47-48)

This myth concerning retarded persons had an inevitable effect on the nature of treatment facilities. Institutions became larger and were now built in remote rural areas "to protect society from the deviant" (Wolfensberger, 1969). In addition, the number of institutions increased rapidly, as can be seen in Figure 10.1.

It was also during this period that sterilization laws were passed. Eugenicists had advocated such laws, promising the "possible improvement of the human breed" (Galton, 1901). The issue first became prominent in meetings of institutional administrators during the early 1900s (Johnson, 1906; Risley, 1905; Barr, 1904). Indiana passed the first state sterilization law in 1907. In 1927 these state statutes received full legal support when the Supreme Court ruled favorably on Virginia's sterilization law. Justice Oliver Wendell Holmes expressed the Court's sentiments with his famous declaration that "Three generations of imbeciles are enough" (*Buck* v. *Bell*, 1927). By 1936, 25 states had passed laws permitting the involuntary and systematic sterilization of retarded men and women (see Deutsch, 1949). Although California was the only state to practice sterilization of retarded individuals on a large scale, sterilization stands out as among the

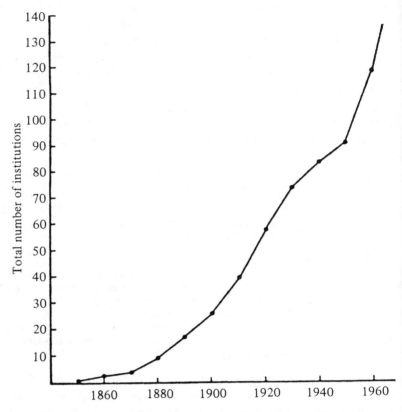

Figure 10.1. Total number of institutions in the United States, 1860–1960. (Baumeister, 1970, with permission)

worst practices to which retarded persons have been subjected (see Davies & Ecob, 1959).

By the mid-1920s, however, societal views toward retarded people shifted again, this time in a more positive direction. Workers began to realize that retardation was not the cause of all social ills, and that there were "good defectives and bad defectives," the good far outnumbering the bad. The leader in this reevaluation was, again, Walter Fernald. In 1919 Fernald published a widely influential study of 646 retarded children who had been released from the Waverly School (later, the Fernald School) in Massachusetts during the previous 25 years. Most of them had been released under administrators' protests – Fernald recalls that "We honestly believed that nearly all of these people should remain in the institution indefinitely" (from Davies, 1930, p. 191). Of the 176 women who had been released, slightly over half (90) had either married, were single and self-supporting, or were living at home and performing work commensurate with their abilities. The other half (86) had died or been readmitted to Waverly or another institution. Outcomes of the males released from the institution were similar. Slightly over half (240 of 470) had made at least a fair adjustment to life outside the institution, whereas the other half had either died, been arrested, or been readmitted. As Fernald summarized, "The survey shows that there are bad defectives and good defectives . . . And it shows much justice in the plea of the well-behaved adult defective to be given a trial outside for apparently a few defectives do not need or deserve life-long segregation" (from Davies, 1930, pp. 200–201).

The years following the 1920s reflect several trends in the care of retarded people. First, as Baumeister (1970) noted, the period from 1915 to 1935 was one of extensive utilization of the large institutions. During this 20-year period, the number of institutional residents rose from 30,000 to 100,000 (all figures approximate). Even when considered in relation to the growing U.S. population, this rise signified a dramatic increase; whereas only 30 of every 100,000 Americans resided in institutions for the retarded in 1915, almost 80 per 100,000 were institutional residents in 1935 (Baumeister, 1970).

Second, the post-1920 period featured the beginnings of community care for retarded people. Faced with growing waiting lists and state legislatures reluctant to allocate more money for institutional care, administrators began to realize that not all retarded individuals could be served by residential facilities. In response, several alternative methods of care were tried. A short (and incomplete) description of some of these innovations follows.

Parole. With the awareness that many retarded individuals could adjust to the community, "parole" from institutions was attempted to a limited degree. For the most part, such extra-institutional care was entrusted to the retarded person's immediate family or other relatives. A study in 1922 (Hoakley, 1922) found that 17 of 26 institutions surveyed had a parole system in operation, although most involved only small numbers of residents. These systems operated throughout the United States.

Early diagnosis and parental counseling. Since much of the impetus for institutional placements came from families unable to handle their retarded children, Walter Fernald instituted his "psychological clinic" at the Waverly facility in 1891. To ensure the early identification of mental retardation, children three or more years behind in school were evaluated on Fernald's (1922) "ten fields of inquiry." This was a multidisciplinary assessment that included a physical exam, family history, personal and developmental histories, information on school progress, and a psychological test. Parents of identified retarded children were then counseled, so they could continue to keep their offspring at home.

Colonies. Begun in New York State in 1908, colonies consisted of small numbers (10–20) of retarded persons living under the supervision of a farmer and his wife. The residents worked on the farm, partially supporting themselves through their labors. Such programs also flourished in more urban areas, with work involving jobs in the local community (see Adams, 1971). As Charles Bernstein, the founder of the system in New York state, noted, residents in colonies "can easily earn sufficient funds to support the unit and in prosperous times have a little surplus for individual savings, and in this way self-respect is engendered in the individual rather than dependency, humiliation and discouragement" (1921, p. 44). Although the numbers of persons served outside of the large institutions were small, community care was a practice closely followed by workers in mental retardation. In light of today's developments, many of these innovations seem farsighted indeed.

Up until very recently, however, most retarded persons under residential care were in large state institutions. We turn now to an analysis of the effects of institutions, leaving recent issues in the care of retarded persons for later in this chapter.

Effects of institutions on retarded residents

Any discussion of the effects of institutions on retarded residents must begin by addressing the common misconception that institutions are all the same. On the contrary, institutions vary widely one from another. In the authors' state of Connecticut, for example, retarded persons reside in large institutions, regional centers (smaller, but still sizable facilities), group homes, community training homes (familylike units in which a licensee houses three or four clients), nursing homes, foster homes, and supervised apartments. Add to this a dizzying array of funding sources and state departments that administer various facilities, and one begins to realize how divergent institutions actually are.

To date, most of the research on the effects of institutions has focused on how variations in their "demographic characteristics" affect the behaviors of retarded residents. These demographics include size of the institution, size of living units, costs per resident, number of professional staff per client, etc. Little attention has been paid to the social and psychological characteristics and practices operating in the institutions studied (Cleland, 1965; Zigler, 1971; Zigler & Balla, 1977).

To illustrate what is meant by these social and psychological features, let us compare two large residential schools in the same state with identical admission practices. Butterfield and Zigler (1965b) described the institutions as follows:

In institution A, every effort is made to provide a noninstitutional (i.e., homelike) environment. School classes, residential units at the younger age levels, and frequent social events are all coeducational. Meals are prepared in the living units, where the residents eat in small groups. Emphasis is placed upon individual responsibility rather than upon external control by the staff.

In institution B, little effort is made to provide a homelike environment for the residents. School classes, all residential units, movies, and most other social events are segregated by sex. Meals are prepared and residents eat in a large central dining room with virtually no individual supervision. Emphasis is upon external control of the residents by the staff, rather than upon inculcating individual responsibility. (pp. 48–49)

Obviously, although these institutions were of the same type and size, the way they treated their residents was indeed different.

Our point is that it is simplistic to assert that large institutions necessarily provide inadequate care or that smaller settings are necessarily better for retarded persons. Although there is a tendency for larger facilities to be more institution-oriented as opposed to resident-oriented in their care practices (King, Raynes, & Tizard, 1971; McCormack, Balla, & Zigler, 1975), "there are excellent large institutions and inadequate community-based facilities" (Balla, 1976, p. 118). Balla's conclusion is borne out by data from numerous studies comparing the institutional practices of large and small settings (e.g., McCormack et al., 1975; Hodapp & Zigler, 1985); in all of these studies, certain small institutions were less resident-oriented than some large institutions.

An additional point concerning demographics is that institutional size within any particular type of institution (e.g., group home, large central institution) does not seem to have an effect on the care of the residents. Comparing 20 group homes ranging in size from 6 to 20 residents, Landesman-Dwyer, Sackett, and Kleinman (1980) found that size had little influence on the amount of interaction between the staff and the residents, even though the ratio of staff to residents was higher in the smaller facilities. This lack of a relationship between size and care practices has also been found in institutions that varied in size from 100 to 1,600 residents (King et al., 1971) and within each of the three types of setting (group home, regional center, large central institution) studied by McCormack et al. (1975). Within a particular category of institution, then, the facility's size, by itself, is of little importance.

In contrast, there is evidence that the social-psychological climate of an institution can affect residents' behavior. For example, comparing the two institutions described earlier, Butterfield and Zigler (1965b) found that residents in the more unenlightened and depriving facility (institution B) had a significantly higher motivation to receive attention from adults. The warmer, more homelike environment of institution A helped make its residents less dependent on adult attention and approval.

In a second, more ambitious study, Balla et al. (1974) investigated the long-term effects of four institutions located in different parts of the country. They attempted a more detailed assessment of each institution by measuring such dimensions as size, number of residents per living unit, cost per resident per day, employee turnover rate, number of direct-care personnel per resident, number of professional staff per resident, and number of volunteer-hours per resident per year. The residents themselves were tested twice within six months of their admission and again after 2.5 years of institutional experience. In addition to the measure of responsiveness to social reinforcement used in previous studies (see Chapter 6), measures of MA, IQ, verbal dependency, extent of imitation of adults, and variability of behavior were also obtained.

Balla et al. found considerable evidence of psychological growth over the 2.5-year period. In all of the institutions, residents became less verbally dependent, less imitative, and more variable in their behavior. IQ level did not change but MA level increased. There were, however, few differences in the residents' behavior due to demographic differences among the institutions. Indeed, the only finding in this regard was that residents in the largest institution were more responsive to social reinforcement than were those in the smaller institutions.

In a later study using many of the same measures, Zigler, Balla, and Kossan (in press) examined the behavioral effects of two large and five small institutions. The facilities were rated not only for demographic traits, but for their social-psychological characteristics. The latter were assessed using King et al.'s (1971) measure, which rates care practices on a scale from *institution-oriented* to *resident-oriented*.

The outcome behaviors of interest were the individual's degree of wariness, imitation, and responsiveness to social reinforcement. As in prior research, MA was found to affect these motivational measures. Residents who had higher MAs were less dependent on adult social reinforcement; they were also less wary and less imitative of adults. Only one other personal variable related to the residents' behavior and this was the number of prior residential placements. The greater the number of previous residences, the more wary of adults the retarded residents became. For the most part, the demographic and social-psychological features of the institutions did not affect the residents' behaviors that were measured.

In addition to examinations of the effects of institutions on personality and motivation, several studies have explored the effects of institutions on the IQs of their retarded residents. In a series of studies performed in England, Clarke and Clarke (1954; also, Clarke, Clarke, & Reiman, 1958) found that the IQ scores of institutionalized retarded children increased over varying lengths of time. However, Zigler and his colleagues found a decline in intelligence over three years of institutional experience in one U.S. sample (Zigler & Williams, 1963), but an increase in IQ in another sample (Zigler, Balla, & Butterfield, 1968). Such inconsistent findings might be attributable to differences in the institutions studied.

Another possibility is that the characteristics of individual residents interact with those of the institution to cause intellectual (and personality) change. For example, in many of the IQ studies to date, the level of deprivation suffered by the retarded individual prior to institutionalization was an important factor affecting IQ change. Those individuals who were most deprived were more likely to show larger IQ gains over several years in the institution, while those from adequate homes showed small gains (Clarke et al., 1958), stayed the same (Balla et al., 1974), or showed slight decreases (Zigler & Williams, 1963). The increase in the IQ scores of deprived individuals occurred even when widely divergent methods were employed to assess preinstitutional deprivation, as in the work of Clarke et al. (who used a 12-item scale) and of Zigler and his colleagues (who used the Preinstitutional Social Deprivation Scale of Zigler, Butterfield, & Goff, 1966).

The preinstitutional history of the retarded individual may even have a more pronounced effect on motivational change than on changes in IQ. For example, Zigler and Williams (1963) found that, while all retarded residents became increasingly motivated to receive adult attention over three years of institutionalization, those from relatively good homes showed a much greater increase than did those from inadequate homes. Zigler, Butterfield, and Capobianco (1970) tested these same individuals seven and ten years later, and again found that the highly deprived residents were less responsive to social reinforcement. In essence, the effects of the residents' preinstitutional histories had lasted over the entire ten-year period. As Zigler and Balla (1977) concluded, "Social deprivation is a phenomenon that, once experienced, is built into the motivational structure of the individual and subsequently mediates his interactions with the environment" (p. 3).

When considering the effects of institutionalization on retarded residents, then, it is important to consider both the social-psychological characteristics of the institutions themselves and the specific traits of the individual (especially preinstitutional history). As Zigler (1971) noted in his review of institutional effects, such a multifactorial view of the effects of institutions "seems preferable to the more common one where institutions for the retarded are seen as equally depriving environments which exert uniform influences on all children" (p. 105).

Deinstitutionalization

From the vantage point of the mid-1980s, it is an understatement to say that institutions for retarded persons are changing. In 1983, Scheerenberger (1983b) found that 80% of residents in large institutions were severely or profoundly retarded, indicating a tremendous decrease in the percentages of mildly and moderately retarded residents from only a decade or so earlier. In addition, although the number of institutions continues to increase, the overall institutionalized retarded population has decreased from approximately 190,000 to 120,000 residents in the period from 1970-71 to 1981-82.

The impetus for these changes in (and calls for the demise of) large institutions comes from a variety of sources (Vitello & Soskin, 1985). First, a series of indictments of large institutions during the 1960s shocked the U.S. public. For example, Blatt and Kaplan (1966) provided a photographic record of the deplorable conditions in several large institutions. Conditions at the Willowbrook facility on Staten Island in New York were brought to public awareness by both political (e.g., Senator Robert F. Kennedy's visit) and media (television reporter Geraldo Rivera's exposé) attention. Second, advocacy groups such as the National Association of Retarded Citizens were effective in exerting pressure to change existing institutions. Third, the 1960s featured a legislative and philosophical movement (to be examined in the next chapter) that mandated services within the "least restrictive environment" for all retarded individuals.

Finally, there was the development of the concept of normalization, the philosophical backbone of both the deinstitutionalization and mainstreaming movements. Normalization is based on the idea that each person has the right to experience a style of life that is normal within his or her own culture. In Western societies, such a lifestyle includes a normal rhythm to one's day (e.g., getting up in the morning, going to bed at an age-appropriate hour at night), to one's year (e.g., vacations, holidays), and to one's life (e.g., school, work), all while living in a humane environment that is conducive to individual development. As originally conceptualized by Nirje (1969), normalization referred primarily to the individual; that is, the retarded person, like all people, should be allowed to live as normal a life as possible.

With a book by Wolfensberger (1972), however, the principle of normalization shifted from the individual to the services provided to that individual. Adherents of normalization began to call for a "normalization of services" to retarded persons. Some even called for an end to large institutions altogether. They argued that such institutions could not provide a normal lifestyle and that all retarded residents could be served in smaller, community-based facilities (e.g., group homes, supervised apartments). Two strong proponents of deinstitutionalization, Menolascino and McGee (1981a), provide a flavor of such thinking: "Currently institutionalized mentally retarded persons are there because of archaic professional views that persistently support social policies designed to maintain institutions regardless of the demonstrable needs and potentials of the mentally retarded persons residing therein" (p. 219).

Probably the best example of the debate among professionals over deinstitutionalization can be found in the arguments over the Partlow facility in Alabama (see Cavalier & McCarver, 1981). Begun in 1971, the so-called Partlow case has actually consisted of a series of court cases (*Wyatt* v. *Stickney*, *Wyatt* v. *Alderholt*, *Wyatt* v. *Hardin*, *Wyatt* v. *Ireland*) lasting over a decade. Legal action began after Alabama's commissioner of mental health, in an effort to dramatize the state's lack of funding for mental health care and to shift funds to community treatment, fired several professionals at Bryce Hospital, a mental health facility. Advocates of Ricky Wyatt, an involuntarily committed Bryce resident, then initiated a class action suit in his behalf. Residents of the Partlow State School, a large mental retardation facility, were subsequently included in the Wyatt proceedings, and eventually their case was considered separately by the court.

U.S. District Court Judge Frank Johnson identified deficiencies in the physical plant and staffing and in the individualized treatment plans of Partlow residents. He ordered the state to follow 49 guidelines, including "staffing ratios for service personnel, individualized habilitation plans for every resident, and stringent admission policies which prohibited admitting borderline or mildly retarded individuals" (Cavalier & McCarver, 1981, p. 210). Alabama's compliance with these 49 guidelines was at issue in the *Wyatt* v. *Hardin* proceedings, the 1978 case in which most of the issues involving deinstitutionalization were discussed, with experts in mental retardation offering strong testimony for each side.

On one side stood the Partlow Committee, who presented a "Motion to Modify" Judge Johnson's original 49 guidelines. The arguments of this group, led by Norman Ellis and including many of the leading experts in the field, mainly concerned the right to treatment (habilitation) and the appropriateness of community-based facilities for all retarded persons. We quote from three parts of the Motion to Modify.

1. Habilitation interpreted to mean deinstitutionalization or return to home/ community living is an unrealistic goal for the majority of residents in Partlow. Indeed, the behavior of many cannot reasonably be expected to improve *significantly* with training, even for living within the sheltered environment of an institution.

2. Residents shall have a right to habilitation, including medical treatment, education and care, suited to their needs regardless of age, degree of retardation or handicapping condition. Residents who fail to improve with extensive education and training efforts will not be subjected to further training or education *per se*. Residents who are not continued in training or education programs will receive a full program of enriching activities. . . . This program [of enrichment] should not be interpreted to mean traditional custodial care. Instead it includes an enriched program of activities that insures the best approximation to normal life that can be achieved taking into account the capabilities of the resident and the degree of restriction needed to protect the life and well-being of the person. It does preclude subjecting such persons to continuing ritualistic training/educational programs which offer the person no reward, neither immediate satisfaction nor long-range improvement.

3. Only a small number of the present Partlow residents can reasonably be expected to adjust to community living. . . . and to place many of those residents in the community would do them a serious injustice. They require protection from ordinary hazards and close supervision in order to insure both their safety and well-being. Further, a group home that met their needs would, in fact, be at least as restrictive as their present residence. (Ellis, Balla, Estes, Warren, Meyers, Hollis, Isaacson, Palk, & Siegel, 1981, pp. 221–222)

On the other side stood those experts, like Menolascino and McGee (1981a, 1981b), who felt that group homes or community residences are appropriate for all retarded individuals. These workers pointed to the conditions at the large facilities and asserted that they could never offer humane care. They interpreted research findings to show that all retarded people, regardless of level, can benefit from intensive treatment, and declared that the Partlow Committee's recommendations amounted to a return to custodial care and a self-fulfilling prophesy for retarded residents of the large institutions. Menolascino and McGee (1981b) concluded that "institutional populations are *not* as developmentally delayed as the Partlow Committee would have us believe; it is also a misconception that those without self-help skills are unable to benefit from developmental services in these [community] programs" (p. 228). Opponents of deinstitutionalization considered Judge Johnson's decision (which was substantially in their favor) as evidence that their arguments were correct.

Clearly, these issues are complicated in nature and emotional in presentation. We are struck, however, by the similarity of the arguments to those made in earlier days. For example, the entire debate over the right to habilitation is reminiscent of the debate over the educational status of the early training schools. Should retarded persons, especially those at the lowest levels of function, be taught or trained or do they mainly require, as Governor Butler said, "good and kind treatment; but not a school"? The position of proponents of deinstitutionalization, in particular, carries the danger of an overoptimism concerning retarded individuals' potential for improvement. This could predispose the field to a series of disappointments in future years, like those that occurred in the late 19th and early 20th centuries.

We are also struck by the emotionalism in the arguments of both sides. Those advocating deinstitutionalization frequently refer to large institutions as "warehouses," and assert that these facilities are able to provide only custodial care and are by their very nature inhumane. These advocates also portray group homes in idealistic terms, asserting that they provide more care, more contact with nonretarded individuals, and a more normal environment. Advocates of institutions, for their part, overstate the amount of change possible in the practices of large institutions, and minimize the extent of the harmful practices that have existed and in some cases continue to exist. All too often, each side lapses into an advocacy or apologist role vis-à-vis group homes or large institutions.

Our view is that the appropriateness of various types of institutional placement for different types of retarded people is an empirical issue. Unfortunately, most of the research needed to answer this question conclusively remains to be done. There are, however, some data available that suggest that neither side is totally correct. For example, several large-scale studies have reported that a substantial portion of retarded people (approximately 20%) who had previously been placed in community settings were returned to the large institutions (see Table 10.1). Although this does not mean that some retarded persons will always have to be in large institutions (especially if group homes can be made to accommodate them), it does imply the present need for these facilities.

Community placement might be more successful if we had a profile of traits which make certain retarded individuals' return to the institution more likely. There are now some indications that one of these traits is maladaptive behavior. For example, Landesman-Dwyer and Sulzbacher (1981) found that 21% of those returned to the large institution from community settings had inflicted physical harm on others, and 19% had destroyed objects or set fires (see also Hill & Bruininks, 1984). A second

Table 10.1. *Recidivism rate for residents released from institutions for the mentally retarded*

	Number released and located	Number returned to institution	Recidivism rate (%)
Willer and Intagliata (1980)	477	168	35
Birenbaum and Re (1979)	63	21	33
Miller et al. (1975)	158	40	25
Baker et al. (1977)	—[a]	—	22
Sutter et al.	77	17	22
Schalock et al. (1981)	166	26	16
Moen et al. (1975)	85	13	15
Bell et al. (1981)	582	—	14
Gollay et al. (1978)	440	58	13
Aninger and Bolinsky (1977)	19	1	5

[a]Not reported.
Source: From Craig and McCarver (1984), with permission.

factor leading to the failure of community placement may be the presence of associated handicaps. Lakin et al. (1983) found that almost half of those persons returned to the large institutions had a handicap such as epilepsy, blindness, deafness, or cerebral palsy in addition to their retardation. A third factor is the individual's level of retardation, as all studies show a preponderance of the lowest-functioning persons (those who are severely or profoundly retarded) remaining in the large facilities (e.g., Cleland et al., 1980).

A second empirical issue concerns the quality of care provided in group homes versus large institutions. Proponents of deinstitutionalization generally assume that "less restrictive environments" such as group homes offer more humane care for retarded residents. As we have pointed out, this assumption is not always true. Within a single type of institution, the equation of "less restrictive" (if defined as smaller) with "better" also does not always hold. In a series of studies examining group homes of from 6 to 20 residents, Landesman-Dwyer and her colleagues (Landesman-Dwyer, 1981; Landesman-Dwyer, Sackett, & Kleinman, 1980; Landesman-Dwyer, Stein, & Sackett, 1978; Landesman-Dwyer & Sulzbacher, 1981) have found several counterintuitive results. For example, greater amounts of positive social behaviors occurred in larger facilities, and residents in specially designed new group homes had less community interaction than those in older buildings not originally built as group homes. Findings of this type cast doubt on the notion that one type of facility is always best for all individuals.

The third and perhaps most persuasive argument for group homes is that residents progress faster than they do in the large institutional setting. Study of this question is complicated by the facts that some residents fail in their community placements (e.g., Hill & Bruininks, 1984), that oftentimes the amount of programming provided the clients differs in the two facilities (Sandler & Thurman, 1981), and that there are difficulties in performing random assignment studies in this area. Another complication is that there are wide variations among different group homes (Balla & Klein, 1976; Butler & Bjaanes, 1977; Landesman-Dwyer, 1981) and different large institutions (Butterfield & Zigler, 1965b).

Despite these caveats, there have now been several studies of the effects of smaller, community-based facilities versus institutional placements. In the most rigorous of these studies, Eyman and Arndt (1979) employed a semilongitudinal design that involved 3,457 institutional and 312 community residents of differing ages. By conducting testing at four yearly intervals, Eyman and Arndt were able to disentangle effects due to the year in which a person was born (i.e., cohort effects) from those due to development. Their study therefore provides a picture of development in both institutional and community-based residents over the life span.

Results showed that on three measures of adaptive behavior, all retarded groups increased in their levels of functioning over time. However, in contrast to expectations, "the quality of the environment did not have a differential effect on developmental growth for the retarded groups studied" (p. 347). The only difference between residents of the two types of facility was that community-based clients were more variable in their acquisition of adaptive behavior than were institutional residents.

The results of other studies, however, have shown that group homes promote development more than do institutional placements, at least in certain areas. Schroeder and Henes (1978) found that language and self-help skills of group-home residents increased more than in institutional residents matched on a number of relevant variables. In a study of retarded persons residing in group homes for varying lengths of time, Kleinberg and Galligan (1983) also pointed to language and self-help skills (such as independent functioning and domestic activities) as areas particularly facilitated by group-home placements. These workers explained the changes as follows: "It appears that deinstitutionalized individuals show changes that primarily represent manifestation of skills already in their repertoire. The new environment provides the opportunity for the manifestation of those skills, not only in the sense of permitting, but also in providing social reinforcement" (pp. 25-26).

Behavioral changes seem to occur in the first few months after movement to the group-home setting. In a study by Cohen, Conroy, Frazer, Snelbecker, and Sprout (1977), for example, all changes found occurred within several weeks after moving to the new facilities. Similarly, Kleinberg and Galligan (1983) reported most change within the first four months after placement in the group home. Depending on the area of functioning, there was subsequently either no change (e.g., the areas of social interaction and domestic activity) or slow deterioration (e.g., language) after this time.

The period directly after movement to a new facility may also be the time when adverse changes occur. Anecdotal reports (e.g., Zigler, 1983) and studies of geriatric (Kasl, 1972) and retarded (Dingman, Tarjan, Eyman, & Miller, 1977) residents previously implied the negative outcomes of moving from one living setting to another, but few studies have examined this phenomenon with respect to deinstitutionalization. Of the few that have, Cohen et al. (1977) found that the lowest-functioning persons in their study (with a mean IQ less than 20) emitted more behaviors – of both a social and antisocial nature – in the first six weeks after transferring from one to another institutional setting. Conversely, the higher-functioning clients (with a mean IQ of 35) showed generalized patterns of withdrawal and decreased behavioral outputs. Such a potentially negative outcome of interinstitutional transfer, the so-called relocation effect (see Craig & McCarver, 1984), constitutes a risk inherent in deinstitutionalization, a risk that becomes especially high if clients are transferred to their new homes without careful, sensitive, and sufficient preparations.

Conclusion

The long debate over the best living settings for retarded people is hardly settled. Up to the present time, the amount of heat – as opposed to light – generated in this debate has been alarming. In an effort to contribute some clarity to these issues, we end this chapter with a middle-ground position based on the following three principles.

Continuum of care

The work of many researchers leads us to believe that a continuum of care is needed with respect to the living environments of retarded persons. Available options should range from family care to placement in large institutions, depending on the characteristics and abilities of particular retarded individuals and their families. This call for a continuum of care is not new; our brief historical overview shows that the beginnings of the concept date back to the early 20th century.

The job is now one of fitting the particular retarded individual to the most appropriate residential alternative, based on the best available knowledge. This being the case, we should make serious efforts to improve each of the alternatives, to make each a suitable dwelling for retarded persons. With regard to large institutions, we feel that these facilities should continue to function, but they must be made better. The practices depicted in Blatt and Kaplan's *Christmas in Purgatory* (1966) all too often continue to exist, and opposition to the deinstitutionalization of all retarded people must not be allowed to become advocacy of inhumane large institutions.

The continued existence of large facilities has recently led to discussions of their functions in future years. Lakin et al. (1983) noted that large institutions will continue to serve as the primary living settings for the lowest-functioning and most seriously handicapped or multihandicapped persons, as stable living alternatives for those whose community placements have deteriorated (e.g., because of antisocial behavior), and as transitional facilities until greater numbers of community residences can be built. However, large institutions may play an even larger role in providing services to retarded individuals. In a conference discussing the future of the Vineland Training School, Marie Crissey and other leaders in the mental retardation field proposed a plan designed to specify the possible functions that could be served by Vineland and other large facilities (Crissey, in press). She emphasized that large facilities were ideally suited to oversee a centralized network of services to retarded persons throughout the life span. They could serve as information and referral sources to parents of retarded children, provide short-term, long-term, and supportive care for retarded people of all ages, and could serve as liaisons to public schools, vocational workshops, hospitals, and other agencies serving retarded people. New generations of professionals could be trained to work with retarded persons (a function that the Vineland Training School has historically performed). Retarded individuals and their families would know that the large institution was a safe haven for them. This knowledge would provide comfort to parents worried about the fate of their deinstitutionalized children as they themselves get older (see Novak, 1980, for a discussion of this issue). This listing of the possible uses of the large institution, so different from the usual concept of the isolated facility, is currently being attempted at Vineland, Elwyn, and some other large facilities.

Need for a historical view

As mentioned earlier, there is a blindness to historical experience in the current deinstitutionalization controversy. In particular, there seems to be an unwarranted optimism concerning the benefits of group home and community-based residences for all retarded people. Overoptimism is not a harmless tendency; once hopes are dashed, it readily leads to pessimism and despair. This is exactly what happened not very long ago, when hope that retarded persons could be made "normal" was suddenly transformed into Fernald's "legend of the feebleminded" (see Zigler & Harter, 1969). We therefore advise caution in claiming that community facilities can or should be appropriate for all retarded people. At the same time, we do not think that the fact that community residences are inappropriate for some retarded individuals in any way lessens the responsibility of states and administrators to make the large institutions more humane. A view based on history counsels caution, but it also implies the need for continuing work to improve each residential alternative.

Normalization of lifestyles for retarded individuals

At present there is an overconcern with the normalization of services for retarded individuals, which has meant getting them into homes, schools, and other facilities that are as much like those used by the nonretarded population as possible. Such concern misses the mark: Our ultimate goal, as outlined in Nirje's (1969) original proposal, should be to allow retarded individuals to live a style of life that is as close as possible to that of the larger society. Such a style of life can be led in a large facility (as in institution A in Butterfield & Zigler, 1965b) or in a group home.

These two concepts – normalization of lifestyle and normalization of services – are too often confused, with proponents of normalized services generally thinking that they are making the lives of retarded individuals more like the lives of the nonretarded by changing the nature of the available services. Although more humane and normalized services often do lead to more normal lives for retarded residents (e.g., Eyman, Demaine, & Lei, 1979), the equation is not perfect. Abuses under the banner of normalization have and continue to exist (Zigler, 1983). Only through a closer examination of what is best for each retarded individual, from both a humanitarian and a developmental standpoint, can we know how best to provide appropriate care. Such is the challenge for professionals in the mental retardation field in the years to come.

11 Mainstreaming

H.L. Mencken once declared that "For every complex issue there is a simple answer, and it is wrong." Such an observation could easily apply to the care and treatment of mentally retarded persons, especially to the current debate over educating retarded children in mainstreamed versus special-education classes. Few issues are characterized by such a complicated interplay of social, political, legal, and educational forces, yet few have been so often oversimplified.

To understand the roots of the mainstreaming debate, let us look briefly at the history of special education in the United States. This is not a long history, since all programs of education for retarded children are relatively new. Until the middle of the 19th century, most retarded and mentally ill people were cared for in their own families. On rare occasions, the local jail or poorhouse might take in a retarded person, but social service institutions as we now know them did not exist.

As we saw in Chapter 10, the 19th century was characterized by an optimistic and benevolent attitude toward bettering the lives of all Americans. Fostered by influential scientific and literary statements on the power of the environment to affect individuals (see Rosen, Clark, & Kivitz, 1976), the climate was right for the establishment of a variety of social services. In keeping with this spirit, the late 19th century witnessed the spread of the universal schooling movement. In towns and cities throughout the country, tax-supported schools were founded to provide a free education to all children. These schools were initially age-graded, but eventually students of similar abilities were taught in the same classes, or "tracked." This practice supposedly increased efficiency in education, a goal furthered by the widespread use of mental tests starting in the 1920s. For the first time, there was an objective way to assess a child's level of mental ability. Curricula appropriate for each level could then be developed, and "tests were adopted as a means of sorting individuals into the differentiated curriculum in preparation for their future social roles" (Lazerson, 1975, p. 47).

223

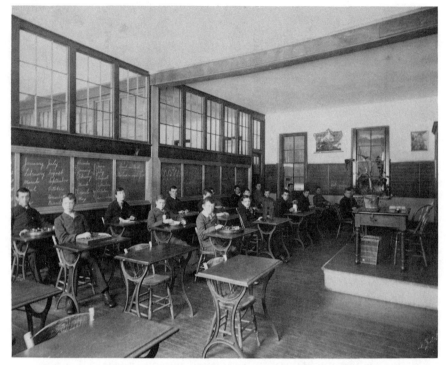

Photo 6. School program, Pennsylvania Institute for Feeble-Minded Children. (Photograph courtesy of Elwyn Institutes, Elwyn, Pennsylvania)

Given these goals of the early schooling movement, special-education classes originated and grew rapidly. Davies and Ecob (1959) reported that New York City and Cleveland first established classes for "problem children" in the 1870s, with Providence originating the first classes specifically for mentally retarded children in 1894. In rapid succession, the cities of Springfield, Mass. (1894), Chicago (1898), Boston (1899), New York (1901), Philadelphia (1901), and Los Angeles (1902) all established classes for retarded children in their school systems. By 1929, Cleveland had over 6% of its elementary school population in special-education classes, Philadelphia 3.5%, and Detroit 2.1% (Lazerson, 1975). By the early 1930s, most educators could agree with Davies and Ecob's statement that "special classes, at first frankly an expedient to rid the school of an overwhelming burden [the instruction of slow-learning children], are now recognized to have a rightful place in the educational system" (1959, p. 173).

Still, there was never an uncritical acceptance of special-education classes, even after they had existed in a school a number of years. Since these classes were smaller and more individualized than regular classes, the public often balked at their cost. As Lazerson (1975) notes,

Where classes did exist, they were usually in the least desirable buildings and rooms. Equipment and materials were scarce, few of the teachers specially trained, and the curriculum a watered down version of what the regular classes did. Parental hostility to classes for mental defectives was high, forcing school systems to resort to such euphemisms as ungraded, opportunity, Binet, and adjustment classes. Finally, the distinctions between mental deficiency, behaviorally disruptive and truant children, and the physically handicapped were frequently ignored, with the special classes dumping grounds for those the system could not accommodate or tolerate. (p. 49)

It is noteworthy that many of these criticisms of special-education classes reappeared in an article by Lloyd Dunn in 1968, which was to become the major theoretical impetus for mainstreaming. According to Dunn, throughout history regular schools and educable (i.e., mildly) retarded children had been forced into "a reluctant mutual recognition of each other" (p. 5, original quotation from Hollingworth, 1923). He pointed to the many "efficacy studies" that demonstrated that educable mentally retarded (EMR) children in special classes did no better academically than they did when placed in regular classrooms. Dunn argued that segregated classes could not provide an education equal to that provided in regular classes, and that contact with nonretarded children would reduce the stigmatization of EMR children. He also pointed to the documented overrepresentation of black and minority children in special classes. Finally, Dunn recognized the many innovations then taking place in the educational system (team teaching, new curricula, increased numbers of support personnel, new educational technology), and argued that "regular school programs are now better able to deal with individual differences in pupils" (p. 10). For each of these reasons – similar academic achievement, labeling, over-representation of minorities in special classes, segregation from nonretarded children, and the schools' ability to handle individual differences – Dunn felt that special classes were not necessary for many educable retarded children. As a strong and cogent argument against special classes, Dunn's article provided the theoretical basis for the entire mainstreaming movement.

Other factors also contributed to the widespread acceptance of mainstreaming. In 1954, the U.S. Supreme Court in *Brown* v. *Board of Education* had proclaimed that racially segregated schools could not be "separate but equal." This reasoning, bolstered by the civil rights struggles of the 1960s, permeated the thinking of special educators (see Blatt, 1979, for an example of this position). A series of court decisions, culminating in the famous *Larry P.* v. *Riles* case in California, ruled against special-class placements for black and minority educable retarded children (for reviews, see H.R. Turnbull, 1978; Vitello & Soskin, 1985). Judicial opinion in these cases fostered the view that children assigned to special-education classes were necessarily doomed; Gottlieb (1981) noted that the "opinion in the *Larry P.* case . . . referred to self-contained classes as 'dead-ends' no less than nine times" (p. 115). Finally, with societal concerns over shrinking resources in the 1970s and 1980s (best illustrated by the defeat of numerous school budgets in referendums during this period), mainstreaming seemed to make sense to many Americans.

However, even more than the Dunn article or the sociopolitical climate, the passing of Public Law 94-142 was the true impetus to the mainstreaming movement in the United States. Known as the Education for All Handicapped Children Act of 1975, this federal law addressed many of the complaints of Dunn and others concerning special education. The law mandated that "a free appropriate public education" was a right for all children, no matter how impaired. It also provided children and their parents the right to due process (especially the right to a hearing over the child's educational placement), declared that children should be placed in the "least restrictive" educational setting, and mandated that every child should have an individualized educational plan (IEP) (see MacMillan, 1982). The Education for All Handicapped Children Act was to become the landmark law in the history of special education.

As concerns mainstreaming, the least restrictive environment provision of Public Law 94-142 was generally translated into a regular-class placement for most EMR children. Indeed, several states have adopted mainstreaming to such an extent that it is almost impossible to find EMR children who are not being mainstreamed for most if not all of their school day (see Caparulo & Zigler, 1983). We now turn to a discussion of the definition and goals of mainstreaming, and an evaluation of whether the practice has accomplished its stated goals.

The definition and goals of mainstreaming

One of the many difficulties in accurately assessing the merits of mainstreaming is the definition of the practice itself. In common parlance, mainstreaming involves the placement of retarded or otherwise handicapped children into classes composed predominantly of nonhandicapped children; the handicapped child is thus entered into the metaphorical main stream of the school environment.

In theory, however, the definition of mainstreaming often involves more than the placement of handicapped children into regular classrooms. Here, for example, is the oft-cited definition of mainstreaming as given by Kaufman, Gottlieb, and Kukic (1975):

Mainstreaming refers to the temporal, instructional and social integration of eligible exceptional children with normal peers. It is based on an ongoing individually determined educational needs assessment requiring clarification of responsibility for coordinated planning and programming by regular and special education administrative, instructional and support personnel. (pp. 40-41)

This definition includes but is not limited to the time that the handicapped child spends in the regular classroom, presumably in social interaction with nonhandicapped children. It also features "instructional integration," a practice that may lead to a curriculum that is more oriented toward academics than to training in life skills. (For a debate over the changing curriculum of special education brought about by mainstreaming, see Blatt, 1979; Childs, 1979; and Warren, 1979.) The Kaufman et al. definition also includes an IEP for each child, and coordinated planning by regular- and special-education personnel.

As might be imagined, mainstreaming is rarely followed in practice as precisely as it has been defined. Indeed, the Kaufman et al. definition has been referred to as the "idealized" (Gottlieb, 1981) or "philosophical" (Gresham, 1985) definition of mainstreaming. Gottlieb (1981) notes that "The mere placement of EMR children in a regular-education program in contact with nonhandicapped peers for an arbitrarily fixed minimum amount of time is defined by the schools as mainstreaming" (p. 116). Along with other workers (e.g., Corman & Gottlieb, 1978; Gresham, in press; Semmel, Gottlieb, & Robinson, 1979), Gottlieb advances the practical criterion that mainstreaming can be considered to occur when the handicapped child is in a regular classroom for at least 50% of the school day. The nature of the classes in which the child participates, the methods of teaching, and the type of social interactions that take place are all explicitly ignored in the practical definition of mainstreaming.

A related issue concerns who should be mainstreamed. Meisel (in press) points out that Public Law 94-142 specifically declared that all handicapped children should be educated with nonhandicapped children *to the extent possible*. Such a provision allows educators to identify which children, under which particular circumstances, are best suited to a mainstreamed placement. The results of some attempts to draw these specifications are shown in Table 11.1. In addition to the need for further refinement and increased empirical support for these guidelines, many other characteristics of the handicapped child must be considered. Zigler and Hall (in press)

Table 11.1. *Proposed guidelines concerning when mainstreaming is appropriate for any individual child*

A child should be mainstreamed	Caution should be used in considering mainstreaming
If the child is young and the problem has been identified rather early in the school year.	If the child is older and the problem has continued unimproved for some time in the regular class.
If the child's problem is mild and not readily apparent outside of the school context.	If the child's problem is severe and pervades other areas of the child's life.
If the child's problem is limited to a single area of functioning.	If the child's problems are multiple (e.g., mild retardation *and* a behavior problem).
If remediation of the child's problem does not require complicated equipment or materials.	If the child's condition requires complicated remedial equipment or teaching methods.
If the child appears to have friends or the ability to develop supportive friendships with normal children.	If the child has had repeated difficulty in developing friendships with nonhandicapped children.
If the regular classroom contains less than 25 or 30 children.	If the regular classroom contains more than 30 or 35 children.
If the child's regular-class teacher appears knowledgeable and willing to deal with the child's problem.	If the child's teacher appears to be unwilling or grossly unable to continue working with the child.
If the child's family appears to be willing and able to deal effectively with his or her problem.	If the child's family appears to lack extensive support for dealing with his or her problem.

Source: From S. R. Forness, "Clinical criteria for mainstreaming mildly handicapped children," *Psychology in the Schools*, 1979, 16, 508–514. Reprinted by permission of the author.

suggested that type of retardation, gender, type and degree of associated handicaps, MA, CA, IQ, and various personality-motivational variables might all enter into the decision to mainstream a particular child. Gresham (1983) argued that assessment of a child's social skills (by way of naturalistic observations, peer sociometric measures, and teacher ratings) should also be used in placement decisions. To date, however, the effects of few of these child characteristics on the outcome of mainstreaming have been investigated.

Given the ambiguity over the definition of mainstreaming, it is not surprising that workers do not agree about the goals that the practice is supposed to achieve. However, from the original Dunn (1968) article, and the Gottlieb (1981) and other reviews, at least the following general goals of the practice can be identified:

1. Equal or better educational attainment compared to handicapped children in special classes;
2. Increase in the social skills of handicapped children through contact with nonhandicapped peers;
3. Reduction of stigmatization from other children, teachers, and from (and of) nonhandicapped family members;
4. More racially integrated educational settings; and
5. Less costly, but equally individualized, instruction.

We now turn to each of these issues in an attempt to evaluate whether mainstreaming has accomplished its implied goals.

Evaluation of the effects of mainstreaming

Educational achievement

Among the most powerful indictments of special-class placements were the findings that EMR children placed in special classrooms fared no better than children in regular classes on a variety of academic tasks (see Kirk, 1964). This criticism was central to Dunn's (1968) argument, and served to place the proponents of special-education classes on the defensive. If EMR children were just as well off academically in regular as in special classes, why spend the extra dollars for special-education teachers and for the higher teacher to student ratios that characterized special classes? Within a sociopolitical climate favoring integration of all pupils and given the belief that curricula could be individualized in regular classes, Dunn's argument seemed especially persuasive.

Reviews of special-class versus mainstreamed placements have generally supported the findings of no differences between the two educational settings (e.g., Semmel et al., 1979). Some reviews (e.g., Corman & Gottlieb, 1978; Kirk; 1964; Semmel et al. 1979) have noted occasional studies that showed better academic achievement for children in mainstreamed than in special classes (usually in reading), but such findings have usually been confounded by the lack of random assignment of subjects. That is, although the children were equated on a number of variables, differences between those in the two types of class may have been due to initial differences between the two groups (Corman & Gottlieb, 1978; Kirk, 1964). In the few studies that have randomly assigned EMR students to either special or mainstream classes (e.g., Budoff & Gottlieb, 1976), few differences have emerged in any areas of academic achievement.

Before leaving the topic of academic achievement, several points should be emphasized. First, as Gottlieb (1981) notes, it may very well be that "an appropriate education for mentally retarded children has not yet been developed" (p. 118). In the studies reviewed by Semmel et al. (1979), for example, the average reading score for the EMR children was equal to a grade-equivalent of 3.8 years, an extremely low level of achievement for any child. A finding of no differences between special and mainstream classes should not be seen as a blanket endorsement of either alternative as an effective educational intervention for EMR children.

Second, it does appear that increased attention from teachers and smaller, more individualized classes may help EMR children academically, regardless of whether such conditions are found in a mainstream or special class. Haring and Krug (1975) compared four special-education classes, two experimental and two control. The experimental classes featured highly structured teaching, charts showing progress, and clear-cut rewards for good performance, while the control classes presented the regular special-class curriculum. In both reading and arithmetic, experimental-class children outperformed control-class children over the period of one school year. Similar results were obtained when features of mainstreamed classes were examined in a large-scale study of 42 Texas school districts (Project Prime). Kaufman, Agard, and Semmel (1978) found that mainstreamed EMR children were more likely to pay attention to academic tasks when in their resource rooms than when they were in their regular classrooms. The environment of the smaller, more individualized resource room seemed to help these children to focus on their school work.

Summarizing these and other mainstreaming studies, Semmel et al. (1979) concluded that "Temporal integration as a defining feature of 'mainstreaming' apparently had no empirical significance. It is likely that participant composition (peers and teachers) of an instructional environment and the nature of the instructional process to which the handicapped child is subjected are more important variables in determining his or her school accomplishments" (p. 240). As Zigler and Muenchow (1979) noted (and we will expand upon this later), the proof of mainstreaming is in its implementation, not in the fact that a child is or is not in a regular classroom.

Social interaction

Dunn's criticism of special-class placement for EMR children emphasized the beneficial effects of social interaction between EMR and nonhandicapped children. He noted that "Homogeneous groupings tend to work to the disadvantage of slow learners and underprivileged" (1968, p. 6), and pointed to court decisions that had overturned the tracking system in several school districts. Dunn's concerns were subsequently addressed in the Kaufman et al. (1975) definition of mainstreaming, particularly in the provision that handicapped children should be "socially integrated" with their nonhandicapped peers.

Implicit in Dunn's argument was the so-called contact hypothesis (Christopoulos & Renz, 1969), the idea that contact between handicapped and nonhandicapped peers would prove beneficial to both groups. The hope was that mainstream classes would foster greater amounts of peer interaction by handicapped children, and would allow them the opportunity to learn from their nonhandicapped peers. The contact hypothesis also led to the belief that the nonhandicapped children would ultimately come to accept their special classmates.

There has now been over a decade of work on various aspects of the contact hypothesis, but controversy still exists as to its merits. With respect to the possibility that handicapped children will improve their social skills through mainstreaming, the results are generally positive. In a study by Gampel, Gottlieb, and Harrison (1974), 26 special-class EMR children (CA = 10 years, IQ = 70) were randomly assigned to special or mainstream classes for the upcoming school year. Researchers then examined the pattern of social interactions occurring in their rooms. An observational scoring system of 12 common classroom behaviors was developed, and each child was observed for a total of 30 minutes over six days. The frequency of 3 of the 12 behaviors, restlessness, negative verbal responses to peer, and negative verbal responses from peer, differed in the two EMR groups. Segregated children were significantly more restless, and had a greater amount of negative responses to and from peers, than did the EMR children in mainstreamed classes. Indeed, compared with a random sample of nonretarded children in these classes, the mainstreamed EMR children looked identical on each of the 12 observed behaviors (see Gampel, Harrison, & Budoff, 1972; Guerin & Szatlocky, 1974; and Grosenick, 1970, for similar results). Although the scoring procedures employed by these authors may have missed important (low-frequency) behaviors of the mainstreamed EMR children (see Corman & Gottlieb, 1978), it appears that "*In situ* observational data indicate that integrated EMR pupils do not display behavioral patterns which distinguish them from their nonhandicapped peers" (Semmel et al. 1979, p. 262).

A second corollary of the contact hypothesis is that EMR children will learn from the nonhandicapped children in mainstream classes. The bulk of this research has focused on imitation, that is, whether EMR children imitate the appropriate social behaviors of their nonhandicapped peers. Reviewing seven studies relating to this question, Gresham (1982) concluded that "there is little empirical evidence to suggest that integration of handicapped subjects into regular classrooms will result in beneficial modeling effects" (p. 426). He further noted that handicapped children can be taught to imitate their nonhandicapped classmates (see Guralnick, 1976; and Snyder, Apolloni, & Cooke, 1977), but that this outcome does not appear automatically. Educational personnel must systematically pave the way for handicapped children to succeed in learning from their peers.

Stigmatization

The third corollary of the contact hypothesis concerns stigmatization, the idea that one becomes a social outcast because of one's status or label (Goffman, 1963). As mentioned in Chapter 1, Mercer (1973a, 1973b) argued that children labeled retarded adopt a particular role when in certain social systems (e.g., school), but not necessarily when in others (e.g., at home). Foreshadowing this argument, Dunn (1968) suggested that the integration of EMR children into mainstream classes might reduce their social stigmatization, that their interactions with "normal" children might help them to be accepted by their classmates.

Unfortunately, this has not happened, a finding derived from several studies that employed sociometric measures of peers. One study illustrates the methodology: Iano, Ayers, Heller, McGettigan, and Walker (1974) asked nonhandicapped children in mainstreamed elementary school classes who they did and did not like best and who they would most and least like to play with. In results consistent with numerous other studies (see Gresham, 1982), Iano et al. found that the nonhandicapped students in the mainstreamed class received the highest mean acceptance rates and the lowest mean rejection rates. EMR children who had formerly been in special classes were least accepted and most rejected by the nonhandicapped children, and a third group, children who had never been identified as EMR but who received resource room help, were intermediate between the EMR and nonhandicapped groups.

Similar findings occur using other methodologies. Surveying a number of studies, Gresham (1982) concluded that examination of actual interactions demonstrated that "nonhandicapped children interact very little with mainstreamed handicapped children" (p. 423). In both attitude and behavior, then, nonhandicapped children tend to ostracize their EMR classmates.

The strength of the low social status held by handicapped children does not appear to be influenced by amount of contact with nonhandicapped children (Goodman, Gottlieb, & Harrison, 1972) or, as mentioned above, by the presence or absence of negative behaviors displayed by the EMR children (Gampel et al., 1974). In fact, it may even be the case that the more contact nonhandicapped children have with EMR children, the less the retarded children are accepted (Gottlieb & Budoff, 1973). As summarized by Corman and Gottlieb (1978), "There is evidence that the low social status of integrated children is not due to the fact that they were previously labeled EMR (Iano et al., 1974), the extent of their exposure to nonretarded peers . . . , nor to the actual frequency of their misbehavior as measured in observation studies (Gampel et al., 1974; Gottlieb et al., 1975)" (p. 271).

Why then do retarded children who attend mainstream classes suffer such a low social status in the eyes of their nonhandicapped classmates? The answer may lie in the teachers' perception of EMR students, a perception that may be subtly communicated to the other children (see Corman & Gottlieb, 1978). For example, Gottlieb, Semmel, and Veldman (1978) found that nonhandicapped children and their teachers rated the behaviors of EMR students in their classes very similarly. The degree to which teachers and nonhandicapped students perceived EMR children as less intelligent predicted the peer acceptance of these children; the degree to which the two groups perceived EMR children as more disruptive was related to the nonhandicapped peers' active rejection of EMR classmates (i.e., the number of times that the nonhandicapped children said that they did not like an EMR child). Such findings suggest the possibility that the opinions of teachers influence how well EMR children are accepted by their nonhandicapped classmates.

Teacher opinions of EMR students are themselves affected by several factors. In a large-scale study of regular-classroom teachers of grades K-12, Larivee and Cook (1979) found that two variables predicted a teacher's attitude toward mainstreaming: the degree of success that the teacher had previously experienced teaching handicapped children, and the amount of supportive services the teacher received. In addition, teachers who taught higher grades (e.g., junior high school and high school) were more negative in their opinions of mainstreaming than were teachers of younger children. Teachers of upper grades felt that they might be less able to succeed in teaching these older retarded children, expressed a need for supportive services, and in general were increasingly uncomfortable with the idea of EMR students in their classrooms.

A final aspect of stigmatization concerns the parents of EMR children in mainstreamed classes. Few studies have as yet tackled this issue, but it does appear that parental views toward the practice are mixed. Turnbull and Turnbull (1978) reported the feelings of one·parent, who concluded that "Mainstreaming, currently fashionable, simply means that *all* kids have an equal shot at mediocre schooling" (Bennett, 1978, p. 164). Other parents are more laudatory, as exemplified by Lockard's (1978) statement that "Mainstreaming has given Gregory [her handicapped son] confidence that he can function in the real world" (p. 528). In one of the few studies in the area, Dunst (1976) found that parents of handicapped children in regular and in segregated classrooms both felt that the respective placements were appropriate for their individual children. Clearly, more work is needed in this area (see also Turnbull & Blacher-Dixon, 1981).

Racial integration

Strongly influenced by the civil rights movement and by the general sociopolitical climate of the 1960s, Dunn (1968) and others hoped that mainstreaming might help to change the pattern of racial segregation in our nation's public schools. Such thinking received further support when Mercer (1974) documented that disproportionate numbers of black and Hispanic children were being labeled retarded compared to the percentages of each group in the general population. Upon diagnosis, these children were routinely placed in self-contained, special-education classrooms. Judicial opinion in the *Larry P., Diana*, and other court cases (see Turnbull, 1977) further bolstered the argument that mainstreaming would lessen the degree of racial segregation in the public schools.

Unfortunately, it does not appear that mainstreaming has solved or even slightly ameliorated the problem of racial segregation. Results from Project Prime showed that mainstream and special-education classrooms were about equally segregated in regard to the race of the students. To quote Gottlieb (1981),

as long as children continue to attend neighborhood schools that are racially segregated, merely switching EMR children from self-contained to mainstreamed classes is not apt to reduce the ethnic imbalance to which EMR children are exposed. Instead, EMR children will attend racially segregated regular classes rather than racially segregated self-contained classes. (p. 121)

Cost and individualized instruction

The final hope of the early adherents of mainstreaming was that the practice would foster instruction as individualized as that which occurs in special-education classes, but at a lower cost. Dunn (1968) pointed to the following changes as events that might prevent mainstreaming from becoming tantamount to depersonalizing the education of EMR children.

1 Changes in school organization, including the greater prevalence of team teaching, flexible grouping, and ungraded classes in public schools.
2 Curricular changes, including "many new and exciting options" for teaching reading and new mathematics curricula.
3 A wider variety of support personnel within the schools to aid classroom teachers (Dunn listed psychologists, guidance counselors, remedial reading specialists, and teachers' aides).
4 Hardware changes, including computerized teaching, teaching machines, and videotape equipment.

According to Dunn, each of these changes in the school system could, conceivably, be used to maximize the amount of services to each individual student within the mainstream classroom.

In regard to the first issue, costs per pupil, it does appear that special-class placements are more expensive than mainstreamed placements. Kakalik, Furry, Thomas, and Carney (1982) reported that, in the elementary years, the education of a handicapped child costs 4.98 times that of a nonhandicapped child, whereas the differential in the high school years is on the order of 2.5 times more (from Vitello & Soskin, 1985). In absolute terms, the costs of educating an EMR child were approximately $3,800 per year and for a severely retarded child $5,900 per year. (These amounts have risen since the Kakalik et al. report.)

However, the hope that the least restrictive environment (i.e., mainstream classrooms) might be more than simply the least expensive environment has not been borne out. In an in-depth study of 150 self-contained and 400 mainstream classes, Kaufman et al. (1978) found that, if anything, special-class instruction might be more individualized. Special-education teachers provided individual instruction for a greater percentage of the time (26.7%) than did mainstream class teachers (12%), and reading instruction was offered for a greater proportion of the day in the special classroom (27% to 16%). Other workers (see Gottlieb, 1981; Leinhardt & Pallay, 1982) have similarly concluded that EMR pupils in mainstream classrooms do not receive any greater amount of individualized instruction than they receive in special classrooms.

Overview and recommendations

In assessing the many effects of mainstreaming, we are left with a mixed set of results. EMR students in special-education and in regular classes

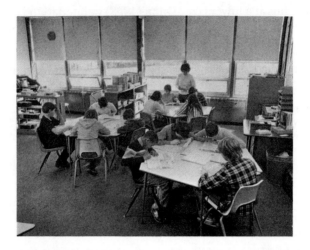

Photo 7. Special-education class. (Photograph courtesy of Elwyn Institutes, Elwyn, Pennsylvania)

appear to do equally well on academic achievement. While mainstreamed students show higher social skills, they are routinely stigmatized by their nonhandicapped peers. Levels of racial segregation are about equal in the two educational settings. Mainstream education costs less than education within self-contained classrooms, but may not be as individualized to the needs of special students. Regular-class teachers feel unprepared to instruct handicapped children, and teacher discomfort increases in the higher grades. Parental assessments of mainstreaming seem mixed. To sum up the data on mainstreaming, "there appears to be no unambiguous answer to the primitive question of whether segregated or integrated placement is superior" (Meyers, MacMillan, & Yoshida, 1980, p. 201).

The murkiness of the mainstreaming issue is further complicated by the historical forces from which the practice arose. As we have indicated, mainstreaming has been based more on a political and philosophical justification than on any scientific evidence regarding the best school placements for children with particular handicaps. Indeed, even Dunn's (1968) persuasive review of the evidence on the ineffectiveness of special-class placements ignored other evidence, equally available at the time, that children in mainstreamed placements were often stigmatized by their nonhandicapped peers (see Kirk, 1964). Mainstreaming is clearly a case in which court opinions, legislation, sociopolitical climates, and other nonscientific factors have been used to support preconceptions about what is or is not best for retarded children. Combined with the fact that mainstreaming is not well defined, does not have clear or agreed-upon goals, and varies in practice from school to school, it is small wonder that the issue remains so confused.

Still, the studies we have reviewed here do suggest some ways to make mainstreaming more effective. First, teachers need to be trained to work with the handicapped children in their mainstream classrooms. In their survey of over 1,800 teachers, Flynn, Gacka, and Sundean (1978) found that the majority of regular-class teachers felt that their standard teacher training had left them ill-equipped to handle the special challenges presented by handicapped children. Although preparation of teachers is an obvious aid to the success of mainstreaming, it is also an area which is often overlooked.

Second, the instruction of teachers of special education needs to be updated. As Sarason and Doris (1979) noted, although public policy now calls for placing handicapped children in the least restrictive environment, teacher training centers continue to educate school personnel in the tradition of the most restrictive alternative.

Finally, there is a need to provide professional supportive services to teachers of mainstreamed classes. In Dunn's (1968) original call for mainstreaming, services such as remedial reading, physical therapy, speech and language intervention, and psychological evaluation and counseling were assumed to be available. Dunn implied that the only way to ensure an individualized and effective education for mainstreamed EMR children is the full utilization of such supportive services. Unfortunately, the provision of these services has generally not been forthcoming. Indeed, Larivee and Cook (1979) found that the attitudes of regular-class teachers toward mainstreaming were related to the degree to which such supportive services were available: Those teachers who received large amounts of supportive services had higher opinions of mainstreaming than those who did not.

The training of regular-class teachers, the retraining of special-education teachers, and the provision of supportive services to teachers of mainstreamed classes all cost money. As Zigler and Muenchow (1979) noted, "any mainstreaming worthy of the name is likely to cost more, not less, than the old special education classes" (p. 994). Unfortunately, as one school superintendent put it, the federal government is "better at mandating than at allocating" when it comes to Public Law 94-142. Federal law now mandates that states serve all handicapped children, but "the federal contribution to the costs of meeting that service and other requirements of PL 94-142 is only a fraction of the costs borne by the states and local agencies" (Education Commission of the States Policy Committee, 1977).

The proof of mainstreaming lies in its implementation. In theory, mainstreaming can have many positive effects on all children, but this policy will be an empty slogan, with many negative effects, if not accompanied by adequate teacher training and support services. In addition, mainstreaming must not be presented as a panacea for handicaps. As Cruickshank (1977) observed, mainstreaming and the concept of the least restrictive environment "will not, in and of itself, solve a single problem of a single child" (p. 193). More work is needed to determine which children, with which particular characteristics, will benefit from mainstreamed placements, and which aspects of all classroom environments do and do not promote development for all students.

Part VI

Conclusion

12   Conclusion

In reviewing this and other books about mental retardation, one realizes that the field has come a long way indeed. A few decades ago there was a small amount of research, much of it of low quality; today the field of mental retardation can compete successfully with any established discipline. Large numbers of gifted and sophisticated workers are making advances on a variety of fronts, and the fruits of their efforts are becoming evident in the more complete understanding of, and ability to intervene with, retarded people.

The hallmark of these advances is specialization. Various workers now concentrate on one or a small set of issues; it is becoming increasingly rare for any one worker to span the field of mental retardation. Thus, we have groups of workers who are interested in early intervention, assessment of treatment effects, definition, classification, prevalence, motivation and personality development, mainstreaming, or institutionalization. Each subfield comprises an extensive array of work, much of it very high in quality.

But the cost of such specialization is often fragmentation. Whereas we as workers in the field now know more about each topic in mental retardation, it becomes increasingly difficult for any one person to know all areas, or even to understand or appreciate the issues in every subfield.

In an effort to bring some cohesion to the mental retardation field, or at least to those topics discussed in this volume, we will now specify some of the book's major themes. All of these themes are general in nature; all cross a number of chapter and topical boundaries. Each also sheds further light on how we have attempted to think about various issues in mental retardation. We follow our discussion of each general theme with our own preliminary ideas as to how each can lead to new research and intervention efforts in future years.

241

Need to go beyond conventional or accepted answers

In our discussions, we have often been struck by the litany of assumptions that those in the field of mental retardation accept uncritically as facts. For example, it is an article of faith to some workers that 3% of the population is retarded, even as a 1% prevalence rate is an equally solid "fact" to other workers. Many feel certain that familial retardation can only be caused by "sociocultural deprivation," that only cognitive deficits need be taken into account when describing the functioning of retarded individuals, that large institutions are necessarily inhumane, or that mainstreamed classes are always the optimal educational placement for retarded children. Some answers that we ourselves have always accepted might also not be true. For example, as discussed in Chapter 5, the commonly accepted 3 to 1 ratio of nonorganically to organically retarded people may not hold up under close scrutiny. In short, there are numerous assumptions that are accepted on faith alone by mental retardation workers.

Whatever one's reaction to any of the conclusions proposed in this book, the amount of conventional (and unchallenged) wisdom concerning mental retardation is disturbing. If, as stated at the beginning of Chapter 1, mental retardation research is to continue to be "vibrant work of high quality" (Zigler, 1977), then workers must not be content to accept uncritically such conventional answers. New theories must continue to be offered, contentions must be challenged, and data must be accumulated that will help refine or even supplant earlier work. To the extent that experts in mental retardation continue to be bound by conventional wisdom, such scientific activity is impossible.

One new proposal is the suggestion to further differentiate the category of organic retardation. So far, we have attempted to subdivide the non-organically retarded category (Chapter 4), but have not yet attempted to differentiate the various etiologies of organic retardation with respect to the psychological characteristics of each. For example, it now seems clear that Down syndrome children show decelerating IQs over time (see Hodapp & Zigler, in press), whereas IQs tend to remain relatively stable for other etiological groups (e.g., cerebral palsy). It may also be the case that the so-called structures of intelligence vary among different etiological groups (just as organically retarded people, as a group, differ in their structures of intelligence compared to familial retarded or nonretarded people). Other psychological phenomena may also vary across different etiological groups. Although further specification of the characteristics of each individual etiology is a painstaking task, the resultant research findings should enhance precision in our thinking about mental retardation.

Other efforts might be aimed at further examining the prevalence of mental retardation in different locales, among different age groups, and in males versus females. The entire issue of the percentage of retarded people who do and do not suffer from organic impairment needs more study, and precise diagnostic criteria for the various types of nonorganic retardation are required. Only through such efforts will the amount of questionable thinking be lessened and work in mental retardation advanced.

Utility of the developmental perspective

An openness to challenge and refinement ought not to imply that workers in mental retardation should have no overriding perspectives that guide their work. Our own perspective is that of development, as described by Piaget and Werner (see Chapter 2). We believe that the best way to conceptualize change over time in retarded children (especially those who do not show organic involvement) is through the lens of normal development, that the sequences, structures, and reactions to environmental events will be similar in retarded and in nonretarded children. The developmental perspective has itself been expanded to include examinations of developments in noncognitive areas and of the influence of the family and of other systems on the child's development.

In support of the developmental perspective, we note that both traditional and expanded versions of developmental theory have had demonstrable applicability to retarded individuals. The many programs of intervention in early cognition and language show the value of Piagetian and Wernerian viewpoints with retarded children, especially those who are severely retarded. These programs would not have been possible without knowledge of the various sequences of normal development described by theorists and researchers in child development. The recent discoveries of specific cognitive prerequisites for certain communicative skills also support the utility of the developmental perspective for guiding early intervention efforts.

The expanded version of the developmental perspective has also proven useful in work with retarded individuals. Thirty years of work on motivation and personality development in retarded persons (see Chapter 6) have demonstrated the need to look beyond cognitive functioning for a comprehensive assessment of functioning in retarded persons. By emphasizing the temporal aspects of the interaction between the child and the environment, Sameroff's transactional model has led to a more complete picture of the environment over time, and the family perspective has led to a focus on the particular makeup of that environment at any one point in time. Each of these efforts has led to an emphasis on the whole child and the whole environment in which that child develops. Each has also served to broaden the view of human development, a perspective that can then be applied to retarded persons.

Future work using the developmental perspective to study mentally retarded children will take several directions. As concerns the traditional developmental perspective, there is a need for evaluation studies on the efficacy of developmentally-based programs in several domains. For example, it remains unclear whether Piagetian-based cognitive programs or linguistic interventions based on the normative sequences of early language development do indeed promote the cognitive or linguistic development of retarded children (see Simeonsson, Cooper, & Scheiner, 1982, for qualified support for the effectiveness of early intervention programs with young severely retarded children; see Dunst & Rheingrover, 1981, for arguments that the effectiveness of such programs remains unclear). Whether such programs promote faster development than could be expected using other programs is unknown. Generalization of new concepts to unique situations must also be assessed using developmentally-based programs. All of this work is necessary to ascertain if a curriculum designed to take advantage of a similar sequence of development in retarded and nonretarded children is the optimal method of intervention with mentally retarded children.

A second area of work arises from the expanded developmental perspective. As mentioned in Chapters 2 and 7, we still know relatively little about the so-called ecology of childhood or about the ongoing transactions of the child and the environment over time. This is especially true with respect to the mentally retarded child. For example, we have some preliminary knowledge about how parents react to the birth and early development of retarded children, but have almost no understanding about how these reactions affect the behaviors of parents toward their offspring. The fathers of retarded children have received little attention, nor have the interactions among father, mother, and child been adequately examined. For example, in a longitudinal study of nonretarded children, Clarke-Stewart (1978) discovered that during the period from 15 to 30 months of age the most likely directions of effects "is mother influencing child, child influencing father and father influencing mother" (p. 476). This type of longitudinal work, examining the transactions of several individuals over time, is almost totally lacking in research involving mentally retarded children.

The status of siblings of retarded children is also in need of more study. Indeed, after reviewing all of the studies in the area, Lobato (1983) concluded that "there are few well-designed empirical studies indicating that, as a group, siblings of handicapped children are actually at risk or exhibit more problems of psychological adjustment" (p. 360) than do other children. Research into the particular mediating factors (e.g., sex, age, birth order) that might make some siblings more at risk is also necessary. Almost totally absent is sibling research that examines effects proceeding in the opposite direction – for example, studies of how nonretarded children promote development in their retarded siblings. In short, we need more and better research on the siblings of retarded and handicapped children.

Finally, many questions remain unexplored concerning the various institutions affecting retarded people. For example, although we know that there is an interaction between the retarded child's degree of preinstitutional social deprivation (PISD) and the effects of institutionalization, is there also an interaction between the child's home situation and the effects of mainstreaming? What are the effects of retarded children themselves on the nonretarded members of a mainstreamed class, or, put another way, do *mainstreamed* classes containing retarded children differ from *mainstream* classes that lack them? We simply do not know the answers to these and similar questions.

Before ending our discussion of the merits and future directions of the developmental perspective, we must also recognize that the developmental perspective is but one of many perspectives one can bring to bear on mental retardation and retarded persons. We have in passing mentioned two viewpoints common in the mental retardation field, the behaviorist and social systems perspectives. Like the developmental perspective, each offers a variety of new and interesting questions for work in mental retardation. Although neither represents our own particular orientation, each is nevertheless part of the "broad and rich array of theoretical formulations" (Zigler, 1977) guiding work in this area.

Need for a humane outlook

We have attempted to emphasize a humane and caring outlook toward retarded individuals throughout this book. Thus our emphasis on treating the retarded individual as a whole person, our focus on greater social competence as the main criterion of successful intervention, and our emphasis on helping the family members of retarded children. The issue of humaneness has also arisen in our discussions of mainstreaming and of deinstitutionalization, as we have attempted to keep ourselves attuned to those practices that are best for retarded individuals.

An argument could be made that one's own views on what constitutes humane care are always subjective, and to an extent this is true. The issue arises most clearly in our discussions of mainstreaming and deinstitution- alization, where proponents of each practice often vigorously oppose dis- senting viewpoints. Our response is twofold. First, we have attempted to look beyond current fads and trends to understand the accumulated history and thinking of workers in mental retardation throughout the past 130 years. In this way, we feel ourselves better prepared to identify exaggerated claims and potentially dangerous promises. Second, through our evaluation of the research evidence, we have tried in each chapter to ascertain what is best for retarded individuals. Thus, we enumerated the five proposed goals of mainstreaming and evaluated the practice according to the avail- able evidence on whether those goals had been achieved. Similarly, our discussion of deinstitutionalization centered around both the purposes of care for retarded people throughout U.S. history, and the effects of living in small-group settings on achieving those purposes. In this way, each topic has been kept, to the extent possible, an empirical issue. We think that by combining a historical analysis with an evaluation of the best available evidence, our conclusions are made more balanced and perhaps more humane.

Our emphasis on a humane outlook toward retarded individuals should not be confused with overoptimism, however. We have tried hard to be realistic and factual. Thus, we have strongly criticized a simplistic envi- ronmentalism in the mental retardation field, even as we realize that, if it were true that small or short-term change in the environment brought about large gains in intelligence, successful intervention with retarded individuals would be easier. Similarly, our evaluation of vitamin and patterning ther- apies has led us to the conclusion that both are ineffective, despite con- tinuing claims and hopes to the contrary. In short, we believe that a fair and realistic evaluation of the research evidence – while not always com- forting – is important to parents and interventionists working with retarded individuals.

Future research will continue to help provide insights into the best ways to care for and intervene with retarded individuals. In the past few years alone, there have been a series of studies attempting to replicate the findings of Harrell et al. (1981) on vitamin therapy, as workers have wanted to know if indeed a cure for mental retardation is imminent. Although each study has shown no effects of this therapy, the interest generated by the possible efficacy of vitamin therapy is instructive. Similarly, research on mainstreaming and deinstitutionalization continues to appear in the major journals on mental retardation. Indeed, much of the "vibrant work of high quality" in the mental retardation field concerns how best to care for and intervene with retarded persons.

The interest of workers in improving the care of retarded people does not imply that such issues are settled, however. It is striking that we still do not know which particular children are and are not most suitable for mainstreamed placements. Similarly, there remains a strong need for more high-quality research into deinstitutionalization. Thus, while we know much about which are and are not the most humane practices and interventions, there is a staggering amount yet to learn.

In addition, the issue of humane care may involve more than research per se. There is a need to expand and improve services to retarded persons. The provision of respite care must be expanded to allow parents short periods away from their retarded children, the effects of Public Law 94–142 must be monitored, and laws must be implemented that will help support the parents and families of mentally retarded children. Negative stereotypes of and behaviors toward retarded people must be combated, as in the current backlash against the placement of group homes in residential neighborhoods (see Vitello & Soskin, 1985). In all of these efforts, research is not enough; we must also endeavor, through legislative and educational means, to improve the lives of retarded individuals.

We can only conclude this book with a mixed verdict concerning the field of mental retardation. There has been great progress but there remains a long way to go. It is true that the field has advanced greatly in the past several decades, and that knowledge about mental retardation is accumulating at an astonishing rate. But it is equally true that a number of important questions remain. Although we have tried to give tentative answers to these questions, much future research and practice are needed for a more complete understanding of mental retardation.

References

Abramowicz, H. K., & Richardson, S. A. (1975). Epidemiology of severe mental retardation in children: Community studies. *American Journal of Mental Deficiency, 80,* 18–39.

Achenbach, T. (1970). Comparison of Stanford-Binet performance of nonretarded and retarded persons matched for MA and sex. *American Journal of Mental Deficiency, 74,* 488–499.

Achenbach, T., & Zigler, E. (1963). Social competence and self-image disparity in psychiatric and nonpsychiatric patients. *Journal of Abnormal and Social Psychology, 67,* 197–205.

Achenbach, T. & Zigler, E. (1968). Cue-learning and problem-learning strategies in normal and retarded children. *Child Development, 39,* 827–848.

Adams, A. (1971). The historical background to services for the mentally retarded. *Mental retardation and its social dimensions.* New York: Columbia University Press.

Adams, J. (1973). Adaptive behavior and measured intelligence in the classification of mental retardation. *American Journal of Mental Deficiency, 78,* 77–81.

Adubato, S. A., Adams, M. K., & Budd, K. S. (1981). Teaching a parent to train a spouse in child management techniques. *Journal of Applied Behavioral Analysis, 14,* 193–205.

Åkesson, H. O. (1961). *Epidemiology and genetics of mental deficiency in a southern Swedish population.* Uppsala: Almqvist & Wiksell.

Åkesson, H. O. (1967). Severe mental deficiency in a population in western Sweden: A preliminary report. *Acta Genetica (Basel), 17,* 243–247.

Als, H. (1977). The newborn communicates. *Journal of Communication, 27,* 66–73.

Aninger, M., & Bolinsky, K. (1977). Levels of independent functioning of retarded adults in apartments. *Mental Retardation, 15,* 12–13.

American Psychiatric Association (1980). *Diagnostic and statistical manual of mental disorders* (3rd ed.). Washington, D.C.: The American Psychiatric Association.

American Psychological Association. *Psychological Abstracts, 1977–1982.* Washington, D.C.: American Psychological Association.

Anderson, S., & Messick, S. (1974). Social competency in young children. *Developmental Psychology, 10,* 282–293.

Arnold, S., Sturgis, E., & Forehand, R. (1977). Training a parent to teach communication skills. *Behavior Modification, 1,* 259–276.

Ashurst, D. I., & Meyers, C. E. (1973). Social system and clinical model in school identification of the educable retarded. In R. K. Eyman, C. E. Meyers, & G. Tarjan (Eds.), *Sociobehavioral studies in mental retardation.* Washington, D.C.: American Association on Mental Deficiency.

Astin, A. W., & Ross, S. (1960). Glutamic acid and human intelligence. *Psychological Bulletin, 57,* 429–434.

Bacher, J. H. (1965). The effect of special class placement on the self-concept, social adjustment, and reading growth of slow learners. *Dissertation Abstracts, 26,* 70–71.

248

Baer, D. M., Peterson, R. F., & Sherman, J. A. (1967). The development of imitation by reinforcing behavioral similarity to a model. *Journal of Experimental Analysis of Behavior*, *10*, 405–416.

Baer, D. M., & Sherman, J. A. (1964). Reinforcement control of generalized imitation in young children. *Journal of Experimental Child Psychology*, *1*, 37–49.

Baker, B. (1984). Intervention with families with young, severely handicapped children. In J. Blacher (Ed.), *Severely handicapped young children and their families: Research in review*. New York: Academic Press.

Baker, B. L., Seltzer, G. B., & Seltzer, M. M. (1977). *As close as possible – Community residences for retarded adults*. Boston: Little, Brown.

Baldwin, A. L. (1947). Changes in parent behavior during pregnancy. *Child Development*, *18*, 29–39.

Balla, D. (1967). *The verbal action of the environment on institutionalized and noninstitutionalized retardates and normal children of two social classes*. Unpublished doctoral dissertation, Yale University.

Balla, D. (1976). Relationship of institution size to quality of care: A review of the literature. *American Journal of Mental Deficiency*, *81*, 117–124.

Balla, D., Butterfield, E. C., & Zigler, E. (1974). Effects of institutionalization on retarded children: A longitudinal, cross-institutional investigation. *American Journal of Mental Deficiency*, *78*, 530–549.

Balla, D., & Klein, M. (1981). Labels for and taxonomies of environments for retarded persons. In H. C. Haywood & J. R. Newbrough (Eds.), *Living environments for developmentally retarded persons*. Baltimore: University Park Press.

Balla, D., McCarthy, E., & Zigler, E. (1971). Some correlates of negative reaction tendencies in institutionalized retarded children. *Journal of Psychology*, *79*, 77–84.

Balla, D., Styfco, S., & Zigler, E. (1971). Use of the opposition concept and outer-directedness in intellectually average, familial retarded, and organically retarded children. *American Journal of Mental Deficiency*, *75*, 863–880.

Balla, D., & Zigler, E. (1964). Discrimination and switching learning in normal, familial retarded, and organic retarded children. *Journal of Abnormal and Social Psychology*, *69*, 664–669.

Balla, D., & Zigler, E. (1971). The therapeutic role of visits and vacations for institutionalized retarded children. *Mental Retardation*, *9*, 7–9.

Balla, D., & Zigler, E. (1975). Pre-institutional social deprivation, responses to social reinforcement and IQ change in institutionalized retarded individuals: A six-year follow-up study. *American Journal of Mental Deficiency*, *80*, 228–230.

Balla, D., & Zigler, E. (1977). The social policy implications of a research program on the effects of institutionalization on retarded persons. In P. Mittler (Ed.), *Research to practice in mental retardation* (Vol. 1). Baltimore: University Park.

Balla, D., & Zigler, E. (1979). Personality development in retarded persons. In N. R. Ellis (Ed.), *Handbook of mental deficiency* (2nd ed.). Hillsdale, N.J.: Erlbaum.

Baller, W., Charles, D., & Miller, E. (1967). Mid-life attainment of the mentally retarded: A longitudinal study. *Genetic Psychology Monographs*, *75*, 235–329.

Barnard, J. D., Christophersen, E. R., & Wolf, M. M. (1976). Parent-mediated treatment of children's self-injurious behavior using overcorrection. *Journal of Pediatric Psychology*, *1*, 56–61.

Barr, M. W. (1904). *Mental defectives: Their history, treatment and training*. Philadelphia: Blakiston.

Bates, E. (1976). *Language and context – The acquisition of pragmatics*. New York: Academic Press.

Bates, E., Camaioni, L., & Volterra, V. (1975). The acquisition of performatives prior to speech. *Merrill-Palmer Quarterly*, *21*, 205–226.

Baumeister, A. (1967). Problems in comparative studies of mental retardates and normals. *American Journal of Mental Deficiency, 71,* 869–875.

Baumeister, A. (1970). American residential institution: Its history and character. In A. A. Baumeister & E. Butterfield (Eds.), *Residential facilities for the mentally retarded.* Chicago: Aldine.

Bayley, N. (1949). Consistency and variability in the growth of intelligence from birth to eighteen years. *Journal of Genetic Psychology, 75,* 165–196.

Bayley, N. (1955). On the growth of intelligence. *American Psychologist, 10,* 805–818.

Bayley, N. (1969). *Bayley Scales of Infant Development: Birth to two years.* New York: Psychological Corporation.

Bayley, N., & Schaefer, E. S. (1964). Correlations of maternal and child behaviors with the development of mental abilities: Data from the Berkeley Growth Study. *Monographs of the Society for Research in Child Development, 29,* (6). (whole 97).

Beckman, P. J. (1983). Influence of selected child characteristics on stress in families of handicapped infants. *American Journal of Mental Deficiency, 88,* 150–156.

Begab, M. J. (1974). The major dilemma of mental retardation: Shall we prevent it? (Some social implications of research in mental retardation). *American Journal of Mental Deficiency, 78,* 519–529.

Bejar, I. I. (1981). Does nutrition cause intelligence? A reanalysis of the Cali experiment. *Intelligence, 5,* 49–68.

Bell, N. J., Schoenrock, C., & Bensberg, G. (1981). Change over time in the community: Findings of a longitudinal study. In R. H. Bruininks, C. E. Meyers, B. B. Sigford, & H. C. Lakin (Eds.), *Deinstitutionalization and community adjustment of mentally retarded people.* Washington: American Association on Mental Deficiency.

Bell, R. Q. (1968). A reinterpretation of the direction of effects in studies of socialization. *Psychological Review, 75,* 81–95.

Bennett, F., McClelland, S., Kriegsman, E., Anarus, L. B., & Sellas, C. J. (1983). Vitamin and mineral supplementation in Down's Syndrome. *Pediatrics, 74,* 707–713.

Bennett, J. M. (1978). Company halt! In A. P. Turnbull & H. R. Turnbull (Eds.), *Parents speak out: Views from the other side of the two-way mirror.* Columbus, Ohio: Merrill.

Berger, J., & Cunningham, C. C. (1983). Development of early vocal behaviors and interactions in Down's Syndrome and nonhandicapped infant–mother pairs. *Developmental Psychology, 19,* 322–331.

Berk, R. A., Bridges, W. I., & Shih, A. (1981). Does IQ really matter? A study of the use of IQ scores for the tracking of the mentally retarded. *American Sociological Review, 46,* 58–71.

Berman, P., Waisman, H., & Graham, F. (1966). Intelligence in treated phenylketonuric children: A developmental study. *Child Development, 37,* 731–747.

Bernstein, C. (1921). Colony care isolation of defective and dependent cases. *American Association of Mental Deficiency Proceedings, 26,* 43–59.

Berrueta-Clement, J., Schweinhart, L., Barnett, W., Epstein, A., & Weikart, D. (1984). *Changed lives: The effects of the Perry Preschool Program on youths through age 19.* Monographs of the High/Scope Educational Research Foundation. Ypsilanti, Mich.: High/Scope.

Bertalannfy, L. von (1968). *General systems theory.* New York: Braziller.

Best, H. (1965). *Public provision for the mentally retarded in the United States.* Worcester, Mass.: Heffernan Press.

Bijou, S. W. (1966). A functional analysis of retarded development. In N. R. Ellis (Ed.), *International review of research in mental retardation* (Vol. 1). New York: Academic Press.

Bijou, S., & Baer, D. (1961). *Child development: A systematic and empirical theory.* New York: Appleton-Century-Crofts.

Bijou, S., & Baer, D. (1967). *Child development: Readings in experimental analysis.* New York: Appleton-Century-Crofts.

Binder, A. (1963). Further considerations on testing the null hypothesis, and the strategy and tactics of investigating theoretical models. *Psychological Review, 70,* 107–115.

Birch, H. G., Richardson, S. A., Baird, D., Horobin, G., & Illsley, R. (1970). *Mental subnormality in the community: A clinical and epidemiological study.* Baltimore: Williams & Wilkins Co.

Birenbaum, A., & Re, M. A. (1979). Resettling mentally retarded adults in the community – almost 4 years later. *American Journal of Mental Deficiency, 83,* 323–329.

Blacher, J. (1984). *Severely handicapped young children and their families.* New York: Academic Press.

Blais, M. (1983). The unusual education of John Sullivan: Can you buy your baby a high IQ? *Tropic Magazine, Miami Herald,* April 10, 12–16; 23.

Blatt, B. (1979). *The family papers: A return to Purgatory.* New York: Longman.

Blatt, B., & Kaplan, F. (1966). *Christmas in Purgatory.* Boston: Allyn & Bacon.

Blomquist, H.-K., Gustavson, K.-H., & Holmgren, G. (1981). Mild mental retardation in children in a northern Swedish county. *Journal of Mental Deficiency Research, 25,* 169–186.

Bloom, L. (1970). *Language development: From form to function in emerging grammars.* Cambridge, Mass.: MIT Press.

Braginsky, D. D., & Braginsky, B. M. (1971). *Hansels and Gretels: Studies of children in institutions for the mentally retarded.* New York: Holt, Rinehart and Winston.

Brainerd, C. J. (1978). *Piaget's theory of intelligence.* Englewood Cliffs, N.J.: Prentice-Hall.

Brazelton, T. B., Koslowski, B., & Main, M. (1974). The origins of reciprocity: The early mother–infant interaction. In M. Lewis and L. A. Rosenblum (Eds.), *The effects of the infant on its caretaker.* New York: Wiley.

Brehony, K. A., Benson, B. A., Solomon, L. J., & Luscomb, R. L. (1980). Parents as behavior modifiers: Intervention for three problem behaviors in a severely retarded child. *Journal of Clinical Child Psychology, 9,* 213–216.

Bricker, W., & Bricker, D. (1974). An early language training strategy. In R. L. Schiefelbusch & L. Lloyd (Eds.), *Language perspectives: Acquisition, retardation, and intervention.* Baltimore: University Park.

Brinley, M. (1983). Raising a superkid. *McCall's,* November, pp. 100–101; 196–201.

Bromwich, R. (1976). Focus on maternal behavior in infant intervention. *American Journal of Orthopsychiatry, 46,* 439–446.

Bromwich, R. (1980). *Working with parents of infants.* Baltimore: University Park.

Bronfenbrenner, U. (1975). Is early intervention effective? In M. Guttentag & E. L. Struening (Eds.), *Handbook of evaluation research* (Vol. 2). Beverly Hills, Calif.: Sage.

Bronfenbrenner, U. (1979). *The ecology of human development.* Cambridge, Mass.: Harvard University Press.

Brooks-Gunn, J., & Lewis, M. (1984). Maternal responsivity in interactions with handicapped infants. *Child Development, 55,* 782–793.

Brown, A. L. (1973). Conservation of number and continuous quantity in normal, bright and retarded children. *Child Development, 44,* 376–379.

Brown, R. (1973). *A first language.* Cambridge, Mass.: Harvard University Press.

Bruner, J. (1978). Learning how to do things with words. In J. Bruner & A. Garton (Eds.), *Human growth and development.* Oxford University Press.

Buck v. *Bell,* 274 U.S. 200 (1927).

Budd, K. S., Green, D. R., & Baer, D. M. (1976). An analysis of multiple misplaced parental social contingencies. *Journal of Applied Behavior Analysis, 9,* 459–470.

Budoff, M., & Gottlieb, J. (1976). Special class EMR students mainstreamed: A study of an aptitude (learning potential) X treatment interaction. *American Journal of Mental Deficiency, 81,* 1–11.

Butler, A. (1915). The feeble-minded: The need of research. *Proceedings of the National Conference of Charities and Correction,* 356–361.

Butler, E. W., & Bjaanes, A. T. (1977). A typology of community care facilities and differential normalization outcomes. In P. Mittler (Ed.), *Research to practice in mental retardation* (Vol. 1). Baltimore: University Park.

Butterfield, E. C., & Zigler, E. (1965a). The effects of success and failure on the discrimination learning of normal and retarded children. *Journal of Abnormal Psychology, 70,* 25–31.

Butterfield, E., & Zigler, E. (1965b). The influence of differing social climates on the effectiveness of social reinforcement in the mentally retarded. *American Journal of Mental Deficiency, 70,* 48–56.

Butterfield, E. C., & Zigler, E. (1970). Preinstitutional social deprivation and IQ changes among institutionalized retarded children. *Journal of Abnormal Psychology, 75,* 83–89.

Byck, M. (1968). Cognitive differences among diagnostic groups of retardates. *American Journal of Mental Deficiency, 73,* 97–101.

Cameron, A., & Storm, T. (1965). Achievement motivation in Canadian Indian middle and working-class children. *Psychological Reports, 16,* 459–463.

Caparulo, B. K. (1979). *Mainstreaming and teachers' attitudes toward mainstreaming: Their influence on the behavior of mildly retarded children.* Unpublished manuscript, Yale University.

Caparulo, B., & Zigler, E. (1983). The effects of mainstreaming on success expectancy and imitation in mildly retarded children. *Peabody Journal of Education, 60,* 85–97.

Carroll, A. W. (1967). The effects of segregated and partially integrated school programs on self-concept and academic achievement of educable mental retardates. *Exceptional Children, 34,* 93–99.

Casey, L. (1978). Development of communicative behavior in autistic children: A parent program using signed speech. *Devereux Forum, 12,* 1–15.

Castaneda, A., McCandless, B. R., & Palermo, D. S. (1956). The Children's Form of the Manifest Anxiety Scale. *Child Development, 27,* 317–326.

Cavalier, A., & McCarver, R. B. (1981). Wyatt v. Stickney and mentally retarded individuals. *Mental Retardation, 19,* 209–214.

Cavalli-Sforza, L. L., & Bodmer, W. F. (1971). *The genetics of human populations.* San Francisco: Freeman.

Childs, R. (1979). A drastic change in curriculum for the educable mentally retarded. *Mental Retardation, 17,* 299–306.

Christopoulos, F., & Renz, P. (1969). A critical examination of special education programs. *Journal of Special Education, 3,* 371–379.

Cicchetti, D. (1984). The emergence of developmental psychopathology. *Child Development, 55,* 1–7.

Cicchetti, D., & Pogge-Hesse, P. (1982). Possible contributions of the study of organically retarded persons to developmental theory. In E. Zigler and D. Balla (Eds.), *Mental retardation: The developmental–difference controversy.* Hillsdale, N.J.: Erlbaum.

Cicchetti, D., & Serafica, F. (1981). The interplay among behavioral systems: Illustration from the study of attachment, affiliation, and wariness in young Down's Syndrome children. *Developmental Psychology, 17,* 326–339.

Cicchetti, D., & Sroufe, L. A. (1976). The relationship between affective and cognitive development in Down's Syndrome infants. *Child Development, 47,* 920–928.

Clarke, A. D. B., & Clarke, A. M. (1954). Cognitive changes in the feeble-minded. *British Journal of Psychology, 45,* 173–179.

Clarke, A. D. B., Clarke, A. M., & Reiman, S. (1958). Cognitive and social changes in the feeble-minded: Three further studies. *British Journal of Psychology, 49,* 144–157.

Clarke, A. M., & Clarke, A. D. B. (1974a). Genetic-environmental interactions in cognitive development. In A. M. Clarke & A. D. B. Clarke (Eds.), *Mental deficiency: The changing outlook* (3rd ed.). New York: Free Press.

Clarke, A. M., & Clarke, A. D. B. (Eds.) (1974b). *Mental deficiency: The changing outlook* (3rd ed.). New York: Free Press.

Clarke, A. M., & Clarke, A. D. B. (1976). *Early experience: Myth and evidence.* London: Open Books.

Clarke-Stewart, K. A. (1978). And Daddy makes three: The father's impact on mother and young child. *Child Development, 49,* 466–478.

Clausen, J. A. (1967). Mental deficiency: Development of a concept. *American Journal of Mental Deficiency, 71,* 727–745.

Cleland, C. (1965). Evidence on the relationship between size and institutional effectiveness: A review and analysis. *American Journal of Mental Deficiency, 70,* 423–431.

Cleland, C., Case, J., & Manaster, G. (1980). IQs and etiologies: The two group approach to mental retardation. *Bulletin of the Psychonomic Society, 15* (6), 413–415.

Coburn, S., Schaltenbrand, W., Mahuren, J., Clausman, R., & Townsend, D. (1983). Effect of megavitamin treatment on mental performance and plasma vitamin B6 concentrations in mentally retarded young adults. *The American Journal of Clinical Nutrition, 38,* 352–355.

Cochran, I. L., & Cleland, C. C. (1963). Manifest anxiety of retardates and normals matched as to academic achievement. *American Journal of Mental Deficiency, 72,* 30–33.

Cohen, H. J., Birch, H. G., & Taft, L. T. (1970). Some considerations for evaluating the Doman-Delacato "patterning" method. *Pediatrics, 45,* 302–314.

Cohen, H., Conroy, J. W., Frazer, D. W., Snelbecker, G. E., & Spreat, S. (1977). Behavioral effects of institutional relocation of mentally retarded residents. *American Journal of Mental Deficiency, 82,* 12–18.

Consortium for Longitudinal Studies. (Ed.), (1983). *As the twig is bent: Lasting effects of preschool programs.* Hillsdale, N.J.: Erlbaum.

Corman, L, & Gottlieb, J. (1978). Mainstreaming mentally retarded children: A review of research. In N. R. Ellis (Ed.), *International Review of Research in Mental Retardation, 9,* 251–275.

Craig, E., & McCarver, R. B. (1984). Community placement and adjustment of deinstitutionalized clients: Issues and findings. In N. R. Ellis (Ed.), *International Review of Research in Mental Retardation, 12,* 95–122.

Crissey, M. S. (in press). Program components of a therapeutic environment: Blueprint for a dream. In M. S. Crissey and M. Rosen (Eds.), *Institutions for the mentally retarded: A changing role in changing times.* Austin, Tex.: Pro-Ed.

Crnic, K., Friedrich, W., & Greenberg, M. (1983). Adaptation of families with mentally retarded children: A model of stress, coping, and family ecology. *American Journal of Mental Deficiency, 88,* 125–138.

Cromwell, R. L. (1963). A social learning approach to mental retardation. In N. R. Ellis (Ed.), *Handbook in mental deficiency.* New York: McGraw-Hill.

Cromwell, R. L., Blashfield, R. K., & Strauss, J. S. (1975). Criteria for classification systems. In N. Hobbs (Ed.), *Issues in the classification of children* (Vol. 1). San Francisco: Jossey-Bass.

Cronbach, L. J. (1975). Five decades of controversy over mental testing. *American Psychologist, 30,* 1–14.

Cronbach, L. J., & Snow, R. E. (1977). *Aptitudes and instructional methods.* New York: Irvington.

Cruickshank, W. M. (1977). Least restrictive placement: Administrative wishful thinking. *Journal of Learning Disabilities, 10,* 14–17.

Cullen, S. M., Cronk, C. E., Pueschel, S. M., Schnell, R. R., & Reed, R. B. (1981). Social development and feeding milestones of young Down Syndrome children. *American Journal of Mental Deficiency, 85,* 410–415.

Culver, M. (1967). *Intergenerational social mobility among families with a severely mentally retarded child.* Unpublished doctoral thesis, University of Illinois.

Cummings, S. T. (1976). The impact of the child's deficiency on the father: A study of fathers of mentally retarded and chronically ill children. *American Journal of Orthopsychiatry, 46,* 246–255.

Cummings, S., Bayley, H., & Rie, H. (1966). Effects of the child's deficiency on the mother: A study of mothers of mentally retarded, chronically ill and neurotic children. *American Journal of Orthopsychiatry, 36,* 595–608.

Curcio, F. (1978). Sensorimotor functioning and communication in mute, autistic children. *Journal of Autism and Childhood Schizophrenia, 8,* 282–292.

Curtiss, S. (1977). *Genie: A psycholinguistic study of a modern-day "wild child."* New York: Academic Press.

Cytryn, L., & Lourie, R. S. (1975). Mental retardation. In A. M. Freeman, H. I. Kaplan, & B. J. Sadock (Eds.), *Comprehensive textbook of psychiatry, 1,* (2nd ed.). Baltimore: Williams and Wilkins.

Czeizel, A., Lányi-Engelmayer, A., Klujber, L., Metnéki, J., & Tusnády, G. (1980). Etiological study of mental retardation in Budapest, Hungary. *American Journal of Mental Deficiency, 85,* 120–128.

Davies, S. P. (1930). *Social control of the mentally deficient.* New York: Crowell.

Davies, S. P., & Ecob, K. C. (1959). The challenge to the schools. In S. P. Davies (Ed.), *The mentally retarded in society.* New York: Columbia University Press.

Davis, A. (1941). American status systems and the socialization of the child. *American Sociological Review, 6,* 234–254.

Delacato, C. H. (1963). *Diagnosis and treatment of speech and reading problems.* Springfield, Ill.: Thomas.

Dennis, W., & Dennis, M. (1940). The effect of cradling practices upon the onset of walking on Hopi children. *Journal of Genetic Psychology, 56,* 77–86.

Deutsch, A. (1949). *The mentally ill in America: A history of their care and treatment from colonial times* (2nd ed.). New York: Columbia University Press.

Dingman, H. F., & Tarjan, G. (1960). Mental retardation and the normal distribution curve. *American Journal of Mental Deficiency, 64,* 991–994.

Dingman, H. F., Tarjan, G., Eyman, R. K., & Miller, C. R. (1964). Epidemiology in hospitals: Some uses of data processing in chronic disease institutions. *American Journal of Mental Deficiency, 68,* 586–593.

Dobson, J. C., Kushida, E., Williamson, M., & Friedman, E. G. (1976). Intellectual performances of 36 phenylketonuria patients and their nonaffected siblings. *Pediatrics, 58,* 53–58.

Dobzhansky, T. (1962). *Mankind evolving: The evolution of the human species.* New Haven, Conn.: Yale University Press.

Doll, E. A. (1953). *Measurement of social competence: A manual for the Vineland social maturity scale.* Minneapolis: Educational Publishers.

Doll, E. E. (1962). A historical survey of research and management of mental retardation in the United States. In E. P. Trapp & P. Himmelstein (Eds.), *Readings on the exceptional child*. New York: Appleton-Century-Crofts.

Doman, G. (1974). *What to do about your brain injured child*. New York: Doubleday.

Doman, R. J., Spitz, E. B., Zucman, E., Delacato, C. H., & Doman, G. (1960). Children with severe brain injuries. *Journal of the American Medical Association, 174*, 219–223.

Drews, E. M. (1962). *The effectiveness of homogeneous and heterogeneous ability grouping in ninth grade English classes with slow, average and superior students*. Unpublished manuscript, Michigan State University.

Drillien, C. M., Jameson, S., & Wilkinson, E. M. (1966). Studies in mental handicap, Part I: Prevalence and distribution by clinical type and severity of defect. *Archives of Disease in Childhood, 41*, 528–538.

Dugdale, R. L. (1877). *The Jukes*. New York: Putnam.

Dugdale, R. L. (1910). *The Jukes: A study in crime, pauperism, disease and heredity*. New York: Putnam.

Dunn, J., & Kendrick, C. (1980). The arrival of a sibling: Changes in patterns of interaction between mother and first-born child. *Journal of Child Psychology and Psychiatry, 21*, 119–132.

Dunn, J., & Kendrick, C. (1981). Interaction between young siblings: Association with the interaction between mother and first-born child. *Developmental Psychology, 17*, 336–343.

Dunn, L. M., (1968). Special education for the mildly retarded–Is much of it justifiable? *Exceptional Children, 35*, 5–22.

Dunst, C. J. (1976). Attitudes of parents with children in contrasting family education programs. *Mental Retardation Bulletin, 4*, (3), 120–132.

Dunst, C. J. (1980a). *A clinical and educational manual for use with the Uzgiris-Hunt Scales for infant psychological development*. Baltimore: University Park.

Dunst, C. J. (1980b). Family, Infant and Preschool Program: Western Carolina Center, Morganton, North Carolina. *New Jersey Journal of School Psychology, 2*, 26–40.

Dunst, C. J. (1982). *Early intervention, social support and institutional avoidance*. Paper presented at the annual meeting of the Southeastern American Association on Mental Deficiency, Louisville, Ky., November.

Dunst, C. J., & Rheingrover, R. M. (1981). An analysis of the efficacy of infant intervention programs with organically handicapped children. *Evaluation and Program Planning, 4*, 287–323.

Edgerton, R. B., Eyman, R. K., & Silverstein, A. B. (1975). Mental retardation system. In N. Hobbs (Ed.), *Issues in the classification of children* (Vol. 2). San Francisco: Jossey-Bass.

Edgerton, R. B., & Sabagh, G. (1962). From mortification to aggrandizement: Changing self-conception in the careers of the mentally retarded. *Psychiatry, 25*, 263–272.

Education Commission of the States Policy Committee. (1977). *Selected statements*, (Pub. 1, 1.) Denver, Colo.: Education Commission of the States, September.

Ellis, N. R. (Ed.), (1963). *Handbook of mental deficiency*. New York: McGraw-Hill.

Ellis, N. R. (1969). A behavior research strategy in mental retardation: Defense and critique. *American Journal of Mental Deficiency, 73*, 557–566.

Ellis, N., Balla, D., Estes, O., Warren, S., Meyers, C. E., Hollis, J., Isaacson, R., Palk, B., & Siegel, P. (1981). Common sense in the habilitation of mentally retarded persons: A reply to Menolascino and McGee. *Mental Retardation, 5*, 221–225.

Ellis, N. R., & Cavalier, A. R. (1982). Research perspectives in mental retardation. In E. Zigler and D. Balla (Eds.), *Mental retardation: The developmental-difference controversy*. Hillsdale, N.J.: Erlbaum.

Ellis, N. R., & Temporowski, P. D. (1983). Vitamin/mineral supplements and intelligence of institutionalized mentally retarded adults. *American Journal of Mental Deficiency, 88,* 211–214.

Ellman, G., Silverstein, C., Zingarelli, G., Schafer, E., & Silverstein, L. (1984). Vitamin-mineral supplement fails to improve IQ of mentally retarded young adults. *American Journal of Mental Deficiency, 88,* 688–691.

Embry, L. (1980). Family support for handicapped preschool children at risk for abuse. In J. Gallagher (Ed.), *New directions for exceptional children, 4.* San Francisco: Jossey-Bass.

Emde, R. N., & Brown, C. (1978). Adaptation to the birth of a Down's Syndrome infant: Grieving and maternal attachment. *Journal of The American Academy of Child Psychiatry, 17,* 299–323.

Erickson, M. (1969). MMPI profiles of parents of young retarded children. *American Journal of Mental Deficiency, 73,* 727–732.

Evans, R. I. (1973). *Jean Piaget: The man and his ideas.* New York: Dutton.

Eyman, R., & Arndt, S. (1979). Life span development of institutionalized and community based mentally retarded residents. *American Journal of Mental Deficiency, 86,* 342–350.

Eyman, R. K., Demaine, G. C., & Lei, T. (1979). Relationship between community environments and residential changes in adaptive behavior: A path model. *American Journal of Mental Deficiency, 83,* 330–338.

Eyman, R. K., & Miller, C. A. (1978). A demographic overview of severe and profound mental retardation. In C. E. Meyers (Ed.), *Quality of life in severely and profoundly mentally retarded people: Research foundations for improvement. Monographs of the American Association on Mental Deficiency, 3,* ix–xii.

Eysenck, H. J. (1971). *The I.Q. argument.* Freeport: Library Press.

Falender, C., & Heber, R. (1975). Mother and child interaction and participation in a longitudinal intervention program. *Developmental Psychology, 11,* 830–836.

Family Support Project. (1983). *Programs to strengthen families.* New Haven, Conn.: Yale University Press and the Family Resource Coalition.

Farber, B. (1959). The effects of a severely mentally retarded child in family systems. *Monographs of Society for Research in Child Development, 24,* No. 2.

Farber, B. (1970). Notes on sociological knowledge about families with mentally retarded children. In M. Schreiber (Ed.), *Social work and mental retardation.* New York: John Day.

Farren, D. C., & Haskins, R. (1980). Reciprocal influence in the social interactions of mothers and three-year-old children from different socioeconomic backgrounds. *Child Development, 51,* 780–791.

Fernald, W. (1912). The burden of feeblemindedness. *Journal of Psycho-Asthenics, 17,* 87–111.

Fernald, W. et al. (1913). Discussion of H. H. Goddard's "The improvability of feebleminded children." *Journal of Psycho-Asthenics, 17,* 126–131.

Fernald, W. (1919). After-care study of the patients discharged from Waverly for a period of twenty-five years. *Ungraded, 5,* 25–31.

Fernald, W. (1922). The inauguration of a state-wide public school mental clinic in Massachusetts. *Mental Hygiene, 6,* 471–486.

Fernald, W. (1924). Thirty years of progress in the care of the feeble-minded. *Proceedings of the American Association for the Study of the Feeble-Minded, 212.*

Field, T. (1978). The three R's of infant–adult interactions: Rhythms, repertoires, and responsivity. *Journal of Pediatric Psychology, 3,* 131–136.

Fischer, K. W. (1980). A theory of cognitive development: The control and construction of a hierarchy of skills. *Psychological Review, 87,* 477–531.

Flavell, J. H. (1963). *The developmental psychology of Jean Piaget.* Princeton: Van Nostrand.

Flavell, J. H. (1977). *Cognitive development*. Englewood Cliffs, N.J.: Prentice-Hall.
Flavell, J. H. (1982). Structures, stages, and sequences in cognitive development. In W. A. Collins (Ed.), *The concept of development: The Minnesota Symposia on Child Psychology*. Hillsdale, N.J.: Erlbaum.
Flynn, J. R., Gacka, R. C., & Sundean, N. (1978). Are classroom teachers prepared for mainstreaming? *Phi Delta Kappan*, *59*, 562.
Følling, A. (1934). Ueber Ausscheidung von Phenlybrenztraubensaure in den Harn als Stoffwechselanomalie in Verbindung mit Imbezillität. *Hoppe Seyler Z. Physiol. Chem.* 227, 169–176.
Forehand, R., Cheney, T., & Yoder, P. (1974). Parent behavior training: Effects on the noncompliance of a deaf child. *Journal of Behavior Therapy and Experimental Psychiatry*, *5*, 281–283.
Fox, A. M. (1975). Families with handicapped children – A challenge to the caring professions. *Community Health*, *6*, 217–223.
Fox, R. A., & Roseen, D. L . (1977). A parent-administered token program for dietary regulation of phenylketonuria. *Journal of Behavior Therapy and Experimental Psychiatry*, *8*, 441–443.
Frazier, J. R., & Schneider, H. (1975). Parental management of inappropriate hyperactivity in a young retarded child. *Journal of Behavior Therapy and Experimental Psychiatry*, *6*, 245–247.
Freeman, R. D. (1967). Controversy over "patterning" as a treatment for brain damage in children. *Journal of the American Medical Association*, *202*, 385–388.
Friedrich, W. L., & Friedrich, W. N. (1981). Psychosocial assets of parents of handicapped and nonhandicapped children. *American Journal of Mental Deficiency*, *85*, 551–553.
Friedrich, W. N. (1979). Predictors of the coping behavior of mothers of handicapped children. *Journal of Consulting and Clinical Psychology*, *47*, 1140–1141.
Furrow, D., Nelson, K., & Benedict, H. (1979). Mothers' speech to children and syntactic development: Some simple relationships. *Journal of Child Language*, *6*, 423–442.
Furth, H. (1969). *Piaget and knowledge*. Englewood Cliffs, N.J.: Prentice-Hall.
Gallagher, J. (1985). The prevalence of mental retardation: Cross-cultural considerations from Sweden and the United States. *Intelligence*, *9*, 97–108.
Gallagher, J., Beckman, P., & Cross, A. (1983). Families of handicapped children: Sources of stress and its amelioration. *Exceptional Children*, *50*, 10–19.
Galton, F. (1901). The possible improvement of the human breed under the existing conditions of law and sentiment. *Nature*, *64*, 659–665.
Gampel, D. H., Gottlieb, J., & Harrison, R. H. (1974). Comparison of classroom behavior of low IQ and nonretarded children. *American Journal of Mental Deficiency*, *79*, 16–21.
Gampel, D. H., Harrison, R. H., & Budoff, M. (1972). An observational study of segregated and integrated EMR children and their nonretarded peers: Can we tell the difference by looking? *Studies in Learning Potential*, *2*, 27.
Garber, H. L. (1975). Intervention in infancy: A developmental approach. In M. Begab & S. A. Richardson (Eds.), *The mentally retarded and society*. Baltimore: University Park.
Garber, H., & Heber, F. R. (1977). The Milwaukee project: Indications of the effectiveness of early intervention in preventing mental retardation. In P. Mittler (Ed.), *Research to practice in mental retardation* (Vol. 1). Baltimore: University Park.
Garber, H., & Heber, R. (1981). The efficacy of early intervention with family rehabilitation. In M. Begab, C. Haywood, & H. Garber (Eds.), *Psychosocial influences in retarded performance*. Baltimore: University Park.
Gardner, H. (1983) *Frames of mind: The theory of multiple intelligences*. New York: Basic.
Gardner, W. I. (1968). Personality characteristics of the mentally retarded: Review and

critique. In H. J. Prehm, I. A. Hamrlynck, & J. E. Crosson (Eds.), *Behavioral research in mental retardation*. Eugene, Oreg.: University of Oregon Press.

Gath, A. (1977). The impact of an abnormal child upon the parents. *British Journal of Psychiatry, 130*, 405–410.

Gath, A. (1978). *Down's Syndrome and the family: The early years*. New York: Academic.

Gerrard, K. R., & Saxon, S. A. (1973). Preparation of a disturbed deaf child for therapy: A case description in behavior shaping. *Journal of Speech and Hearing Disorders, 38*, 502–509.

Goddard, H. H. (1913a). The improvability of feeble-minded children. *Journal of Psycho-Asthenics, 17*, 121–126.

Goddard. H. H. (1913b). *The Kallikak family: A study in the heredity of feeble-mindedness*. New York: Macmillan.

Goffman, E. (1963). *Stigma*. Englewood Cliffs, N.J.: Prentice-Hall.

Goldberg, S. (1977). Social competence in infancy: A model of parent–infant interaction. *Merrill-Palmer Quarterly, 23*, 163–177.

Gollay, E., Freedman, R., Wyngaarden, M., & Kurz, N. (1978). *Coming back: The community experiences of deinstitutionalized mentally retarded people*. Cambridge: Abt.

Goodman, H., Gottlieb, J., & Harrison, R. H. (1972). Social acceptance of EMRs integrated into a nongraded elementary school. *American Journal of Mental Deficiency, 76*, 412–417.

Gordon, D. A., & MacLean, W. E. (1977). Developmental analysis of outerdirectedness in institutionalized EMR children. *American Journal of Mental Deficiency, 81*, 508–511.

Gorlow, L., Butler, A., & Guthrie, G. (1963). Correlates of self-attitudes of retardates. *American Journal of Mental Deficiency, 67*, 549–554.

Gottesman, I. I. (1963). Genetic aspects of intelligent behavior. In N. Ellis (Ed.), *Handbook of mental deficiency*. New York: McGraw-Hill.

Gottesman, I. I. (1968). Biogenetics of race and class. In M. Deutch, I. Katz, & A. R. Jensen (Eds.), *Social class, race and psychological development*. New York: Holt, Rinehart & Winston.

Gottfried, A. W., & Brody, N. (1975). Interrelationships between and correlates of psychometric and Piagetian scales of sensorimotor intelligence. *Developmental Psychology, 11*, 379–387.

Gottlieb, J. (1981). Mainstreaming: Fulfilling the promise? *American Journal of Mental Deficiency, 86*, 115–126.

Gottlieb, J., & Budoff, M. (1973). Social acceptability of retarded children in nongraded schools differing in architecture. *American Journal of Mental Deficiency, 78*, 15–19.

Gottlieb, J., Semmel, M. I., & Veldman, D. J. (1978). Correlates of social status among mainstreamed mentally retarded children. *Journal of Educational Psychology, 70*, 396–405.

Granat, K., & Granat, S. (1973). Below-average intelligence and mental retardation. *American Journal of Mental Deficiency, 78*, 27–32.

Granat, K., & Granat, S. (1978). Adjustment of intellectually below-average men not identified as mentally retarded. *Scandinavian Journal of Psychology, 19*, 41–51.

Grant, D. A. (1962). Testing the null hypothesis and the strategy and tactics of investigating theoretical models. *Psychological Review, 69*, 54–61.

Gray, S. W. (1977). Home-based programs for mothers of young children. In P. Mittler (Ed.) *Research to practice in mental retardation* (Vol. 1). Baltimore: University Park.

Greenfield, P., & Smith, J. (1976). *The structure of communication in early language development*. New York: Academic Press.

Greenspan, S. (1979). Social intelligence in the retarded. In N. Ellis (Ed.), *Handbook of mental deficiency, psychological theory and research*. (2nd ed.). Hillsdale, N.J.: Erlbaum.

Gresham, F. (1982). Misguided mainstreaming: The case for social skills training for handicapped children. *Exceptional Children*, *48*, 422–433.

Gresham, F. (1983). Social skills assessment as a component of mainstreaming placement decisions. *Exceptional Children*, *49*, 331–336.

Gresham, F. (1985). The effects of social skills training on the success of mainstreaming. In J. Meisel (Ed.), *The consequences of mainstreaming handicapped children*. Hillsdale, N.J.: Erlbaum.

Groff, M. G., & Linden, K. W. (1982). The WISC-R factor score profiles of cultural-familial mentally retarded and nonretarded youth. *American Journal of Mental Deficiency*, *87*, 147–152.

Grosenick, J. K. (1970). Assessing the reintegration of exceptional children into regular classes. *Teaching Exceptional Children*, *2*, 113–119.

Gross, A. M., Eudy, C., & Drabman, R. S. (1982). Training parents to be physical therapists with their physically handicapped child. *Journal of Behavioral Medicine*, *5*, 321–327.

Grossman, F. K. (1972). *Brothers and sisters of retarded children*. Syracuse, N.Y.: Syracuse University Press.

Grossman, H. J. (Ed.), (1973). *Manual on terminology and classification in mental retardation*. Washington, D.C.: American Association on Mental Deficiency Special Publication series no. 2.

Grossman, H. J. (Ed.), (1977). *Manual on terminology and classification in mental retardation* (Rev. ed.). Washington, D.C.: American Association on Mental Deficiency.

Grossman, H. J. (Ed.), (1983). *Manual on terminology and classification in mental retardation* (3rd rev.). Washington, D.C.: American Association on Mental Deficiency.

Gruen, G., Ottinger, D., & Ollendick, T. (1974). Probability learning in retarded children with differing histories of success and failure in school. *American Journal of Mental Deficiency*, *79*, 417–423.

Gruen, G., Ottinger, D., & Zigler, E. (1970). Pre-institutional social deprivation and IQ changes among institutionalized retarded children. *Journal of Abnormal Psychology*, *3*, 133–142.

Gruen, G. E., & Zigler, E. (1968). Expectancy of success and the probability learning of middle-class, lower-class, and retarded children. *Journal of Abnormal Psychology*, *73*, 343–352.

Gruenberg, E. (1964). Epidemiology. In H. A. Stevens & R. Heber (Eds.), *Mental retardation*. Chicago: University of Chicago Press.

Gruenberg, E. (1966). Epidemiology of mental illness. *International Journal of Psychiatry*, *2*, 79–134.

Grunewald, K. (1979). Mentally retarded children and young people in Sweden. *Acta Pediatrica Scandinavia Supplement*, *275*, 75–84.

Guerin, G., & Szatlocky, K. (1974). Integration programs for the mentally retarded. *Exceptional Children*, *41*, 173–179.

Guilford, J. P. (1956). The structure of intellect. *Psychological Bulletin*, *53*, 267–293.

Guralnick, M. J. (1976). The value of integrating handicapped and nonhandicapped preschool children. *American Journal of Orthopsychiatry*, *46*, 236–245.

Gustavson, K.-H., Hagberg, B., Hagberg, G., & Sars, K. (1977). Severe mental retardation in a Swedish county. II. Etiologic and pathogenetic aspects of children born 1959–1970. *Neuropädiatrie*, *8*, 293–304.

Gustavson, K.-H., Holmgren, G., Jonsell, R., & Blomquist, H.-K. (1977). Severe mental retardation in children in a northern Swedish county. *Journal of Mental Deficiency Research*, *21*, 161–179.

Guthrie, R., & Susi, A. A. (1963). Simple phenylalanine method for detecting phenylketonuria in large populations of newborn infants. *Pediatrics*, *32*, 338–343.

Hagamen, M. B. (1980). Family adaptation to the diagnosis of mental retardation in a child and strategies of intervention. In L. Szymaniski & P. Tanguay (Eds.), *Emotional disorders of mentally retarded persons*. Baltimore: University Park.

Hagberg, B., Hagberg, G., Lewerth, A., & Lindberg, U. (1981a). Mild mental retardation in Swedish school children. I. Prevalence. *Acta Pediatrica Scandinavia, 70*, 1–8.

Hagberg, B., Hagberg, G., Lewerth, A., & Lindberg, U. (1981b). Mild mental retardation in Swedish school children. II. Etiologic and pathogenic aspects. *Acta Pediatrica Scandinavia, 70*, 445–452.

Haring, N. G., & Brown, L. J. (1976). *Teaching the severely handicapped*. New York: Grune & Stratton.

Haring, N., & Krug, D. (1975). Placement in regular programs: Procedures and results. *Exceptional Children, 41*, 413–417.

Harrell, R., Capp, R., Davis, D., Peerless, J., & Ravitz, L. (1981). Can nutritional supplements help mentally retarded children? *Proceedings of the National Academy of Science, 78*, 574–578.

Harris, S. (1975). Teaching language to nonverbal children, with emphasis on problems of generalization. *Psychological Bulletin, 82*, 565–580.

Harrison, R. H., & Budoff, H. (1972). Demographic, historical and ability correlates of the Laurelton self-concept scale in an EMR sample. *American Journal of Mental Deficiency, 76*, 460–480.

Harter, S. (1967). Mental age, IQ, and motivational factors in the discrimination learning set performance of normal and retarded children. *Journal of Experimental Child Psychology, 5*, 123–141.

Harter, S., & Zigler, E. (1968). Effectiveness of adult and peer reinforcement on the performance of institutionalized and noninstitutionalized retardates. *Journal of Abnormal Psychology, 73*, 144–149.

Harter, S., & Zigler, E. (1974). The assessment of effectance motivation in normal and retarded children. *Developmental Psychology, 10*, 169–180.

Haskell, P. H. (1944). Mental deficiency over a hundred years. *American Journal of Psychiatry, 100*, 107–118.

Havighurst, F. J. (1970). Minority subcultures and the law effect. *American Psychologist, 25*, 313–322.

Hayden, A. H., & Haring, N. G. (1976). Early intervention for high risk infants and young children: Programs for Down's syndrome children. In T. D. Tjossem (Ed.), *Intervention strategies for high risk infants and young children*. Baltimore: University Park.

Haywood, H. C. (Ed.) (1970a). *Socio-cultural aspects of mental retardation: Proceedings of the Peabody-NIMH Conference*. New York: Appleton-Century-Crofts.

Haywood, H. C. (1970b). Some perspectives on social-cultural aspects of mental retardation. In H. C. Haywood (Ed.), *Socio-cultural aspects of mental retardation: Proceedings of the Peabody-NIMH Conference*. New York: Appleton-Century-Crofts.

Haywood, H. C. (1979). What happened to mild and moderate retardation? *American Journal of Mental Deficiency, 83*, 429–431.

Haywood, H. C., Meyers, E., & Switzky, H. N. (1982). Mental retardation. *Annual Review of Psychology, 33*, 309–342.

Heber, R. (1957). *Expectancy and expectancy changes in normal and mentally retarded boys*. Unpublished doctoral dissertation, George Peabody College for Teachers.

Heber, R. (1959). A manual on terminology and classification in mental retardation. *American Journal of Mental Deficiency, 56*, Monograph Supplement (Rev.).

Heber, R. (1961). Modifications in the manual on terminology and classification in mental retardation. *American Journal of Mental Deficiency, 65*, 499–500.

Heber, R. (1964). Personality. In H. A. Stevens & R. Heber (Eds.), *Mental retardation: A review of research.* Chicago: University of Chicago Press.

Heber, R. (1970). *Epidemiology of mental retardation.* Springfield, Ill.: Thomas.

Hechinger, F. (1984). Blacks found to benefit from preschooling. *New York Times,* September 11.

Heller, K., Holtzman, W., & Messick, S. (Eds.), (1982). *Placing children in special education: A strategy for equity.* Washington, D.C.: National Academy Press.

Hill, B., & Bruininks, R. H. (1984). Maladaptive behavior of mentally retarded individuals in residential facilities. *American Journal of Mental Deficiency, 88,* 380–387.

Hirsh, E. A. (1959). The adaptive significance of commonly described behavior of the mentally retarded. *American Journal of Mental Deficiency, 63,* 639–646.

Hoakley, P. (1922). Extra-institutional care for the feebleminded. *Proceedings of The American Association For The Study of The Feebleminded, 27,* 117–134.

Hobbs, N. (1975). *The futures of children.* San Francisco: Jossey-Bass.

Hodapp, R. (1982). Effects of hospitalization on young children: Implications of two theories. *Children's Health Care, 10,* 83–86.

Hodapp, R., & Goldfield, E. (1983). The use of mother–infant games as therapy with delayed children. *Early Child Development and Care, 13,* 27–32.

Hodapp, R., & Goldfield, E. (1985). Self and other regulation during the infancy period. *Developmental Review, 5,* 274–288.

Hodapp, R., Goldfield, E., & Boyatzis, C. (1984). The use and effectiveness of maternal scaffolding in mother–infant games. *Child Development, 55,* 772–781.

Hodapp, R., & Mueller, E. (1982). Early social development. In B. Wolman (Ed.), *Handbook of developmental psychology.* Englewood Cliffs, N.J.: Prentice-Hall.

Hodapp, R., & Zigler, E. (1985). Placement decisions and their effects on severely retarded individuals. *Mental Retardation, 23,* 125–130.

Hodapp, R., & Zigler, E. (in press). Applying the developmental perspective to individuals with Down Syndrome. In D. Cicchetti & M. Beeghly (Eds.), *Down Syndrome: The developmental perspective.* Cambridge, Mass.: Harvard University Press.

Hohmann, M., Banet, B., & Weikart, D. P. (1979). *Young children in action: A manual for preschool educators.* Ypsilanti, Mich.: High/Scope Educational Research Foundation.

Hollingworth, L. S. (1923). *The psychology of subnormal children.* New York: Macmillan.

Holroyd, J., & McArthur, D. (1976). Mental retardation and stress on the parents: A contrast between Down's syndrome and childhood autism. *American Journal of Mental Deficiency, 80,* 431–436.

Holtzman, N. A., Meek, A. G., & Mellits, E. D. (1974). Neonatal screening for phenylketonuria. I. Effectiveness. *Journal of the American Medical Association, 229,* 667–670.

Hottel, J. V. (1960). *The influence of age and intelligence on independence conformity behavior of children.* Unpublished doctoral dissertation, George Peabody College for Teachers.

Hunt, J. McV. (1961). *Intelligence and experience.* New York: Ronald Press.

Hunt, J. McV. (1971). Parent and child centers: Their basis in the behavioral and educational sciences. *American Journal of Orthopsychiatry, 41,* 13–38.

Iano, R. P., Ayers, D., Heller, H. B., McGettigan, J. F., & Walker, V. S. (1974). Sociometric status of retarded children in an integrative program. *Exceptional Children, 40,* 267–271.

Inhelder, B. (1968). *The diagnosis of reasoning in the mentally retarded* (W. B. Stephens, trans.). New York: Day.

Jensen, A. R. (1969). How much can we boost IQ and scholastic achievement? *Harvard Educational Review, 39,* 1–123.

Jensen, A. R. (1974). Cumulative deficit: A testable hypothesis. *Developmental Psychology, 10,* 996–1019.

Jensen, A. R. (1977). Cumulative deficit in IQ of blacks in the rural south. *Developmental Psychology, 13*, 184–191.

Jensen, A. R. (1980). *Bias in mental testing*. New York: Free Press.

Jensen, A. R. (1981a). *Straight talk about mental tests*. New York: Free Press.

Jensen, A. R. (1981b). Raising the IQ: The Ramey and Haskins study. *Intelligence, 5*, 29–40.

Jensen, A. R. (1982). The debunking of scientific fossils and straw persons (review of S. J. Gould, *The mismeasure of man*). *Contemporary Education Review, 1*, 121–135.

Jervis, G. A. (1963). The clinical picture. In F. L. Lyman (ed.), *Phenylketonuria*. Springfield, Ill.: Thomas.

Johnson, A. (1906). The segregation and permanent detention of the feeble-minded. *Journal of Psycho-Asthenics, 10*, 230–233.

Johnson, M. R., Whitman, T. L., & Barloon-Noble, R. (1978). A home-based program for a preschool behaviorally disturbed child with parents as therapists. *Journal of Behavior Therapy and Experimental Psychiatry, 9*, 65–70.

Johnson, S. M., & Brown, R. A. (1969). Producing behavior change in parents of disturbed children. *Journal of Child Psychology and Psychiatry, 10*, 107–121.

Jones, O. H. M. (1980). Prelinguistic communication skills in Down's syndrome infants. In T. Field, S. Goldberg, D. Stern, & A. Sostek (Eds.), *High-risk infants and children: Interactions with adults and peers*. New York: Academic Press.

Jonsson, G., & Kalveston, A. L. (1964). *222 Stockholm boys*. Uppsala: Almqvist & Wiksell.

Junkala, J. (1977). Teacher assessments and team decisions. *Exceptional Children, 44*, 32–38.

Kagan, J., & Klein, R. (1973). Cross-cultural perspectives on early development. *American Psychologist, 28*, 947–961.

Kahn, J. (1977). Piaget's theory of cognitive development and its relationship to severely and profoundly retarded children. In P. Mittler (Ed.), *Research to practice in mental retardation*. (Vol. 2). Baltimore: University Park Press.

Kahn, J. V. (1975). Relationship of Piaget's sensorimotor period to language acquisitions of profoundly retarded children. *American Journal of Mental Deficiency, 79*, 640–643.

Kakalik, J. S., Furry, W. S., Thomas, M. A., & Carney, M. F. (1982). *The cost of special education: Summary of study findings*. Santa Monica, Calif.: The Rand Corporation.

Kamin, L. G. (1974). *The science and politics of IQ*. New York: Wiley.

Kasl, S. V. (1972). Physical and mental health effects of involuntary relocation and institutionalization on the elderly: A review. *American Journal of Public Health, 62*, 377–384.

Katz, P., & Zigler, E. (1967). Self-image disparity: A developmental approach. *Journal of Personality and Social Psychology, 5*, 186–195.

Kaufman, A. S. (1979). *Intelligent testing with the WISC-R*. New York: Wiley.

Kaufman, A. S., & Kaufman, N. L. (1972). Tests built from Piaget's and Gessell's tasks as predictors of school achievement. *Child Development, 43*, 521–535.

Kaufman, M. J., Agard, J. A., & Semmel, M. I. (1978). *Mainstreaming: Learners and their environment*. Baltimore: University Park.

Kaufman, M. J., Gottlieb, J., Agard, J., & Kukic, M. (1975). Mainstreaming: Toward an explanation of the construct. In E. L. Meyer, G. A. Vergason, & R. J. Whelan (Eds.), *Alternatives for teaching exceptional children*. Denver, Colo.: Love.

Kaye, K. (1982). *The mental and social life of babies*. Chicago: University of Chicago Press.

Keating, D. P. (1975). Precocious cognitive development at the level of formal operations. *Child Development, 46*, 276–280.

Kennedy Foundation (1981). *Mild mental retardation: A comparative analysis of the U.S. and Sweden*. Unpublished manuscript, Joseph P. Kennedy Foundation.

Kerlin, I. N. (1892). President's annual address. *Proceedings and addresses of the Association of Medical Officers of American Institutions for Idiotic and Feeble-Minded Persons. Sixteenth Session*: 274–285. Reprinted 1964. New York: Johnson Reprint Corporation.

Kessen, W. (1962). Stage and structure in the study of children. In W. Kessen and C. Kuhlman (Eds.), *Thought in the young child. Monographs of the Society for Research in Child Development, 27*, 53–70.

Kier, R. J., Styfco, S. J., & Zigler, E. (1977). Success expectancies and the probability learning of children of low and middle socioeconomic status. *Developmental Psychology, 13*, 444–449.

Kier, R. J., & Zigler, E. (1969). *Probability learning strategies of lower and middle-class children and the expectancy of success hypothesis.* Unpublished manuscript, Yale University.

Kimble, G., Garmezy, N., & Zigler, E. (1984). *Principles of general psychology* (5th ed.). New York: Wiley.

King, R. D., Raynes, N. V., & Tizard, J. (1971). *Patterns of residential care: Sociological studies in institutions for handicapped children.* London: Routledge and Kegan Paul.

Kirk, S.A. (1964). Research in education. In H. A. Stevens & R. Heber (Eds.), *Mental Retardation.* Chicago: University of Chicago Press.

Kleinberg, J., & Galligan, B. (1983). Effects of deinstitutionalization on adaptive behavior of mentally retarded adults. *American Journal of Mental Deficiency, 88*, 21–27.

Knobloch, H., & Pasamanick, B. (1961). Genetics of mental disease: 2. Some thoughts in the inheritance of intelligence. *American Journal of Orthopsychiatry, 31*, 454–473.

Kohlberg, L. (1969). Stage and sequence: The cognitive-developmental approach to socialization. In D. Goslin (Ed.), *Handbook of socialization theory and research.* Chicago: Rand McNally.

Kohlberg, L., & Zigler, E. (1967). The impact of cognitive maturity on the development of sex-role attitudes in the years four to eight. *Genetic Psychology Monographs, 75*, 80–165.

Kopp, C., & McCall, R. (1982). Predicting later mental performance for normal, at risk, and handicapped infants. In P. Baltes & O. Brim (Eds.), *Life-span development and behavior, 4*, New York: Academic Press.

Kounin, J. (1941a). Experimental studies of rigidity: I. The measurement of rigidity in normal and feebleminded persons. *Character and Personality, 9*, 251–272.

Kounin, J. (1941b). Experimental studies of rigidity: II. The explanatory power of the concept of rigidity as applied to feeble-mindedness. *Character and Personality, 9*, 273–282.

Kounin, J. S. (1948). The meaning of rigidity: A reply to Heinz Werner. *Psychological Review, 55*, 157–166.

Kraft, I. (1961). Edouard Seguin and the 19th Century moral treatment of idiots. *Bulletin of the History of Medicine, 35*, 393–418.

Krietler, S., Zigler, E., & Kreitler, H. (1984). Curiosity and demographic factors as determinants of children's probability learning. *Journal of Genetic Psychology, 145*, 61–75.

Kugel, R. B. (1967). Familial mental retardation–Fact or fancy? In J. Hellmuth (Ed.), *Disadvantaged child* (Vol. 1). New York: Brunner/Mazel.

Kushlick, A., & Blunden, R. (1974). The epidemiology of mental subnormality. In A. M. Clarke & A. D. B. Clarke (Eds.), *Mental deficiency: The changing outlook* (3rd ed.). New York: Free Press.

Labov, W. (1970). The logic of nonstandard English. In F. Williams (Ed.), *Language and poverty.* Chicago: Markham.

Lakin, K., Hill, B., Hauber, F., Bruininks, R., & Heal, L. (1983). New admissions and readmissions to a national sample of public residential facilities. *American Journal of Mental Deficiency, 88*, 13–20.

Lamb, M. (1978). Influences of the child on marital quality and family interaction during the prenatal, perinatal, and infancy periods. In R. Lerner & G. Spanier (Eds.), *Child influences on marital and family interaction.* New York: Academic Press.

Landesman-Dwyer, S. (1981). Living in the community. *American Journal of Mental Deficiency, 86,* 223–234.

Landesman-Dwyer, S., Sackett, G. P., & Kleinman, J. S. (1980). Relationship of size to residential and staff behavior in small community residences. *American Journal of Mental Deficiency, 85,* 6–17.

Landesman-Dwyer, S., Stein, J. G., & Sackett, G. P. (1978). A behavioral and ecological study of group homes. In G. P. Sackett (Ed.), *Observing behavior, 1. Theory and application in mental retardation.* Baltimore: University Park.

Landesman-Dwyer, S., & Sulzbacher, F. (1981). Residential placement and adaptation of severely and profoundly retarded individuals. In R. Bruininks, C. Meyers, C. Stiedard, & K. Lakin (Eds.), *Deinstitutionalization and community adjustment of mentally retarded people.* Washington, D.C.: American Association on Mental Deficiency.

Lane, H. (1976). *The wild boy of Aveyron.* Cambridge, Mass.: Harvard University Press.

Larivee, B., & Cook, L. (1979). Mainstreaming: A study of the variables affecting teacher attitude, *Journal of Special Education, 13,* 315–324.

Larry P. v. *Riles,* 343 F. Supp. 1306, aff'd 502 F 2d 963 (9th Cir., 1974); now in trial on merits.

Laurendeau, M., & Pinard, A. (1962). *Causal thinking in the child.* New York: International Universities Press.

Lazar, I., Darlington, R., Murray, H., Royce, J., & Snipper, A. (1982). *Lasting effects of early education. Monographs of the Society for Research in Child Development.* Serial No. 195, *Vol. 47.*

Lazerson, M. (1975). Educational institutions and mental subnormality: Notes on writing a history. In M. Begab & S. Richardson (Eds.), *The mentally retarded and society.* Baltimore: University Park.

Leahy, R., Balla, D., & Zigler, E. (1982). Role taking, self-image, and imitation in retarded and nonretarded individuals. *American Journal of Mental Deficiency, 86,* 372–379.

Legg, C., Sherick, I., & Wadland, W. (1975). Reaction of preschool children to the birth of a sibling. *Child Psychiatry & Human Development, 5,* 5–39.

Leinhardt, G., & Pallay, A. (1982). Restrictive educational settings: Exile or haven? *Review of Educational Research, 52,* 557–578.

Leland, H. (1969). The relationship between "intelligence" and mental retardation. *American Journal of Mental Deficiency, 73,* 533–535.

Leland, H., Shellhaas, M., Nihira, K., & Foster, R. (1967). Adaptive behavior: A new dimension in the classification of the mentally retarded. *Mental Retardation Abstracts, 4,* 359–387.

Lemkau, P. V., & Imre, P. D. (1969). Results of a field epidemiologic study. *American Journal of Mental Deficiency, 73,* 858–863.

Lenneberg, E. (1967). *Biological foundations of language.* New York: Wiley.

Leonard, L. B. (1975). Relational meaning and the facilitation of slow-learning children's language. *American Journal of Mental Deficiency, 80,* 180–185.

Lewin, K. (1936). *A dynamic theory of personality.* New York: McGraw-Hill.

Lewis, E. (1933). Types of mental deficiency and their social significance. *Journal of Mental Science, 79,* 298–304.

Lewis, M. (Ed.), (1976). *The origins of intelligence.* New York: Plenum.

Li, C. C. (1971). A tale of two thermos bottles: Properties of a genetic model of human intelligence. In R. Cancro (Ed.), *Intelligence and environmental influences.* New York: Grune & Stratton.

Lipman, R. S., & Griffith, B. C. (1960). Effects of anxiety level on concept formation: A test of drive theory. *American Journal of Mental Deficiency, 65*, 342–348.

Lobato, D. (1983). Siblings of handicapped children: A review. *Journal of Autism and Developmental Disorders, 13*, 347–364.

Lockard, G. (1978). Mainstreaming: One child's experience. *Phi Delta Kappan, 59*, 527–528.

Locke, A. (1979). *Action, gesture, symbol.* New York: Academic Press.

Louttit, R. T. (1965). Chemical facilitation of intelligence among the mentally retarded. *American Journal of Mental Deficiency, 69*, 495–501.

Lubbs, H. A. (1969). A marker-X chromosome. *American Journal of Human Genetics, 21*, 231–244.

Lubs, M. L. E., & Maes, J. (1977). Recurrence risk in mental retardation. In P. Mittler (Ed.), *Research to practice in mental retardation* (Vol. 3). Baltimore: University Park.

Lucito, L. J. (1959). *A comparison of independence-conformity behavior of intellectually bright and dull children.* Unpublished doctoral dissertation, University of Illinois.

Lustman, N., & Zigler, E. (1982). Imitation by institutionalized and noninstitutionalized mentally retarded and non-retarded children. *American Journal of Mental Deficiency, 87*, 252–258.

MacDonald, J. D., & Blott, J. P. (1974). Environmental language intervention: A rationale for diagnostic and training strategy through rules, context and generalization. *Journal of Speech and Hearing Disorders, 39*, 395–415.

MacMillan, D. L. (1969). Motivational differences: Cultural-familial retardates vs. normal subjects on expectancy for failure. *American Journal of Mental Deficiency, 74*, 254–258.

MacMillan, D. L. (1977). *Mental Retardation in school and society.* Boston: Little, Brown.

MacMillan, D. L. (1982). *Mental retardation in school and society* (2nd ed.). Boston: Little, Brown.

MacMillan, D. L., & Keogh, B. K. (1971). Normal and retarded children's expectancy for failure. *Developmental Psychology, 4*, 343–348.

MacMillan, D. L., & Knopf, E. D. (1971). Effect of instructional set on perceptions of event outcomes by EMR and nonretarded children. *American Journal of Mental Deficiency, 76*, 185–189.

MacMillan, D. L., & Meyers, C. E. (1980). *Larry P.:* An educational interpretation. *School Psychology Review, 9*, 136–148.

MacMillan, D. L., & Wright, D. (1974). Outerdirectedness in children of three ages as a function of experimentally induced success and failure. *Journal of Educational Psychology, 68*, 919–925.

Mahoney, G., & Snow, K. (1983). The relationship of sensorimotor functioning to children's responses to early language training. *Mental Retardation, 6*, 248–254.

Malpass, L. F., Marh, S., & Palmero, D. S. (1960). Responses of retarded children to the Children's Manifest Anxiety Scale. *Journal of Educational Psychology, 51*, 305–308.

Marfo, K. (1984). Interactions between mothers and their mentally retarded children: Integration of research findings. *Journal of Applied Developmental Psychology, 5*, 45–69.

Masland, R. L., Sarason, S. B., & Gladwin, T. (1958). *Mental subnormality.* New York: Basic.

Maslow, A. (1948). Cognition of the particular and of the generic. *Psychology Review, 55*, 22–48.

Matin, M. A., Sylvester, P. E., Edwards, O., & Dickerson, J. W. T. (1981). Vitamin and zinc status in Down Syndrome. *Journal of Mental Deficiency Research, 25*, 121–126.

Mautner, H. (1959). *Mental retardation: Its care, treatment and physiological base.* Elmsford, N.Y.: Pergamon.

McCall, R. B. (1979). Qualitative transitions in behavioral development in the first three years. In M. H. Bornstein & W. Kessen (Eds.), *Psychological development from infancy*. Hillsdale, N. J.: Erlbaum.

McCandless, B. R. (1970). Modeling and power in cognitive development. In H. C. Haywood (Ed.), *Social-cultural aspects of mental retardation: Proceedings of the Peabody NIMH Conference*. New York: Appleton-Century-Crofts.

McCarver, R. B., & Craig, E. M. (1974). Placement of the retarded in the community: Prognosis and outcome. *International Review of Research in Mental Retardation, 7*, 145–207.

McClelland, D. C. (1973). Testing for competence rather than intelligence. *American Psychologist, 28*, 1–14.

McCormick, M., Balla, D., & Zigler, E. (1975). Resident care practices in institutions for retarded persons: A cross-institutional, cross-cultural study. *American Journal of Mental Deficiency, 80*, 1–17.

McCurley, R., Mackay, D. N., & Scally, B. (1972). The life expectancy of the mentally subnormal under community and hospital care. *American Journal of Mental Deficiency, 16*, 57–67.

McKinney, J. P., & Keel, T. (1963). Effects of increased mothering on behavior of severely retarded boys. *American Journal of Mental Deficiency, 67*, 556–562.

McLean, J., & Snyder-McLean, L. (1978). *A transactional approach to early language training*. Columbus, Ohio: Merrill.

Meisel, J. (in press). *Mainstreaming: A review of current research and practice*. Hillsdale, N.J.: Erlbaum.

Menolascino, F. J., & McGee, J. J. (1981a). The new institutions: Last ditch arguments. *Mental Retardation, 19*, 215–220.

Menolascino, F. J., & McGee, J. J. (1981b). Rejoinder to the Partlow Committee. *Mental Retardation, 19*, 227–230.

Mercer, J. (1973a). *Labeling the mentally retarded*. Berkeley: University of California Press.

Mercer, J. (1973b). The myth of three percent prevalence. In C. E. Meyers (Ed.), *Sociobehavioral studies in mental retardation. Monographs of the American Association on Mental Deficiency. 1*.

Mercer, J. R. (1974). *The eligibles and the labeled*. Berkeley: University of California Press.

Meyers, C. E., MacMillan, D. L., & Yoshida, R. K. (1980). Regular class education of EMR students, from efficacy to mainstreaming: A review of issues and research. In J. Gottlieb (Ed.), *Educating mentally retarded persons in the mainstream*. Baltimore: University Park.

Miller, J., & Yoder, D. (1974). An ontogenetic language teaching strategy for retarded children. In R. Schiefelbusch and L. Lloyd (Eds.), *Language perspectives: Acquisition, retardation and intervention*. Baltimore: University Park.

Miller, S. I., Miller, P., Kim, M., Kutz, N., Lozier, J., & Misenheimer, B. (1975). Foster home adjustment of retardates. *The Indian Journal of Social Work, 36*, 145–154.

Mischel, W. (1968). *Personality and assessment*. New York: Wiley.

Moen, M., Bogen, D., & Aanes, D. (1975). Follow-up of mentally retarded adults successfully placed in community group homes. *Hospital and Community Psychiatry, 26*, 754–756.

Moore, B. L., & Bailey, J. S. (1973). Social punishment in the modification of a pre-school child's "autistic-like" behavior with a mother as therapist. *Journal of Applied Behavior Analysis, 6*, 498–507.

Moser, H. W., Young, D., & Efron, M. L. (1967). Diagnosis and treatment of maple sugar urine disease. In G. A. Jervis (Ed.), *Mental retardation*. Springfield, Ill.: Thomas.

Mundy, P., Siebert, J. M., & Hogan, A. E. (1984). Relationship between sensorimotor and early communication abilities in developmentally delayed children. *Merrill-Palmer Quarterly, 30*, 33–48.

Neman, R. (1975). A reply to Zigler and Seitz. *American Journal of Mental Deficiency, 79,* 493–505.

Neman, R., Roos, P., McCann, B. M., Menolascino, F., & Heal, L. W. (1974). Experimental evaluation of sensorimotor patterning used with mentally retarded children. *American Journal of Mental Deficiency, 79,* (4), 372–384.

Nirje, B. (1969). The normalization principle and its human management implications. In R. Kugel and W. Wolfensberger (Eds.), *Changing patterns in residential services for the mentally retarded.* Washington, D.C.: Government Printing Office.

North, A. F. (1979). Health services in Head Start. In E. Zigler and J. Valentine (Eds.), *Project Head Start: A legacy of the war on poverty.* New York: Free Press.

Novak, A. (1980). Backlash to the deinstitutionalization movement. In A. Novak & L. Heal (Eds.), *Integration of developmentally disabled individuals into the community.* Baltimore: Brooks.

Oates, S. (1977). *With malice toward none: The life of Abraham Lincoln.* New York: Harper & Row.

Ollendick, T., Balla, D., & Zigler, E. (1971). Expectancy of success and the probability learning of retarded children. *Journal of Abnormal Psychology, 77,* 275–281.

Ollendick, T., & Gruen, G. (1971). Level of achievement and probability in children. *Developmental Psychology, 4,* 486.

Overton, W., & Reese, H. (1973). Models of development: Methodological implications. In J. Nesselroad & H. Reese (Eds.), *Life span developmental psychology.* New York: Academic Press.

Page, E. (1972). Miracle in Milwaukee: Raising the IQ. *Educational Researcher, 1,* 8–10, 15–16.

Parke, R. D. (1979). Perspectives in father–infant development. In J. D. Osofsky (Ed.), *Handbook of infant development.* New York: Wiley.

Penrose, L. S. (1963). *The biology of mental defect.* London: Sidgwick & Jackson.

Piaget, J. (1954). *The construction of reality in the child.* New York: Ballantine.

Piaget, J. (1956). The general problem of the psychobiological development of the child. *Discussions on Child Development, 4,* 3–27.

Piaget, J. (1962). *Play, dreams and imitation in childhood.* New York: Norton.

Piaget, J. (1966). *Origins of intelligence in children.* New York: International Universities Press.

Piaget, J. (1981). *Intelligence and affectivity: Their relationship during child development.* Palo Alto, Calif.: Annual Reviews Inc.

Plenderleith, M. (1956). Discrimination learning and discrimination reversal learning in normal and feebleminded children. *Journal of Genetic Psychology, 88,* 107–112.

Plomin, R., & DeFries, J. C. (1980). Genetics and intelligence: Recent data. *Intelligence, 4,* 15–24.

Podolsky, C. (1964). *The relation of chronological age and mental age to the performance of school age normals and retardates in selected learning tasks.* Unpublished doctoral dissertation, New York University.

Polloway, E. A., & Smith, J. D. (1983). Changes in mild mental retardation: Population, programs, and perspectives. *Exceptional Children, 50,* 149–159.

President's Committee on Mental Retardation. (1973). *MR–72: Islands of excellence.* Washington, D.C.: Government Printing Office.

Provence, S., & Naylor, A. (1983). *Working with disadvantaged parents and children: Scientific issues and practice.* New Haven, Conn.: Yale University Press.

Pryer, M. W., & Cassel, R. H. (1962). The Children's Manifest Anxiety Scale: Reliability with aments. *American Journal of Mental Deficiency, 66,* 860.

Raiten, D. J., & Massaro, T. F. (in press). Nutrition and developmental disabilities: An examination of the orthomolecular hypothesis. In D. Cohen & A. Donnellan (Eds.), *Handbook of autism and disorders of atypical development.* New York: Wiley.

Raloff, J. (1982). Childhood lead: Worrisome national levels. *Science News, 121,* 88.

Ramey, C., & Campbell, F. (1977). Prevention of developmental retardation in high risk children. In P. Mittler (Ed.), *Research to practice in mental retardation* (Vol. 1). Baltimore: University Park.

Ramey, C., & Campbell, F. (1979). Early childhood education for disadvantaged children: The effects on psychological processes. *American Journal of Mental Deficiency, 83,* 645–648.

Ramey, C., Campbell, F., & Finkelstein, N. (1984). Course and structure of intellectual development in children at high risk for developmental retardation. In P. Brooks, R. Sperber, & C. McCauley (Eds.), *Learning and cognition in the mentally retarded.* Hillsdale, N.J.: Erlbaum.

Ramey, C., Dorval, B., & Baker-Ward, L. (in press). Group daycare and socially disadvantaged families: Effects on the child and the family. In S. Kilmer (Ed.), *Advances in early education and daycare.* Greenwich, Conn.: JAI Press.

Ramey, C. T., & Finkelstein, N. W. (1981). Psychosocial mental retardation: A biological and social coalescence. In M. J. Begab, H. C. Haywood, & H. Garber (Eds.), *Psychosocial influences in retarded performance* (Vol. 1). *Issues and theories in development.* Baltimore: University Park.

Ramey, C., & Haskins, R. (1981a). Causes and treatment of school failure: Insights from the Carolina Abecedarian Project. In M. J. Begab, H. Garber, & H. C. Haywood (Eds.), *Prevention of retarded development in psychosocially disadvantaged children.* Baltimore: University Park.

Ramey, C., & Haskins, R. (1981b). The modification of intelligence through early experience. *Intelligence, 5,* 5–19.

Ramey, C., & Haskins, R. (1981c). Early education, intellectual development, and school performance: A reply to Arthur Jensen and J. McVicker Hunt. *Intelligence, 5,* 41–48.

Ramey, C., MacPhee, D., & Yeates, K. O. (1982) Preventing developmental retardation: A general systems model. In L. Bond & J. Joffee (Eds.), *Facilitating infant and early childhood development.* Hanover, N.H.: University Press of New England.

Ramey, C., & Smith, B. (1977). Assessing the intellectual consequences of early intervention with high risk infants. *American Journal of Mental Deficiency, 81,* 315–324.

Reed, E. W., & Reed, S. C. (1965). *Mental retardation: A family study.* Philadelphia: Saunders.

Reese, H. (1961). Manifest anxiety and achievement test performance. *Journal of Educational Psychology, 52,* 132–135.

Reese, H., & Overton, W. (1970). Models of development and theories of development. In L. R. Goulet & P. Baltes (Eds.), *Life span development psychology: Research and theory.* New York: Academic Press.

Reschly, D. J. (1981). Evaluation of the effects of SOMPA measures on classification of students as mildly retarded. *American Journal of Mental Deficiency, 86,* 16–20.

Reschly, D., & Jipson, F. (1976). Ethnicity, geographic locale, age, sex, and urban rural residence as variables in the prevalence of mild retardation. *American Journal of Mental Deficiency, 81,* 154–161.

Rescorla, L., Provence, S., & Naylor, A. (1982). The Yale Child Welfare Research Program: Description and results. In E. Zigler & E. Gordon (Eds.), *Daycare: Scientific and social policy issues.* Boston: Auburn House.

Richards, I. D. G., & McIntoch, H. T. (1973). Spina bifida survivors and their parents: A study of problems and services. *Developmental Medicine and Child Neurology, 15,* 292–304.

Richards, L. E. (1935). *Samuel Gridley Howe.* New York: Appleton-Century.

Richardson, S. A. (1981). Family characteristics associated with mild mental retardation. In M. H. Begab, H. C. Haywood, & H. L. Garber (Eds.), *Psychosocial influences in retarded performance* (Vol. 2). Baltimore: University Park.

Risley, S. D. (1905). Is asexualization ever justifiable in the case of imbecile children? *Journal of Psycho-Asthenics, 9,* 92–98.

Robbins, M. P., & Glass, G. V. (1969). The Doman-Delacato rationale: A critical analysis. In J. Hellmuth (Ed.), *Educational Therapy.* Seattle: Special Child Publications.

Robinson, H. B., & Robinson, N. M. (1965). *The mentally retarded child: A psychological approach.* New York: McGraw-Hill.

Robinson, N. (1980). Editor's note: Terminology, classification, and description in mental retardation research. *American Journal of Mental Deficiency, 65,* 107.

Robinson, N., & Robinson, H. (1976). *The mentally retarded child* (2nd ed.). New York: McGraw-Hill.

Rodgers, S. (1977). Characteristics of the social development of profoundly retarded children. *Child Development, 48,* 837–843.

Rondal, J. (1977). Maternal speech to normal and Down syndrome children. In P. Mittler (Ed.), *Research to practice in mental retardation* (Vol. 2). Baltimore: University Park.

Rosen, M., Clark, G. R., & Kivitz, M. S. (1976). *The history of mental retardation* (Vol. 1.). Baltimore: University Park.

Rosen, M., Diggory, J. C., & Werlinsky, B. (1966). Goal setting and expectancy of success in institutionalized and noninstitutionalized mental subnormals. *American Journal of Mental Deficiency, 71,* 249–255.

Rothbaum, F. (1976). *Imitation of parents and strange adults on objective and subjective tasks.* Unpublished doctoral dissertation, Yale University.

Ruble, D. N., & Nakamura, C. (1973). Outerdirectedness as a problem solving approach in relation to developmental level and selected task variables. *Child Development, 44,* 519–528.

Ruebush, B. K. (1963). Anxiety. In H. W. Stevens, J. Kagan, & C. Spiker (Eds.), *Child psychology.* Chicago: University of Chicago Press.

Rutter, M. (1979). Maternal deprivation, 1972–1978: New findings, new concepts, new approaches. *Child Development, 50,* 283–305.

Rutter, M., Tizard, J., & Whitmore, K. (Eds.) (1970). *Education, health & behavior.* London: Longmans.

Sailor, W., Guess, D., & Baer, D. (1973). Functional language for verbally deficient children. *Mental Retardation, 11,* 27–35.

Sameroff, A. (1975). Early influences on development: Fact or fancy? *Merrill-Palmer Quarterly, 21,* 267-294.

Sanders, B., Zigler, E., & Butterfield, E. C. (1968). Outer-directedness in the discrimination learning of normal and mentally retarded children. *Journal of Abnormal Psychology, 73,* 368–375.

Sandler, A., & Thurman, K. S. (1981). Status of community placement research: Effects on retarded citizens. *Education and Training of the Mentally Retarded, 16,* 245–251.

Sarason, S. B., Davidson, K. S., Lighthall, F. F., Waite, R. R., & Ruebush, B. K. (1980). *Anxiety in elementary school children.* New York: Wiley.

Sarason, S. B., & Doris, J. (1979). *Educational handicap, public policy, and social history: A broadened perspective on mental retardation.* New York: Park Press.

Sarason, S. B., & Gladwin, T. (1958). Psychological and cultural problems in mental subnormality: A review of research. *Genetic Psychology Monographs, 57,* 3–290.

Scarr, S., & Carter-Saltzman, L. (1982). Genetics and intelligence. In R. Sternberg (Ed.), *Handbook of human intelligence.* Cambridge University Press.

Scarr, S., & Weinberg, R. A. (1976). IQ test performance of black children adopted by white families. *American Psychologist, 31*, 726–739.

Scarr, S., & Weinberg, R. A. (1978). The influence of family background on intellectual attainment. *American Sociological Review, 43*, 642–692.

Scarr, S., & Weinberg, R. (1979). Intellectual similarities in adoptive and biological related families of adolescents. In L. Willerman & R. G. Turner (Eds.), *Readings about individual and group difference*. San Francisco: Freeman.

Scarr, S., & Yee, D. (1980). Heritability and educational policy: Genetic and environmental effects on IQ, aptitude, and achievement. *Educational Psychologist, 15*, 1–22.

Scarr-Salapatek, S. (1974). Genetics and the development of intelligence. In F. Horowitz, E. M. Hetherington, S. Scarr-Salapatek, & J. Siegel (Eds.), *Review of child development research* (Vol. 4). Chicago: University of Chicago Press.

Scarr-Salapatek, S. (1975). An evolutionary perspective on infant intelligence: Species patterns and individual variations. In M. Lewis (Ed.), *Origins of intelligence*. New York: Plenum.

Scarr-Salapatek, S. (1976). Unknowns in the IQ equation. In N. J. Block & G. Dworkin (Eds.), *The IQ controversy*. New York: Pantheon.

Schalock, R. L., Harper, R. S., & Genung, T. (1981). Community placement and program success. *American Journal of Mental Deficiency, 85*, 478–488.

Scheerenberger, R. C. (1983a). *A history of mental retardation*. Baltimore: Brooks.

Scheerenberger, R. C. (1983b). *Public residential services for the mentally retarded: 1982*. Washington, D.C.: National Association of Superintendents of Public Residential Facilities for the Mentally Retarded.

Schlesinger, I. (1971). Production of utterances in language acquisition. In D. Slobin (Ed.), *The ontogenesis of grammar*. New York: Academic Press.

Schroeder, S. R., & Henes, C. (1978). Assessment of progress of institutionalized and deinstitutionalized retarded adults: A matched control comparison. *Mental Retardation, 16*, 147–148.

Schroeder, S., Mulick, J., & Schroeder, C. (1979). Management of severe behavior problems of the retarded. In N. R. Ellis (Ed.), *Handbook of mental deficiency* (2nd ed.). Hillsdale, N.J.: Erlbaum.

Schweinhart, L. J., & Weikart, D. P. (1980). *Young children grow up: The effects of the Perry Preschool Program on youths through age 15. Monographs of the High/Scope Educational Research Foundation, 7*, Ypsilanti, Mich.: High/Scope.

Schweinhart, L. J., & Weikart, D. P. (1981). Perry Preschool effects nine years later: What do they mean? In M. Begab, H. C. Haywood, & H. L. Garber (Eds.), *Psychological influences in retarded performance*. Baltimore: University Park.

Schweinhart, L. J., & Weikart, D. P. (1983). The effects of Perry Preschool Program on youths through age 15 – a summary in Consortium for Longitudinal Studies. In Consortium for Longitudinal Studies (Ed.), *As the twig is bent: Lasting effects of preschool programs*. Hillsdale, N.J.: Erlbaum.

Seguin, E. (1866). *Idiocy and its treatment by the physiological method*. New York: William Wood.

Seibert, J. M., & Oller, D. K. (1981). Linguistic pragmatics and language intervention strategies. *Journal of Autism & Developmental Disorders, 11*, 75–88.

Seitz, V., Apfel, N., & Efron, C. (1978). Longterm effects of early intervention: The New Haven Project. In B. Brown (Ed.), *Found: Long term gains for early intervention*. Boulder, Colo.: Westview Press.

Seitz, V., Apfel, N. H., & Rosenbaum, L. (1981). Projects Head Start and Follow-Through: A longitudinal evaluation of adolescents. In M. J. Begab, H. Garber, & H. C. Haywood

(Eds.), *Prevention of retarded development in psychosocially disadvantaged children.* Baltimore: University Park.

Seitz, V., Rosenbaum, L., & Apfel, N. (1983). *Day care as family intervention.* Paper Presented at the Biennial Meeting of the Society for Research in Child Development, Detroit, Mich.

Seitz, V., Rosenbaum, L., & Apfel, N. (1985). Effects of family support intervention: A ten year follow-up. *Child Development, 56,* 376–391.

Sells, C. J., & Bennett, F. C. (1977). Prevention of mental retardation: The role of medicine. *American Journal of Mental Deficiency, 82,* (2), 117–129.

Semmel, M., Gottlieb, J., & Robinson, N. (1979). Mainstreaming: Perspectives on educating handicapped children in the public school. In D. C. Berliner (Ed.), *Review of research in education.* Washington, D.C.: American Educational Research Association.

Shallenberger, P., & Zigler, E. (1961). Negative reaction tendencies, and cosatiation effects in normal and feebleminded children. *Journal of Abnormal and Social Psychology, 63,* 20–26.

Shirley, M. M. (1931). *The first two years: I. Locomotor development.* Minneapolis: University of Minnesota Press.

Shultz, T., & Zigler, E. (1970). Emotional concomitants of visual mastery in infants: The effects of stimulus movement on smiling and vocalizing. *Journal of Experimental Child Psychology, 10,* 390–402.

Siebert, J., & Oller, D. K. (1981). Linguistic pragmatics and language intervention strategies. *Journal of Autism and Developmental Disorders, 11,* 75–88.

Siegel, P. S., & Foshee, J. G. (1960). Molar variability in the mentally defective. *Journal of Abnormal and Social Psychology, 61,* 141–143.

Silverstein, A. B. (1970). The measurement of intelligence. In N. R. Ellis (Ed.), *International review of research in retardation* (Vol. 4). New York: Academic Press.

Silverstein, A. B. (1973). Note on prevalence. *American Journal of Mental Deficiency, 77,* 380–382.

Silverstein, A. B. (1982). Note on the constancy of IQ. *American Journal of Mental Deficiency, 87,* 227–228.

Silverstein, A. B., & Owens, E. P. (1968). Factor structure of the social deprivation scale for mongoloid retardates. *American Journal of Mental Deficiency, 73,* 315–317.

Simeonsson, R. J., Cooper, D. H., & Scheiner, A. P. (1982). A review and analysis of the effectiveness of early intervention programs. *Pediatrics, 69,* 635–641.

Skeels, H. (1966). Adult status of children with contrasting early life experiences: A follow-up study. *Monographs of the Society for Research in Child Development, 31,* (No. 105), 1–65.

Skeels, H., Updergraff, R., Wellman, D. L., & Williams, H. M. A. (1938). A study of environmental stimulation. *University of Iowa Study of Child Welfare, 15,* No. 4.

Skodak, M., & Skeels, H. (1949). A final follow-up study of one hundred adopted children. *Journal of Genetic Psychology, 74,* 84–125.

Slater, E., & Cowie, V. (1971). *Genetics of mental disorders.* New York: Oxford University Press.

Sloan, W. (1963). Four score and seven. *American Journal of Mental Deficiency, 68,* 6–14.

Smith, G., Spiker, D., Peterson, C., Cicchetti, D., & Justine, P. (1984). Use of megadoses of vitamins with minerals in Down syndrome. *Journal of Pediatrics, 105,* 228–234.

Smith, J. D. & Polloway, E. A. (1979). The dimension of adaptive behavior in mental retardation research: An analysis of recent practices. *American Journal of Mental Deficiency, 84,* 203–206.

Snow, R. E. (1978). Theory and method for research on aptitude processes. *Intelligence, 2,* 225–278.

Snyder, L. S. (1978). Communicative and cognitive abilities and disabilities in the sensori-motor period. *Merrill-Palmer Quarterly, 24,* 161–180.

Snyder, L., Apolloni, T., & Cooke, T. P. (1977). Integrated settings at the early childhood level: The non-retarded peers. *Exceptional Children, 43,* 262–266.

Solnit, A. J. (1976). Discussion in D. M. Klaus & J. H. Kennell, *Maternal-infant bonding.* St. Louis: Mosby.

Solnit, A.J., & Stark, M. H. (1961). Mourning and the birth of a defective child. *The Psychoanalytic Study of the Child, 16,* 523–537.

Sontag, L., Baker, C., & Nelson, V. (1958). Mental growth and personality development: A longitudinal study. *Monographs of the Society for Research in Child Development, 23* (2 Serial No. 68).

Sparrow, S. S., & Cicchetti, D. V. (1978). Behavior rating inventory for moderately, severely, and profoundly retarded persons. *American Journal of Mental Deficiency, 82,* 365–374.

Sparrow, S., & Zigler, E. (1978). Evaluation of patterning treatment for retarded children. *Pediatrics, 62,* 137–150.

Spearman, C. (1927). *The abilities of man.* New York: Macmillan.

Spence, K. W. (1958). A theory of emotionally-based drive (D) and its relation to performance in simple learning situations. *American Psychologist, 13,* 131–141.

Spiker, D. (1982). Parent involvement in early intervention activities with their children with Down's Syndrome. *Education and Training of the Mentally Retarded, 17,* 24–29.

Spitz, H. (1963). Field theory in mental deficiency. In N. R. Ellis (Ed.), *Handbook of mental deficiency.* New York: McGraw-Hill.

Spitz, R. A. (1945). Hospitalism: An inquiry into the genesis of psychiatric conditions in early childhood. *Psychoanalytic Study of the Child, 1,* 54–74.

Spitz, R. A. (1946). Hospitalism: A follow-up report. *Psychoanalytic Study of the Child, 2,* 113–117.

Spitz, R. A., & Wolf, K. M. (1946). Anaclitic depression. *The Psychoanalytic Study of the Child, 2,* 313–342.

Stern, D. (1974). Mother and infant at play: The dyadic interaction involving facial, vocal and gaze behaviors. In M. Lewis & L. A. Rosenblum (Eds.), *The effect of the infant on its caretaker.* New York: Wiley.

Sternberg, R. (1981a). Cognitive-behavioral approaches to the training of intelligence in the retarded. *Journal of Special Education, 15,* 165–183.

Sternberg, R. (1981b). The nature of intelligence. *New York University Education Quarterly, 12,* 10–17.

Sternberg, R. J., Conway, B. E., Ketron, J. L., & Bernstein, M. (1981). People's conception of intelligence. *Journal of Personality and Social Psychology, 41,* 37–55.

Sternberg, R. J., & Salter, W. (1982). Conceptions of intelligence. In R. Sternberg (Ed.), *Handbook of human intelligence.* Cambridge University Press.

Stevenson, H. W., & Fabel, L. (1961). The effect of social reinforcement on the performance of institutionalized and noninstitutionalized normal and feebleminded children. *Journal of Personality, 29,* 136–147.

Stevenson, H. W., & Weir, M. W. (1959). The variables affecting children's performance in a probability learning task. *Journal of Experimental Psychology, 57,* 403–412.

Stevenson, H. W., & Weir, M. W. (1968). The role of age and verbalization in probability learning. *American Journal of Psychology, 76,* 299–305.

Stevenson, H. W., & Zigler, E. (1957). Discrimination learning and rigidity in normal and feebleminded individuals. *Journal of Personality, 25,* 699–711.

Stevenson, H. W., & Zigler, E. (1958). Probability learning in children. *Journal of Experimental Psychology, 56,* 185–192.

Suelzle, M., & Keenan, V. (1981). Changes in family support networks over the life cycle of mentally retarded persons. *American Journal of Mental Deficiency, 86,* 267–274.

Sutter, P., Mayeda, T., Call, T., Yanagi, G., & Yee, S. (1980). Comparison of successful and unsuccessful community-placed mentally retarded persons. *American Journal of Mental Deficiency, 85,* 262–267.

Switzky, H., Rotatori, A. F., Miller, T., & Freagon, S. (1979). The developmental model and its implications for assessment and instruction for the severely/profoundly handicapped. *Mental Retardation, 17,* 167–170.

Tarjan, G. (1970). Some thoughts on socio-cultural retardation. In H. C. Haywood (Ed.), *Social-cultural aspects of mental retardation: Proceedings of the Peabody-NIMH Conference.* New York: Appleton-Century-Crofts.

Tarjan, G., & Benson, F. (1953). Report on the pilot study at Pacific Colony. *American Journal of Mental Deficiency, 57,* 453–462.

Tarjan, G., Wright, S., Eyman, R., & Keeran, C. (1973). Natural history of mental retardation: Some aspects of epidemiology. *American Journal of Mental Deficiency, 77,* 369–379.

Tarjan, G., Wright, S., Kramer, M., Person, P. H., Jr., & Morgan, R. (1958). The natural history of mental deficiency in a state hospital: I. Probabilities of release and death by age, intelligence quotient, and diagnosis. *American Journal of Disease of Children, 96,* 64–70.

Taylor, J. A. (1963). Drive theory and manifest anxiety. In M. T. Mednich & S. A. Mednich (Eds.), *Research in personality.* New York: Holt, Rinehart & Winston.

Terman, L. M., & Merrill, M. A. (1973). *Stanford-Binet Intelligence Scale: 1972 Norms Edition.* Boston: Houghton Mifflin.

Terrell, G., Jr., Durkin, K., & Wiesley, M. (1959). Social class and the nature of all incentive in discrimination learning. *Journal of Abnormal and Social Psychology, 59,* 270–272.

Tew, B. J., Payne, H., & Lawrence, K. M. (1974). Must a family with a handicapped child be a handicapped family? *Developmental Medicine & Child Neurology, 16,* 95–98.

Thiessen, D. (1972). *Gene organization and behavior.* New York: Random House.

Towne, R. C., Joiner, L. M., & Schurr, T. (1967). *The effect of special class placement on the self-concept and academic ability of the mentally retarded. A time series experiment.* Paper presented at meetings of the Council for Exceptional Children, St. Louis, Mo.

Trickett, P. K., Apfel, N. H., Rosenbaum, L. K., & Zigler, E. (1982). A five year follow-up of participants in the Yale Child Welfare Research Program. In E. Zigler & E. Gordon (Eds.), *Daycare: Scientific and social policy issues.* Boston: Auburn House.

Tuddenham, R. D. (1971). Theoretical regularities and individual idiosyncracies. In D. Green, M. Ford, & G. Flamer (Eds.), *Measurement and Piaget.* New York: McGraw-Hill.

Turnbull, A., & Blacher-Dixon, J. (1981). Preschool mainstreaming: An empirical and conceptual review. In P. Strain & M. M. Keer (Eds.), *Mainstreaming handicapped children: Research and instructional perspectives.* New York: Academic Press.

Turnbull, A., & Turnbull, H. R. (1972). Parent involvement in the education of handicapped children: A critique. *Mental Retardation, 20,* 115–122.

Turnbull, A., & Turnbull, H. R. (1978). *Parents speak out: Views from the other side of the two-way mirror.* Columbus, Ohio: Merrill.

Turnbull, H. R. (1977). Mainstreaming emotionally disturbed children: Legal implications. In A. T. Pappanikov (Ed.), *Mainstreaming emotionally disturbed children.* Syracuse, N.Y.: Syracuse University Press.

Turnbull, H. R. (1978). The past and future impact of court decisions in special education. *Phi Delta Kappan, 59,* 523–527.

Turner, G., & Turner, B. (1974). X-linked mental retardation. *Journal of Medical Genetics, 11,* 109–113.

Turnure, J. E. (1970a). Children's reactions to distractors in a learning situation. *Developmental Psychology, 2*, 115–122.

Turnure, J. E. (1970b). Reactions to physical and social distractors by moderately retarded, institutionalized children. *Journal of Special Education, 4*, 283–294.

Turnure, J. E., & Zigler, E. (1964). Outer-directedness in the problem-solving of normal and retarded children. *Journal of Abnormal and Social Psychology, 69*, 427–436.

United States Census of Population and Housing. (1981). Washington, D.C.: Government Printing Office.

Uzgiris, I. C. (1970). Sociocultural factors in cognitive development. In H. C. Haywood (Ed.), *Social-cultural aspects of mental retardation: Proceedings of the Peabody-NIMH conference.* New York: Appleton-Century-Crofts.

Uzgiris, I., & Hunt, J. (1975). *Assessment in infancy: Ordinal scales of psychological development.* Urbana, Ill.: University of Illinois Press.

Valente, M., & Tarjan, G. (1974). Etiologic factors in mental retardation. In G. Tarjan (Ed.), *Mental retardation.* New York: Insight Communications.

Vandenberg, S. G. (1971). The genetics of intelligence. In L. C. Deighton (Ed.), *Encyclopedia of education* (Vol. 2). New York: Macmillan.

Vernon, P. E. (1971). *The structure of human abilities.* London: Methuen.

Vernon, P. (1979). *Intelligence: Heredity and environment.* San Francisco: Freeman.

Vietze, P. M., Abernathy, S. R., Ashe, M. L., & Faulstich, G. (1978). Contingent interaction between mothers and their developmentally delayed infants. In G. D. Sackett (Ed.), *Observing behavior* (Vol. 1). Baltimore: University Park.

Vitello, S. J., & Soskin, R. (1985). *Mental retardation: Its social and legal context.* Englewood Cliffs, N.J.: Prentice-Hall.

Vogel, W., Broverman, D. M., Draguns, J. G., & Klaiber, E. (1966). The role of glutamic acid in cognitive behaviors. *Psychological Bulletin, 65* (6), 367–382.

Wagner, R. K., & Sternberg, R. J. (in press). Alternative conceptions of intelligence and their implications for education. *Review of Education Research.*

Wallin, J. E. (1958). Prevalence of mental retardation. *School and Society, 86*, 55–56.

Warren, S. A. (1979). What is wrong with mainstreaming? A comment on drastic change. *Mental Retardation, 17*, 301–303.

Warshaw, R. (1982). The minds of children. *Philadelphia Magazine*, April, pp. 120–124; 180–189.

Watson, R. I., & Midslarsky, E. (1979). Reactions of mothers with mentally retarded children: A social perspective. *Psychological Reports, 45*, 309–310.

Weathers, C. (1983). Effects of nutritional supplementation on IQ and certain other variables associated with Down Syndrome. *American Journal of Mental Deficiency, 88*, 214–217.

Weaver, J. (1966). *The effects of motivation-hygiene orientation and interpersonal reaction tendencies in intellectually subnormal children.* Unpublished doctoral dissertation, George Peabody College for Teachers.

Weaver, S. J., Balla, D., & Zigler, E. (1971). Social approach and avoidance tendencies of institutionalized retarded and noninstitutionalized retarded and normal children. *Journal of Experimental Research in Personality, 5*, 98–110.

Wechsler, D. (1974). *Manual for Wechsler Intelligence for Children – Revised.* New York: Psychological Corporation.

Weir, M. W. (1962). Effects of age and instruction on children's probability learning. *Child Development, 33*, 729–735.

Weisz, J. (1978). Transcontextual validity in developmental research. *Child Development, 49*, 1–12.

Weisz, J. (1982). Learned helplessness and the retarded child. In E. Zigler & D. Balla (Eds.), *Mental retardation: The developmental-difference controversy.* Hillsdale, N.J.: Erlbaum.

Weisz, J. R., Yeates, K. D., & Zigler, E. (1982). Piagetian evidence and the developmental-difference controversy. In E. Zigler & D. Balla (Eds.), *Mental retardation: The developmental-difference controversy*. Hillsdale, N.J.: Erlbaum.

Weisz, J., & Zigler, E. (1979). Cognitive development in retarded and nonretarded persons: Piagetian tests of the similar structure hypothesis. *Psychological Bulletin, 86*, 831–851.

Werner, H. (1948). *Comparative psychology of mental development* (rev. ed.). New York: Follett.

Werner, H. (1957). The concept of development from a comparative and organismic point of view. In D. Harris (Ed.), *The concept of development*. Minneapolis: University of Minnesota Press.

Werner, H., & Kaplan, B. (1963). *Symbol formation*. New York: Wiley.

White, A. J. R. (1982). Outpatient treatment of oppositional noneating in a deaf retarded boy. *Journal of Behavior Therapy and Experimental Psychiatry, 13*, 251–255.

White, R. (1959). Motivation reconsidered: The concept of competence. *Psychological Review, 66*, 297–333.

White, S. H. (1984). Studies of developing mentality. (Review of H. Werner, *Comparative Psychology of Mental Development*.) *Contemporary Psychology, 29*, 199–202.

White, W. D., & Wolfensberger, W. (1969). The evolution of dehumanization in our institutions. *Mental Retardation, 7*, 5–9.

Whitman, T., & Scibak, J. (1979). Behavior modification research with the severely and profoundly retarded. In N. R. Ellis (Ed.), *Handbook of mental deficiency* (2nd ed.). Hillsdale, N.J.: Erlbaum.

Whitney, E. (1956). Mental Deficiency – 1955. *American Journal of Mental Deficiency, 60*, 676–683.

Wildman, R. W., & Simon, S. J. (1978). An indirect method for increasing the rate of social interaction in an autistic child. *Journal of Clinical Psychology, 43*, 144–149.

Willer, B., & Intagliata, J. (1980). *Deinstitutionalization of mentally retarded persons in New York State (Final Report)*. New York: Office of Human Development, U.S. Department of Health and Human Services, Region II.

Willerman, L. (1979). *The psychology of individual and group differences*. San Francisco: Freeman.

Williams, R. J. (1956). *Biochemical individuality: The basis for the genetotrophic concept*. Austin, Tex.: University of Texas Press.

Wilmarth, A. W. (1902). Report of a committee on feeble-minded and epileptic. *Proceedings of the National Conference on Charities and Correction*, 152–161.

Wiltz, N. A., & Gordon, S. B. (1974). Parental modification of a child's behavior in an experimental residence. *Journal of Behavior Therapy and Experimental Psychiatry, 5*, 107–109.

Windle, C. (1962). Prognosis of mental subnormals. *American Journal of Mental Deficiency, 66*. (Monograph Supplement to No. 5).

Wohlhueter, M., & Sindberg, R. M. (1975). Longitudinal development of object permanence in mentally retarded children: An exploratory study. *American Journal of Mental Deficiency, 79*, 513–518.

Wolfensberger, W. (1969). The origin and nature of our institutional models. In R. B. Kugel & W. Wolfensberger (Eds.), *Changing patterns in residential services for the mentally retarded*. Washington, D.C.: Government Printing Office.

Wolfensberger, W. (1972). *The principle of normalization in human services*. Toronto: National Institute on Mental Retardation.

Wolfensberger, W., & Menolascino, F. (1968). Basic considerations in evaluating ability of drugs to stimulate cognitive development in retardates. *American Journal of Mental Deficiency, 73*, 414–423.

Wood, D., Bruner, J., & Ross, G. (1976). The role of tutoring in problem solving. *Journal of Child Psychology and Psychiatry, 17,* 89–100.

Woodward, W. (1959). The behavior of idiots interpreted by Piaget's theory of sensory-motor development. *British Journal of Educational Psychology, 29,* 60–71.

Woodward, W. (1979). Piaget's theory and the study of mental retardation. In N. R. Ellis (Ed.), *Handbook of mental deficiency research* (2nd ed.). Hillsdale, N.J.: Erlbaum.

Woolf, L. I. (1970). Phenylketonuria and phenylalaninemia. In J. Wortis (Ed.), *Mental retardation and developmental disabilities* (Vol. 2), 29–45.

Woolf, L. I., & Vulliamy, D. G. (1951). Phenylketonuria with a study of the effect upon it of glutamic acid. *Archives of Disabilities of Childhood, 26,* 487–494.

Wyatt v. *Aderholt,* 503 F 2nd 1305 (5th cir). 1974.

Wyatt v. *Hardin.* Civil Action No. 3195-N, 1978.

Wyatt v. *Ireland,* No. 3195 (N.D. Ala. Oct. 25, 1979).

Wyatt v. *Stickney* 325 F Supp. 781, 784 (M.D. Ala. 1971).

Yando, R., Seitz, V., & Zigler E. (1978). *Imitation: A developmental perspective.* Hillsdale, N.J.: Erlbaum.

Yando, R., & Zigler, E. (1971). Outerdirectedness in the problem-solving of institutionalized and noninstitutionalized normal and retarded children. *Developmental Psychology, 4,* 277–288.

Yannett, H. (1953). The progress of medical research in the field of mental deficiency. *American Journal of Mental Deficiency, 57,* 447–452.

Yarrow, L. J. (1964). Separation from parents during early childhood. In M. L. Hoffman & L. W. Hoffman (Eds.), *Review of child development research* (Vol. 2). New York: Russell Sage Foundation.

Yarrow, L. J., Morgan, G. A., Jennings, K. D., Harmon, R. J., & Gaiter, J. L. (1982). Infants' persistence at tasks: Relationships to cognitive functioning and early experience. *Infant Behavior and Development, 5,* 131–141.

Zigler, E. (1958). *The effect of preinstitutional social deprivation on the performance of feebleminded children.* Unpublished doctoral dissertation. University of Texas.

Zigler, E. (1961). Social deprivation and rigidity in the performance of feebleminded children. *Journal of Abnormal and Social Psychology, 62,* 413–421.

Zigler, E. (1962). Social deprivation in familial and organic retardates. *Psychological Reports, 10,* 370.

Zigler, E. (1963a). Metatheoretical issues in developmental psychology. In M. Marx (Ed.), *Theories in contemporary psychology.* New York: Macmillan.

Zigler, E. (1963b). Rigidity and social reinforcement effects on the performance of institutionalized and noninstitutionalized normal and retarded children. *Journal of Personality, 31,* 258–269.

Zigler, E. (1963c). Rigidity in the feebleminded. In E. P. Trapp & P. Himelstein (Eds.), *Readings on the exceptional child.* New York: Appleton-Century-Crofts.

Zigler, E. (1963d). Social reinforcement and the child. *American Journal of Orthopsychiatry, 33,* 614–623.

Zigler, E. (1964). The effect of social reinforcement on normal and socially deprived children. *Journal of Genetic Psychology, 104,* 235–242.

Zigler, E. (1966a). Mental retardation: Current issues and approaches. In L. W. Hoffman & M. L. Hoffman (Eds.), *Review of child development research* (Vol. 2). New York: Russell Sage.

Zigler, E. (1966b). Motivational determinants in the performance of feebleminded children. *American Journal of Orthopsychiatry, 36,* 848–856.

Zigler, E. (1967). Familial mental retardation: A continuing dilemma. *Science, 155,* 292–298.

Zigler, E. (1969). Developmental versus difference theories of mental retardation and the problem of motivation. *American Journal of Mental Deficiency, 73*, 536–556.

Zigler, E. (1970a). Level of aspiration and the probability learning of middle- and lower-class children. *Developmental Psychology, 3*, 133–142.

Zigler, E. (1970b). The environmental mystique: Training the intellect versus development of the child. *Childhood Education, 46*, 402–412.

Zigler, E. (1970c). The nature–nurture issue reconsidered. In H. C. Haywood (Ed.), *Socialcultural aspects of mental retardation: Proceedings of the Peabody-NIMH conference.* New York: Appleton-Century-Crofts.

Zigler, E. (1971). The retarded child as a whole person. In H. E. Adams & W. K. Boardman (Eds.), *Advances in experimental clinical psychology.* New York: Pergamon.

Zigler, E. (1973). Why retarded children do not perform up to the level of their ability. In R. M. Allen, A. D. Cortazzo, & R. Toister (Eds.), *Theories of cognitive development: Implications for the mentally retarded.* Coral Gables, Fla.: University of Miami Press.

Zigler, E. (1977). Twenty years of mental retardation research. *Mental Retardation, 14*, 51–53.

Zigler, E. (1978). National crisis in mental retardation research. An editorial. *American Journal of Mental Deficiency, 83*, 1–8.

Zigler, E. (1981). A plea to end the use of patterning treatment with retarded children. *American Journal of Orthopsychiatry, 51*, 388–390.

Zigler, E. (1983). *Conference summary and final thoughts.* Speech given at Elwyn Institutes' Graduate Symposium on Mental Retardation. June.

Zigler, E. (1984). A developmental theory of mental retardation. In B. Blatt & R. Morris (Eds.), *Perspectives in special education: Personal orientations* (Vol. 1). Santa Monica, Calif.: Scott Foresman.

Zigler, E., & Balla, D. (1972). Developmental course of responsiveness to social reinforcement in normal children and institutionalized retarded children. *Developmental Psychology, 6*, 66–73.

Zigler, E., & Balla, D. (1977). The impact of institutionalized experience on the behavior and development of retarded persons. *American Journal of Mental Deficiency, 82*, 1–11.

Zigler, E., & Balla, D. (1979). Personality development in retarded individuals. In N. P. Ellis (Ed.), *Handbook of mental deficiency* (2nd ed.). Hillsdale, N.J.: Erlbaum.

Zigler, E., & Balla, D. (1982a). Issues in personality motivation in mentally retarded persons. In M. J. Begab, H. D. Haywood, & H. Garber (Eds.), *Psychosocial influences in retarded performance* (Vol. 1). Baltimore: University Park.

Zigler, E., & Balla, D. (1982b). Motivational and personality factors in the performance of the retarded. In E. Zigler & D. Balla (Eds.), *Mental retardation: The developmental-difference controversy.* Hillsdale, N.J.: Erlbaum.

Zigler, E., & Balla, D. (1982c). Personality determinants in the behavior of the retarded. In E. Zigler, M. Lamb, & I. Child (Eds.), *Social and personality development* (2nd ed.). New York: Oxford University Press, 238–245.

Zigler, E., & Balla, D. (1982d). Rigidity: A resilient concept. In E. Zigler & D. Balla (Eds.), *Mental retardation: The developmental–difference controversy.* Hillsdale, N.J.: Erlbaum.

Zigler, E., & Balla, D. (1982e). Selecting outcome variables in evaluations of early childhood special education programs. *Topics in Early Childhood Special Education, 1*, 11–22.

Zigler, E., Balla, D., & Butterfield, E. C. (1968). A longitudinal investigation of the relationship between preinstitutional social deprivation and social motivation in institutionalized retardates. *Journal of Personality and Social Psychology, 10*, 437–445.

Zigler, E., Balla, D., & Hodapp, R. (1984). On the definition and classification of mental retardation. *American Journal of Mental Deficiency, 89*, 215–230.

Zigler, E., Balla, D., & Kossan, N. (in press). Effects of types of institutionalization on some non-intellective correlates of retarded persons' behavior. *American Journal of Mental Deficiency.*

Zigler, E., Balla, D., & Styfco, S. J. (1980). New directions for the study of the effects of institutionalized retarded persons. In *Proceedings of the NICHD Conference on Learning and Cognition in the mentally retarded.* Nashville, Tenn.: September 16–18.

Zigler, E., Balla, D., & Watson, N. (1972). Developmental and experimental determinants of self-image disparity in institutionalized and noninstitutionalized retarded and normal children. *Journal of Personality and Social Psychology, 23,* 81–87.

Zigler, E., & Berman, W. (1983). Discerning the future of early childhood intervention. *American Psychologist, 38,* 894–906.

Zigler, E., & Butterfield, E. C. (1966). Rigidity in the retarded: A further test of the Lewin-Kounin formulation. *Journal of Abnormal Psychology, 71,* 224–231.

Zigler, E., & Butterfield, E. C. (1968). Motivational aspects of changes in IQ test performance of culturally deprived nursery school children. *Child Development, 39,* 1–14.

Zigler, E., Butterfield, E. C., & Capobianco, F. (1970). Institutionalization and the effectiveness of social reinforcement: A five- and eight-year follow-up study. *Developmental Psychology, 3,* 255–263.

Zigler, E., Butterfield, E. C., & Goff, G. A. (1966). A measure of preinstitutional social deprivation for institutionalized retardates. *American Journal of Mental Deficiency, 70,* 873–885.

Zigler, E., & Child, I. L. (1969). Socialization. In G. Lindzey & E. Aronson (Eds.), *The handbook of social psychology* (2nd ed.). Reading, Mass: Addison-Wesley.

Zigler, E., & deLabry, J. (1962). Concept-switching in middle-class, lower-class, and retarded children. *Journal of Abnormal and Social Psychology, 65,* 267–273.

Zigler, E., & Glick, M. (in press). *A developmental approach to adult psychopathology.* New York: Wiley.

Zigler, E., & Hall, N. (in press). Mainstreaming and the philosophy of normalization. In J. Meisel (Ed.), *Mainstreaming: A review of current research and practice.* Hillsdale, N.J.: Erlbaum.

Zigler, E., & Harter, S. (1968). The effectiveness of adult and peer reinforcement on the performance of institutionalized and noninstitutionalized retardates. *Journal of Abnormal Psychology, 73,* 368–375.

Zigler, E., & Harter, S. (1969). Socialization of the mentally retarded. In D. A. Goslin & D. C. Glass (Eds.), *Handbook of socialization theory and research.* New York: Rand McNally.

Zigler, E., Hodgden, L., & Stevenson, I. I. (1958). The effect of support on the performance of normal and feebleminded children. *Journal of Personality, 26,* 106–122.

Zigler, E., & Kanzer, P. (1962). The effectiveness of two classes of verbal reinforcers on the performance of middle- and lower-class children. *Journal of Personality, 30,* 157–163.

Zigler, E., Lamb, M., & Child, I. (Eds.), (1982). *Socialization and personality development.* (2nd ed.). New York: Oxford University Press.

Zigler, E., Levine, J., & Gould, L. (1966a). Cognitive processes in the development of children's appreciation of humor. *Child Development, 37,* 507–518.

Zigler, E., Levine, J., & Gould, L. (1966b). The humor response of normal, institutionalized retarded and noninstitutionalized retarded children. *American Journal of Mental Deficiency, 71,* 427–480.

Zigler, E., Levine, J., & Gould, L. (1967). Cognitive challenge as a factor in children's humor appreciation. *Journal of Personality and Social Psychology, 6,* 332–336.

Zigler, E., & Muenchow, S. (1979). Mainstreaming: The proof is in the implementation. *American Psychologist, 34,* 993–996.

Zigler, E., & Phillips, L. (1961a). Psychiatric diagnosis: A critique. *Journal of Abnormal and Social Psychology, 63*, 607–618.

Zigler, E., & Phillips, L. (1961b). Psychiatric diagnosis and symptomatology. *Journal of Abnormal and Social Psychology, 63*, 69–75.

Zigler, E., & Seitz, V. (1975). "An experimental evaluation of sensorimotor patterning": A critique. *American Journal of Mental Deficiency, 79*, (5), 483–492.

Zigler, E., & Seitz, V. (1982). Future research on socialization and personality development. In E. Zigler, I. Child, & M. Lamb (Eds.), *Socialization and personality development* (2nd ed.). New York: Oxford University Press.

Zigler, E., & Trickett, P. (1978). IQ, social competence, and evaluation of early childhood intervention programs. *American Psychologist, 33*, 789–798.

Zigler, E., & Unell, E. (1962). Concept-switching in normal and feebleminded children as a function of reinforcement. *American Journal of Mental Deficiency, 66*, 651–657.

Zigler, E., & Valentine, J. (Eds.), (1979). *Project Head Start: A legacy of the war on poverty.* New York: Free Press.

Zigler, E., & Williams, J. (1963). Institutionalization and the effectiveness of social reinforcement: A three year follow-up study. *Journal of Abnormal Social Psychology, 66*, 197–205.

Zigler, E., & Yando, R. (1972). Outerdirectedness and imitative behavior of institutionalized and noninstitutionalized younger and older children. *Child Development, 43*, 413–425.

Author index

Subject index